Building Data Capacity for Patient-Centered Outcomes Research

Priorities for the Next Decade

Committee on Building Data Capacity for
Patient-Centered Outcomes Research:
An Agenda for 2021 to 2030

Committee on National Statistics
Division of Behavioral and Social Sciences and Education

Board on Health Care Services
Health and Medicine Division

Computer Science and Telecommunications Board
Division on Engineering and Physical Sciences

A Consensus Study Report of

The National Academies of
SCIENCES · ENGINEERING · MEDICINE

THE NATIONAL ACADEMIES PRESS
Washington, DC
www.nap.edu

THE NATIONAL ACADEMIES PRESS   500 Fifth Street, NW   Washington, DC 20001

This activity was supported by a contract between the National Academy of Sciences and the U.S. Department of Health and Human Services (award # HHSP233201400020B/75P00120F37102). Any opinions, findings, conclusions, or recommendations expressed in this publication do not necessarily reflect the views of any organization or agency that provided support for the project.

International Standard Book Number-13: 978-0-309-28711-1
International Standard Book Number-10: 0-309-28711-1
Digital Object Identifier: https://doi.org/10.17226/26489
Library of Congress Control Number: 2022941427

Additional copies of this publication are available from the National Academies Press, 500 Fifth Street, NW, Keck 360, Washington, DC 20001; (800) 624-6242 or (202) 334-3313; http://www.nap.edu.

Copyright 2022 by the National Academy of Sciences. All rights reserved.

Printed in the United States of America

Suggested citation: National Academies of Sciences, Engineering, and Medicine. (2022). *Building Data Capacity for Patient-Centered Outcomes Research: Priorities for the Next Decade*. Washington, DC: The National Academies Press. https://doi.org/10.17226/26489.

The National Academies of
SCIENCES · ENGINEERING · MEDICINE

The **National Academy of Sciences** was established in 1863 by an Act of Congress, signed by President Lincoln, as a private, nongovernmental institution to advise the nation on issues related to science and technology. Members are elected by their peers for outstanding contributions to research. Dr. Marcia McNutt is president.

The **National Academy of Engineering** was established in 1964 under the charter of the National Academy of Sciences to bring the practices of engineering to advising the nation. Members are elected by their peers for extraordinary contributions to engineering. Dr. John L. Anderson is president.

The **National Academy of Medicine** (formerly the Institute of Medicine) was established in 1970 under the charter of the National Academy of Sciences to advise the nation on medical and health issues. Members are elected by their peers for distinguished contributions to medicine and health. Dr. Victor J. Dzau is president.

The three Academies work together as the **National Academies of Sciences, Engineering, and Medicine** to provide independent, objective analysis and advice to the nation and conduct other activities to solve complex problems and inform public policy decisions. The National Academies also encourage education and research, recognize outstanding contributions to knowledge, and increase public understanding in matters of science, engineering, and medicine.

Learn more about the National Academies of Sciences, Engineering, and Medicine at **www.nationalacademies.org**.

The National Academies of
SCIENCES · ENGINEERING · MEDICINE

Consensus Study Reports published by the National Academies of Sciences, Engineering, and Medicine document the evidence-based consensus on the study's statement of task by an authoring committee of experts. Reports typically include findings, conclusions, and recommendations based on information gathered by the committee and the committee's deliberations. Each report has been subjected to a rigorous and independent peer-review process and it represents the position of the National Academies on the statement of task.

Proceedings published by the National Academies of Sciences, Engineering, and Medicine chronicle the presentations and discussions at a workshop, symposium, or other event convened by the National Academies. The statements and opinions contained in proceedings are those of the participants and are not endorsed by other participants, the planning committee, or the National Academies.

For information about other products and activities of the National Academies, please visit www.nationalacademies.org/about/whatwedo.

**COMMITTEE ON BUILDING DATA CAPACITY FOR
PATIENT-CENTERED OUTCOMES RESEARCH:
AN AGENDA FOR 2021 TO 2030**

GEORGE ISHAM (*Chair*), HealthPartners Institute
JOHN F.P. BRIDGES, The Ohio State University
JULIE BYNUM, University of Michigan
ANGELA DOBES, IBD Plexus, Crohn's & Colitis Foundation
DEBORAH ESTRIN, Cornell Tech
OLUWADAMILOLA FAYANJU, The University of Pennsylvania
CONSTANTINE GATSONIS, Brown University
ROBERT GOERGE, Chapin Hall, University of Chicago
GEORGE HRIPCSAK, Columbia University
LISA IEZZONI, Massachusetts General Hospital
S. CLAIBORNE JOHNSTON, The University of Texas at Austin
MIGUEL MARINO, Oregon Health & Science University
ELIZABETH McGLYNN, Kaiser Permanente
DAVID MELTZER, University of Chicago
PAUL TANG, Stanford University and Palo Alto Medical Foundation

KRISZTINA MARTON, *Study Director*
CRYSTAL BELL, *Associate Program Officer*
RUTH COOPER, *Associate Program Officer*
REBECCA KRONE, *Program Coordinator*
BRIAN HARRIS-KOJETIN, *Director, Committee on National Statistics*
SHARYL NASS, *Director, Board on Health Care Services*
JON EISENBERG, *Senior Board Director, Computer Science and
   Telecommunications Board*

SAUL RIVAS (*National Academy of Medicine Fellow*), University of
   Texas Rio Grande Valley

COMMITTEE ON NATIONAL STATISTICS

ROBERT M. GROVES (*Chair*), Georgetown University
LAWRENCE D. BOBO, Harvard University
ANNE C. CASE, Princeton University, emerita
MICK P. COUPER, University of Michigan
JANET M. CURRIE, Princeton University
DIANA FARRELL, JPMorgan Chase Institute, Washington, DC
ROBERT GOERGE, Chapin Hall at the University of Chicago
ERICA L. GROSHEN, Cornell University
HILARY HOYNES, University of California, Berkeley
DANIEL KIFER, The Pennsylvania State University
SHARON LOHR, Arizona State University, emerita
JEROME P. REITER, Duke University
JUDITH A. SELTZER, University of California, Los Angeles, emerita
C. MATTHEW SNIPP, Stanford University
ELIZABETH A. STUART, Johns Hopkins University
JEANNETTE WING, Columbia University

BRIAN HARRIS-KOJETIN, *Director*
MELISSA CHIU, *Deputy Director*
CONSTANCE F. CITRO, *Senior Scholar*

BOARD ON HEALTH CARE SERVICES

DAVID BLUMENTHAL (*Chair*), The Commonwealth Fund
ANDREW BINDMAN, Kaiser Foundation Health Plan, Inc.
NIRANJAN BOSE, Gates Ventures
MELINDA J. BEEUWKES BUNTIN, Vanderbilt University School of Medicine
NEIL S. CALMAN, The Institute for Family Health
PAUL CHUNG, Kaiser Permanente School of Medicine
PATRICIA M. DAVIDSON, Johns Hopkins University School of Nursing
MARTHA DAVIGLUS, University of Illinois at Chicago
JENNIFER E. DeVOE, Oregon Health & Science University
R. ADAMS DUDLEY, University of Minnesota
RICHARD G. FRANK, Harvard Medical School
TERRY FULMER, John A. Hartford Foundation
CINDY GILLESPIE, Arkansas Department of Human Services
ELMER HUERTA, The George Washington University Cancer Center
SHARON INOUYE, Harvard Medical School
JOHN LUMPKIN, Blue Cross Blue Shield of North Carolina Foundation
FAITH MITCHELL, The Urban Institute
DAVID B. PRYOR, Ascension Health
TRISH RILEY, National Academy for State Health Policy
WILLIAM SAGE, The University of Texas at Austin
HARDEEP SINGH, Baylor College of Medicine

SHARYL NASS, *Director*

COMPUTER SCIENCE AND TELECOMMUNICATIONS BOARD

LAURA HAAS (*Chair*), University of Massachusetts, Amherst
DAVID CULLER, University of California, Berkeley
ERIC HORVITZ, Microsoft Corporation
CHARLES ISBELL, Georgia Institute of Technology
BETH MYNATT, Georgia Institute of Technology
CRAIG PARTRIDGE, Colorado State University
DANIELA RUS, Massachusetts Institute of Technology
FRED B. SCHNEIDER, Cornell University
MARGO SELTZER, University of British Columbia
NAMBIRAJAN SESHADRI, University of California, San Diego
MOSHE VARDI, Rice University

JON EISENBERG, *Senior Board Director*

Acknowledgments

This Consensus Study Report was reviewed in draft form by individuals chosen for their diverse perspectives and technical expertise. The purpose of this independent review is to provide candid and critical comments that will assist the National Academies of Sciences, Engineering, and Medicine in making each published report as sound as possible and to ensure that it meets the institutional standards for quality, objectivity, evidence, and responsiveness to the study charge. The review comments and draft manuscript remain confidential to protect the integrity of the deliberative process.

We thank the following individuals for their review of this report: David Cella, Department of Medical Social Sciences, Northwestern University; Steven B. Cohen, Division for Statistical and Data Sciences, RTI International; Abel N. Kho, Institute for Public Health and Medicine Center for Health Information Partnerships, Feinberg School of Medicine, Northwestern University; Marsha Lillie-Blanton, Milken Institute School of Public Health, The George Washington University; Jennifer H. Madans, National Center for Health Statistics (retired) and Center for Inclusive Policy; Deven McGraw, Ciitizen Corporation; Ellen R. Meara, Department of Health Policy and Management, Harvard T.H. Chan School of Public Health; Jodi B. Segal, Center for Drug Safety and Effectiveness, Johns Hopkins University School of Medicine and Bloomberg School of Public Health; Joe V. Selby, Office of Director, Patient-Centered Outcomes Research Institute (retired); and Nigam H. Shah, Stanford Medicine, Stanford University.

Although the reviewers listed above provided many constructive comments and suggestions, they were not asked to endorse the conclusions of this report, nor did they see the final draft before its release. The review of this report was overseen by Andrew B. Bindman, chief medical officer, Kaiser Foundation Health Plan and Hospitals, and Alicia L. Carriquiry, Department of Statistics, Iowa State University. They were responsible for making certain that an independent examination of this report was carried out in accordance with the standards of the National Academies and that all review comments were carefully considered. Responsibility for the final content rests entirely with the authoring committee and the National Academies.

Contents

Summary 1

1 Committee Charge and Process 11
2 Background on the PCOR Data Infrastructure and the Office of
  the Secretary PCOR Trust Fund 17
3 Priority Areas for the PCOR Data Infrastructure 35

Appendixes

A Biographical Sketches of Committee Members 53
B Building Data Capacity for Patient-Centered Outcomes Research:
  Interim Report 1–Looking Ahead at Data Needs 59
C Building Data Capacity for Patient-Centered Outcomes Research:
  Interim Report 2–Data Standards, Methods, and Policy 149
D Building Data Capacity for Patient-Centered Outcomes Research:
  Interim Report 3–A Comprehensive Ecosystem for PCOR 237
E Office of the Secretary PCOR Trust Fund Project Portfolio 335

Boxes, Figures, and Tables

BOXES

1-1 Statement of Task, 12
2-1 Key Data Infrastructure Functionalities in the Existing Strategic Framework for PCOR, 22
2-2 Building Blocks of the PCOR Data Infrastructure, 23
2-3 Key Themes That Emerged from the Stakeholder Prioritization Activity Commissioned by ASPE in 2020, 24
2-4 2020 Office of the Secretary PCOR Trust Fund Projects in Three HHS Priority Areas, 31

FIGURES

2-1 Office of the Secretary PCOR Trust Fund strategic framework for the PCOR data infrastructure, 21
2-2 Relationship between thematic areas funded and the five PCOR data infrastructure functionalities, 29
3-1 Framework for the role of enhanced data infrastructure and effective project management in improving health, 51

TABLES

2-1 Number of Office of the Secretary PCOR Trust Fund Projects by Data Infrastructure Functionality Addressed, 25

2-2   Products Produced by Office of the Secretary PCOR Trust Fund Projects, 26
2-3   Examples of Products Produced by Office of the Secretary PCOR Trust Fund Projects, 27
2-4   Examples of HHS Secretarial Priorities and Office of the Secretary PCOR Trust Fund Projects, 28

Summary

The Office of the Assistant Secretary for Planning and Evaluation (ASPE), in partnership with other agencies and divisions of the U.S. Department of Health and Human Services, coordinates a portfolio of projects that build data capacity for conducting patient-centered outcomes research (PCOR). PCOR focuses on producing scientific evidence on the effectiveness of prevention and treatment options to inform the health care decisions of patients, families, and health care providers, taking into consideration the preferences, values, and questions patients face when making health care choices. The data infrastructure includes data sources and functionalities that support the research.

ASPE asked the National Academies of Sciences, Engineering, and Medicine to appoint a consensus study committee to identify issues critical to the continued development of the data infrastructure for PCOR. The committee's work will contribute to ASPE's development of a strategic plan that will guide its work related to PCOR data capacity over the next decade. This report summarizes the committee's findings and conclusions in the areas that could benefit from being prioritized as part of ASPE's work over the next decade. The report also offers input on strengthening the overall framework for building the data infrastructure over the coming years.

The committee's primary information-gathering mechanisms for this study were three workshops, which focused on obtaining broad inputs from data users and other stakeholders on topics that the committee and ASPE had jointly determined to be particularly relevant to the strategic planning. The topics included (1) data user needs; (2) data standards, methods, and policies; and (3) collaborations, data linkages, and interoperability of electronic databases. The committee has issued three interim reports, which contain conclusions based on the three workshops. The full text of these reports is included in Appendixes B through D and can be consulted for additional details on the discussions that took place at the workshops.

This report is the final product of the committee's work and represents a synthesis of all of the committee's information-gathering activities, its review of additional documentation about the data infrastructure, its deliberations, and its integrated judgment of the input received. The report's conclusions reflect the conclusions of the interim reports, but they are further integrated and combined here as part of a more holistic and streamlined discussion.

Below we summarize the insights and overall conclusions reached by the committee at the end of the study. Due to the complex nature and many important elements of the data infrastructure, the conclusions cover a lot of ground. However, the committee would like to highlight two overarching conclusions, which provide additional context for the more detailed conclusions. First, the committee concluded that the PCOR data infrastructure in the next decade would benefit from a broader focus on people and communities (Conclusion 3-1). Using this lens will support further development of the infrastructure by highlighting data gaps (e.g., about a person's context beyond a clinical setting, or new types of data), taking a longitudinal perspective, linking fragmented datasets (e.g., different types of data from a variety of sources and over time), identifying the questions that matter most to people, and advancing research methods that enable this broader focus.

Second, the committee concluded that greater attention to how the uses of the PCOR data infrastructure are shaping knowledge, practice, and policy can meaningfully inform future investments in the infrastructure (Conclusion 3-27). This requires a more dynamic perspective, expanding the voices that provide guidance, finding the right balance between protecting privacy and advancing knowledge, and proactively identifying areas of investment to ensure that the right work gets done.

FOCUS ON THE PERSON AS A WHOLE

The committee noted the importance of taking a holistic view of an individual's health rather than limiting the perspective, and the data acquired, to that captured about an individual in a clinical setting. Accordingly, the committee believes that broadening the focus of the PCOR data infrastructure from *patient*-centered to *person*-centered would enhance the goals and data requirements needed to conduct meaningful outcomes research. Everything that has been learned about the contributions of social determinants of health indicates that ignoring the health impacts of where individuals live, work, and play also impedes meaningful understanding of important intervention targets to improve health. In other words, expanding the focus from populations to include information about the characteristics of their communities would be of further benefit. A person-centered approach incorporates into the data critical influences beyond the health care processes when people are patients.

The distinction between a person-centered approach and a patient-centered one is not intended to imply that the roles of patient and person are necessarily separate but rather to underscore the broader context that might be missed when the focus is exclusively on the person as a patient. This shift in perspective could be transformative for both research and health care.

> CONCLUSION 3-1: Broadening the focus from the patient to the person more generally and from populations to communities would enable a more comprehensive approach to the data infrastructure and a better understanding of the outcomes that matter to people.

INCLUDING HIGH-PRIORITY TYPES OF DATA IN THE DATA INFRASTRUCTURE

The committee identified several emerging data needs and stakeholder priorities that are not well met by the current data infrastructure. A theme that emerged from the workshops was the magnitude of the gaps in the data that are available to better understand and address health disparities. The cost of care and its impact on the quality and length of life of people in the United States emerged as another topic area suffering from substantial gaps in the available information. The workshops also highlighted the need for and the underutilized potential in performing linkages to existing mortality data. This might be an area where enhancements to linkages in the data infrastructure could have a high impact and be particularly feasible.

> CONCLUSION 3-2: A variety of data types were identified that are less likely to be available or easily accessible in the PCOR data infrastructure, including data on mortality, cost of care, social determinants of health, and disability status, as well as other characteristics of people associated with disparities in health outcomes. Increased attention to filling gaps in the availability of these data will enhance the utility of the infrastructure for answering questions that matter to people and will enable research on potential intervention targets.

A fundamental reason for the data limitations that make it difficult to answer questions important for PCOR is that most of the data available for research are collected for payment or treatment purposes rather than for research. While ongoing work focused on increasing the usefulness and availability of these data for research is crucial, opportunities also exist to incorporate additional and newer data sources into the data platforms used for research.

> CONCLUSION 3-3: An area with opportunities for additional expansion is the collection of patient- and person-generated data and the routine integration of these data into data platforms that can be used both for research and for other purposes, including regulatory decision making and to inform shared decision making.

> CONCLUSION 3-4: Patient-directed disease registries can be a source of in-depth, longitudinal, prospective clinical and patient-reported data that are not available from other data sources.

The usefulness of the data and the data infrastructure could be further enhanced by adopting a longitudinal perspective on a person's journey through the health care system and through life events that have a relevance to health more broadly.

> CONCLUSION 3-5: Assembling a comprehensive longitudinal record of individuals' health journeys, which also includes the social context of their lives to the extent possible, would facilitate more far-reaching outcomes research.

ADDRESSING FRAGMENTATION

The data that exist for PCOR are collected and curated in a variety of databases across a fragmented health system. These data silos are a major barrier to research as well as to increasing the usefulness of the information available for decision making more broadly. Several areas of promising work aimed at overcoming these barriers could result in a better integrated data infrastructure.

> CONCLUSION 3-6: The data available for PCOR are fragmented across a variety of databases. Expanding data linkages could greatly increase the usefulness of these data for research.

> CONCLUSION 3-7: Collaboration among federal agencies and between federal agencies and other partners to address barriers that hinder data linkages, such as the limitations associated with the lack of unique health identifiers and patient or person matching, will improve the PCOR data infrastructure. The usefulness of data available for

PCOR could further be increased by sharing and adopting best practices among the states concerning the collection of data, data quality, and ease of access.

DATA NOT DESIGNED TO ADVANCE KNOWLEDGE

Given that the PCOR data infrastructure relies mostly on data that were not collected primarily for research purposes, developing standards for clinical data and enhancing the interoperability of data systems would facilitate the use of data for research. ASPE has an important role to play in this area.

> CONCLUSION 3-8: Standards are most useful when their development is driven by their potential uses and a clear concept of the value they can contribute.

> CONCLUSION 3-9: Taking an international perspective is important for the development of a PCOR data infrastructure; in particular, the infrastructure focused on standards would benefit from building on work that happens internationally.

> CONCLUSION 3-10: ASPE, in collaboration with other partners and stakeholders, could add significant value in the area of standards for PCOR by:
> - continuing to promote the development of a data infrastructure and an implementation strategy that facilitate the use of standards and access to the data;
> - convening stakeholder meetings to enhance communication and work toward developing a common language for standards;
> - facilitating access to the data and collaborations with existing organizations working in this area;
> - leading efforts to catalogue and exemplify data standards and analytic standards for a holistic view of individuals' health; and
> - increasing consistency in the use of standards for data interoperability and element definitions.

> CONCLUSION 3-11: Prioritizing projects that address fidelity or use of standards may convey greater value for the PCOR infrastructure than developing new standards.

GOVERNING DATA ACCESS

Data access and privacy considerations were a recurring theme during the committee's information-gathering activities. At the same time, it appears that relatively few projects have been funded in this area.

CONCLUSION 3-12: This is an opportune time to revisit and update the legislation and rules governing data privacy and the sharing of data for research.

CONCLUSION 3-13: Governance challenges that create barriers to developing the PCOR infrastructure can be found at all levels of the system. Data availability could be increased by exploring challenges at the local level, including variable interpretations of federal laws and regulations, and by identifying approaches to address those challenges.

DATA ACCESS OPTIONS

While a variety of mechanisms exist for accessing PCOR-relevant data, these processes could all benefit from additional streamlining to facilitate data use. One theme that emerged from stakeholder input was the importance of being transparent about how the data will be used, building trust, and working closely with patient groups and communities. Stakeholder input also highlighted reasons why some organizations might be reluctant to share data, pointing toward considerations necessary for successful data sharing agreements.

CONCLUSION 3-14: Investments in identifying mechanisms for facilitating the ability of researchers, patients, and other people to access data will contribute to increased use of the PCOR infrastructure.

CONCLUSION 3-15: Building and maintaining trust among the people and communities whose data are being sought for research is essential for producing high-quality data, and patient groups can be helpful partners in these efforts. Including representatives of patients and other people in the research process to understand how to measure health impacts that matter to individuals is an important component in building trust. Providing value back to data donors, such as through the sharing of research results, could help underscore the importance and benefits of the information to stakeholders, including individuals, families, clinicians, and communities, in addition to enabling them to use the information in ways they find relevant. These uses could play a particularly important role in reducing health disparities, complementing research efforts in this area.

CONCLUSION 3-16: Successful data sharing partnerships across health care systems and government agencies require participant trust, clear evidence of mutual benefit, and the ability to control risk.

ADVANCING RESEARCH PRACTICES AND ANALYTIC METHODS

Advances in the methods used for PCOR have led to renewed interest in aspects of how the research is carried out. The committee identified some areas that could benefit from additional attention in the coming years.

CONCLUSION 3-17: PCOR products would be enhanced by investing in methods that are essential for the conduct of PCOR, such as including persons throughout the research continuum, addressing problems of missing data, improving study designs, ensuring appropriate inference from methods utilizing observational data, and addressing structural bias in data systems and studies.

CONCLUSION 3-18: Applying best practices to the analytic methods used in PCOR is important to facilitate the reliability and reproducibility of study results.

CONCLUSION 3-19: The results of PCOR are only replicable and most useful when the underlying data and comprehensive research documentation (such as analytic code) are made available for use by others.

PROJECT SELECTION TO SUPPORT THE DATA INFRASTRUCTURE FRAMEWORK

In addition to the conclusions about specific aspects of the PCOR data infrastructure that could benefit from more work in the years ahead, the committee also offers several big-picture observations on project selection. Among the types of projects most likely to enable the data infrastructure to make progress are two general categories of projects that have a high expected return on investment.

CONCLUSION 3-20: The development of the data infrastructure might be enhanced and critical gaps could be filled by proactively identifying necessary projects in areas that examine the overall framework for the

PCOR data infrastructure, particularly in the context of broader issues such as the balance between privacy and increased data use.

CONCLUSION 3-21: Investments in areas unlikely to be funded or developed by other entities may have a particularly high value.

CONCLUSION 3-22: Investments in projects that have potential use and application beyond the condition or disease for which they are proposed will accelerate the use of the infrastructure.

DISSEMINATION OF RESULTS AND USE OF THE DATA INFRASTRUCTURE

Over the years, increasing efforts have been made to disseminate information about the PCOR data infrastructure and PCOR studies. The discussions with stakeholders, however, revealed that awareness of the work could be further increased by additional attention to dissemination.

CONCLUSION 3-23: There is a need to increase awareness among all stakeholders about new data infrastructure developments funded by the Office of the Secretary PCOR Trust Fund. Increased awareness will enhance the efficiency and effectiveness of research, which in turn will increase the impact of the investments made in infrastructure development.

CONCLUSION 3-24: Investments in implementing and disseminating infrastructure tools and products will accelerate the achievement of overall PCOR infrastructure goals.

CONCLUSION 3-25: Dissemination and translation of the research findings could be greatly enhanced by using forms of communication that are relevant to those outside the research community.

UPDATING THE DATA INFRASTRUCTURE FRAMEWORK

While it is clear that the projects funded through the Office of the Secretary PCOR Trust Fund (OS-PCORTF) are well targeted toward further developing and enhancing key aspects of the PCOR data infrastructure, that infrastructure has not reached its full potential. It is not yet able to provide data that can answer the questions that matter to people and enable them to make informed decisions. While ASPE regularly obtains additional input from others, such as researchers and patient advocates, the lack of their representation on the OS-PCORTF Leadership Council likely limits input

SUMMARY 9

on data infrastructure needs. The committee's work identified several ways in which the overall approach to thinking about the data infrastructure could be strengthened.

CONCLUSION 3-26: Explicitly focusing on improved health as the goal of the PCOR infrastructure may be a useful way to prioritize projects and target infrastructure investments.

Finally, the committee's work underscored the need for additional feedback and metrics that would enable ASPE to assess the impact of the investments in the data infrastructure.

CONCLUSION 3-27: A tighter feedback loop with the external end users and developers of evidence would enhance the value of data infrastructure investments. Examining what evidence was generated due to ASPE interventions and identifying what impact it had on policy and knowledge would also help close the gaps observed in realizing the potential of the PCOR data infrastructure.

1

Committee Charge and Process

ISSUES FOR THE COMMITTEE

The Office of the Assistant Secretary for Planning and Evaluation (ASPE), in partnership with other agencies and divisions of the U.S. Department of Health and Human Services (HHS), coordinates a portfolio of projects that build data capacity for conducting patient-centered outcomes research (PCOR). PCOR focuses on producing scientific evidence on the effectiveness of prevention and treatment options to inform the health care decisions of patients, families, and health care providers, taking into consideration the preferences, values, and questions people face when making health care choices. The data infrastructure includes data sources and functionalities that support the research.

ASPE asked the National Academies of Sciences, Engineering, and Medicine to appoint a consensus study committee and identify issues critical to building data capacity for PCOR and for generating new evidence to inform health care decisions. The input provided by the committee will contribute to ASPE's strategic planning for its work related to the data infrastructure over the next decade. The study is part of a broader initiative by ASPE intended to update the strategic plan in light of the reauthorization of the PCOR Trust Fund and the recent advances achieved in health information technology and interoperability tools. Box 1-1 shows the committee's Statement of Task.

The study is a collaboration of three units of the National Academies: the Committee on National Statistics, the Board on Health Care Services, and the Computer Science and Telecommunications Board. The consensus

> **BOX 1-1**
> **Statement of Task**
>
> The National Academies will appoint an ad hoc committee to conduct a series of three one-day public workshops and develop conclusions to help guide the data capacity development for patient-centered research from 2021 through 2030. Each workshop will seek input from key stakeholders on topics relevant to the committee charge, and the specific focus of each workshop will be determined by the committee in consultation with ASPE. As part of its activities, the committee will also
>
> - Consider the published review of the history and trajectory of the Office of the Secretary Patient-Centered Outcomes Research Trust Fund (OS-PCORTF) portfolio of investments and the OS-PCORTF roadmap;
> - Assess anticipated changes to health care priorities and priorities for health data and their impact on building data capacity into the foreseeable future, as identified by ASPE;
> - Evaluate the feasibility and utility of developing a phased-in approach to building the interoperable data capacity for patient-centered outcomes research with existing databases in HHS, other Federal Departments and the private sector in a phased approach, such as projects identified in the Cures Act Title III Section 4003 (Interoperability);
> - Consider other existing legislation, regulations, and the like, as deemed relevant; and
> - Receive input from individuals or groups that represent stakeholders, including patients and their caregivers or families and their health care providers.
>
> The committee will issue interim reports after each public workshop with conclusions, and will produce a final written report with findings and conclusions to help guide a future course to continue building the data capacity for patient-centered research. All reports will follow institutional guidelines and be subject to the National Academies review procedures prior to release.

study committee had a diverse membership, its 15 members including experts with decades of experience as well as emerging leaders in the broad fields of (1) PCOR; (2) research methods, statistics, and demography; (3) computer science and data infrastructure; and (4) patient engagement and patient perspectives. Appendix A contains the biographical sketches of the committee members.

WORKSHOPS AND OTHER INFORMATION-GATHERING ACTIVITIES

To obtain a thorough understanding of the PCOR data infrastructure, the committee met with ASPE and other HHS staff and reviewed background documentation, such as the Office of the Secretary PCOR Trust Fund (OS-PCORTF) project portfolio, annual reports, and reviews completed by other entities. As part of its information-gathering activities, the committee also organized three workshops to collect input from stakeholders on aspects of the charge developed in consultation with ASPE. The workshops focused on key topics that the committee believed would be particularly useful for the strategic planning and would benefit from broad input from a variety of data users and other stakeholders. The three topics were (1) data user needs; (2) data standards, methods, and policies; and (3) collaborations, data linkages, and interoperability of electronic databases.

The first workshop, focused on looking ahead at data user needs over the next decade, was held on May 3, 2021. The committee's goal for this event was to bring together researchers and representatives of patient organizations to understand the needs of these two important data user groups. Specifically, the goals of the workshop were:

- Provide a high-level overview of the types of data included in the data infrastructure for PCOR.
- Identify key questions that stakeholders are most likely to want answered going forward, including general themes that cut across health conditions and circumstances.
- Discuss the implications of the broadened statutory scope for PCOR.
- Identify gaps in what stakeholders need and what the infrastructure allows. Consider both limitations in the existing data and improvements that could be made to new data collections.
- Discuss what questions cannot be answered and who is not served by the current PCOR data infrastructure.
- Discuss what matters HHS is best positioned to address and how the agency could maximize resources available for the PCOR data infrastructure (representing four percent of the PCOR Trust Fund) in the context of HHS's public mission, authorities, programs, and data resources.

The second workshop, held on May 24, 2021, focused on developments in the areas of data standards, methods, and policies relevant to PCOR. The committee's goal for this event was to bring together researchers and policy experts to

- Identify data standards and methods that can make the PCOR data infrastructure more useful for research and other data needs;
- Identify data policies that are needed to facilitate the continued development and operation of the PCOR data infrastructure; and
- Discuss what HHS is best positioned to address and support, and how the agency could maximize resources available for the PCOR data infrastructure (representing four percent of the PCOR Trust Fund), in the context of the HHS public mission, authorities, programs, and data resources.

The third workshop, held on June 14, 2021, focused on ways of enhancing collaborations, data linkages, and the interoperability of electronic databases to make the PCOR data infrastructure more useful in the years ahead. The goals of the workshop were to

- Discuss how research and data collaborations can evolve to meet PCOR and data capacity challenges, and how HHS can support effective research and data collaborations;
- Identify barriers and potential solutions to the access and use of linked public data, and to the access and use of linked public and private/proprietary data; and
- Discuss the feasibility and utility of developing a phased-in approach to building the interoperable data capacity for PCOR with existing databases in HHS, in other federal departments, and in the private sector.

Prior to each workshop, information about the event was disseminated through National Academies mailing lists and on the project website. To collect additional stakeholder input, members of the public were invited to provide comments on topics related to the workshop (or any other topic related to the committee's charge), using a public input form available on the National Academies website.

The discussions and committee conclusions from the workshops were summarized in a series of interim reports. The interim reports have been published as stand-alone reports and are also included as appendixes to this report (see Appendixes B, C, and D). The appendixes contain additional details about the presenters, the input received, and the committee's interim conclusions. Recordings of the workshops and the presentation slides are available on the National Academies website at www.nationalacademies.org/PCORData.

OVERVIEW OF THE REPORT

This report contains the committee's overall findings and conclusions from the study. The findings and conclusions are based on the committee's deliberations and integrated judgment on the materials reviewed and input received from all sources, including the workshops. The report's conclusions reflect the conclusions of the interim reports, but they are further integrated here as part of a more holistic and streamlined discussion. In other words, some of the conclusions from the interim reports are included without substantive changes, while others have been combined and reworded primarily to present them in a more concise way. The final report also includes a few overarching findings and conclusions that do not appear as specific conclusions in any of the three interim reports, resulting instead from the committee's subsequent deliberations that reflected on everything that was learned. Throughout the report, we included references to specific sections of the interim reports (Appendixes B, C, and D) that provide a more in-depth discussion of the topics covered in the final report.

Chapter 2 describes the PCOR data infrastructure and the OS-PCORTF. Chapter 3 discusses the committee's conclusions concerning those aspects of the PCOR data infrastructure that emerged as areas that could particularly benefit from being prioritized as part of ASPE's work over the next decade. The topics covered in the final report reflect the topics covered in the three interim reports, with an effort to offer integrated conclusions on the themes that overlapped across the workshops. Chapter 3 also offers additional conclusions on strengthening the overall framework for building the data infrastructure based on the committee's collective judgment and deliberations on the input received. Appendix A contains biographical sketches of the committee members. Appendixes B, C, and D include the previously published interim reports. Appendix E contains a list and details on the data infrastructure projects funded through the OS-PCORTF.

2

Background on the PCOR Data Infrastructure and Office of the Secretary PCOR Trust Fund

This chapter provides an overview of the patient-centered outcomes research (PCOR) data infrastructure and the PCOR Trust Fund. A brief historical overview of the program's origins and relevant legislation is followed by a discussion of the current state and elements of the data infrastructure, as well as the framework used by the Assistant Secretary for Planning and Evaluation (ASPE) to organize its activities in this area. The chapter also describes the data infrastructure projects and products that have been funded from the Office of the Secretary PCOR Trust Fund (OS-PCORTF) over the years, including prior evaluations of these efforts.

HISTORY OF THE PCOR TRUST FUND

Between 2003 and 2010, three laws were enacted that facilitated the expansion of research on the outcomes and effectiveness of treatments and interventions used in health care in a broad sense. In 2003, the Medicare Prescription Drug, Improvement, and Modernization Act provided authorization for the Agency for Healthcare Research and Quality (AHRQ) to support research comparing the outcomes and effectiveness of treatments and clinical approaches and to disseminate the findings from this research. In 2009, the American Recovery and Reinvestment Act provided additional funding to AHRQ, the National Institutes of Health, and the U.S. Department of Health and Human Services (HHS) for research that compares the effectiveness of medical options. In 2010, the Patient Protection and Affordable Care Act provided further authorization for research that assists patients, clinicians, purchasers, and policy makers in making informed health decisions.

The PCOR Trust Fund within the Department of the Treasury was established by Congress in 2010. The goals of the PCOR Trust Fund are to fund PCOR, disseminate research findings, and build data capacity for PCOR. The bulk of the PCOR Trust Fund funding (around 80 percent of it), which is focused on research, is made available through the Patient-Centered Outcomes Research Institute (PCORI). PCORI is a nongovernmental organization established by Congress with the mandate to improve the quality and relevance of evidence available to help patients, caregivers, clinicians, employers, insurers, and policy makers make better-informed health decisions.[1] Approximately 16 percent of the PCOR Trust Fund is allocated for disseminating research findings, incorporating findings into clinical practice, and training researchers in PCOR. The agency coordinating this work is AHRQ.

The remaining funding, which constitutes four percent of the PCOR Trust Fund, is allocated for building data capacity for PCOR. ASPE, under delegation of authority by the Secretary of HHS, coordinates across relevant federal health programs to build data capacity for PCOR, including administering the OS-PCORTF. Specifically, Section 937(f) of the Public Health Service Act instructed the Secretary of HHS to

> ... provide for the coordination of relevant Federal health programs to build data capacity for comparative clinical effectiveness research, including the development and use of clinical registries and health outcomes research networks, in order to develop and maintain a comprehensive, interoperable data network to collect, link, and analyze data on outcomes and effectiveness from multiple sources including electronic health records.[2]

In 2020, the PCOR Trust Fund was reauthorized through 2029, as part of H.R.1865 of the Further Consolidated Appropriations Act. The most recent statute specified intellectual and developmental disabilities, as well as maternal mortality, as research priorities. The statute also called for PCOR studies to include consideration of the full range of outcomes data, including potential burdens and economic impacts. Specifically, the law states the following:

> Research shall be designed, as appropriate, to take into account and capture the full range of clinical and patient-centered outcomes relevant to, and that meet the needs of, patients, clinicians, purchasers, and policy-

---

[1] https://www.pcori.org/about/about-pcori.
[2] https://aspe.hhs.gov/collaborations-committees-advisory-groups/os-pcortf/about-os-pcortf.

makers in making informed health decisions. In addition to the relative health outcomes and clinical effectiveness, clinical and patient-centered outcomes shall include the potential burdens and economic impacts of the utilization of medical treatments, items, and services on different stakeholders and decision-makers respectively. These potential burdens and economic impacts include medical out-of-pocket costs, including health plan benefit and formulary design, non-medical costs to the patient and family, including caregiving, effects on future costs of care, workplace productivity and absenteeism, and healthcare utilization.[3]

This National Academies of Sciences, Engineering, and Medicine study is focused on issues relevant to continued work on the PCOR data infrastructure. In other words, it is focused on priorities for the use of the OS-PCORTF, or the four percent of the funding that is allocated for HHS to conduct work related to the data infrastructure for PCOR.

ENABLING DATA INFRASTRUCTURE FOR PCOR AND ASPE'S STRATEGIC FRAMEWORK

As the coordinator for the PCOR data infrastructure investment portfolio across HHS agencies, ASPE guides the strategic framework and vision for PCOR data infrastructure, sets funding priorities in collaboration with agencies and departmental leaders, and coordinates interagency workgroups. ASPE's work is assisted by a Leadership Council for the OS-PCORTF, which includes representatives of several other HHS agencies, including the following:

- Administration for Children and Families;
- Administration for Community Living;
- Assistant Secretary for Preparedness and Response;
- Agency for Healthcare Research and Quality;
- Centers for Disease Control and Prevention;
- Centers for Medicare & Medicaid Services;
- Food and Drug Administration;
- Health Resources and Services Administration;
- National Institutes of Health;
- Office of the Chief Technology Officer;
- Office of the National Coordinator for Health Information Technology; and
- Substance Abuse and Mental Health Services Administration.

---

[3] https://www.ssa.gov/OP_Home/ssact/title11/1181.htm.

The agencies that are represented on the Leadership Council bring a variety of perspectives linked with their missions, which include (1) producing data, (2) conducting or funding research, or (3) making evidence-based decisions. The Leadership Council provides input on priorities for the portfolio, including projects to fund.

Using a strategic plan and agency leadership as guides, the OS-PCORTF approach to building data capacity has been characterized by incremental, modular investments. ASPE and its partners conduct an annual review of the progress that has been made and set priorities for the following year, based on statutory priorities and the need to build toward desired functionalities. The current framework for building data capacity is organized according to five data infrastructure goals. These five goals enable functionalities to collect, link, and analyze data for patient-centered research.

Figure 2-1 is a visual representation of the framework that has guided the PCOR data infrastructure portfolio in recent years (as discussed, the reauthorization presents an opportunity for a new strategic direction). The diagram was developed in an attempt to operationalize the mandate for the OS-PCORTF and guide decision making. Definitions for the key terminology used for the framework are provided on the right hand side of the figure. The bottom row shows potential sources of data for PCOR studies, feeding into the PCOR data infrastructure. Data collected as part of clinical care includes data collected for health care delivery and for billing purposes. Examples of primary data collected as part of research studies include data from clinical trials and national health surveys. Other examples of data sources include Medicare or Medicaid claims data, quality or outcomes data collected by health care providers for the purposes of improving health care value, Food and Drug Administration data on the safety of medications and medical devices, and Centers for Disease Control and Prevention data on births and deaths provided by state public health authorities.

The framework describes the relationship between the data sources and major functionalities (middle row), including the "pillars" or core research functions and focus areas that support the research. The key functionalities are described in further detail in Box 2-1. The major building blocks are the services, standards, policies, and governance that enable the use of the data for research, described in Box 2-2. The top row shows the key data users and contributors of data.

The work of HHS agencies toward building data capacity for PCOR is guided by strategic planning that has continuously evolved over the years. The work evolves based on changes in legislation, new priorities in public health and medical care, new HHS policies, strategic opportunities, and the evolving data infrastructure needs of stakeholders.

To gather input on challenges and priorities for the PCOR data infrastructure, in 2020 ASPE commissioned a study centered on an "online

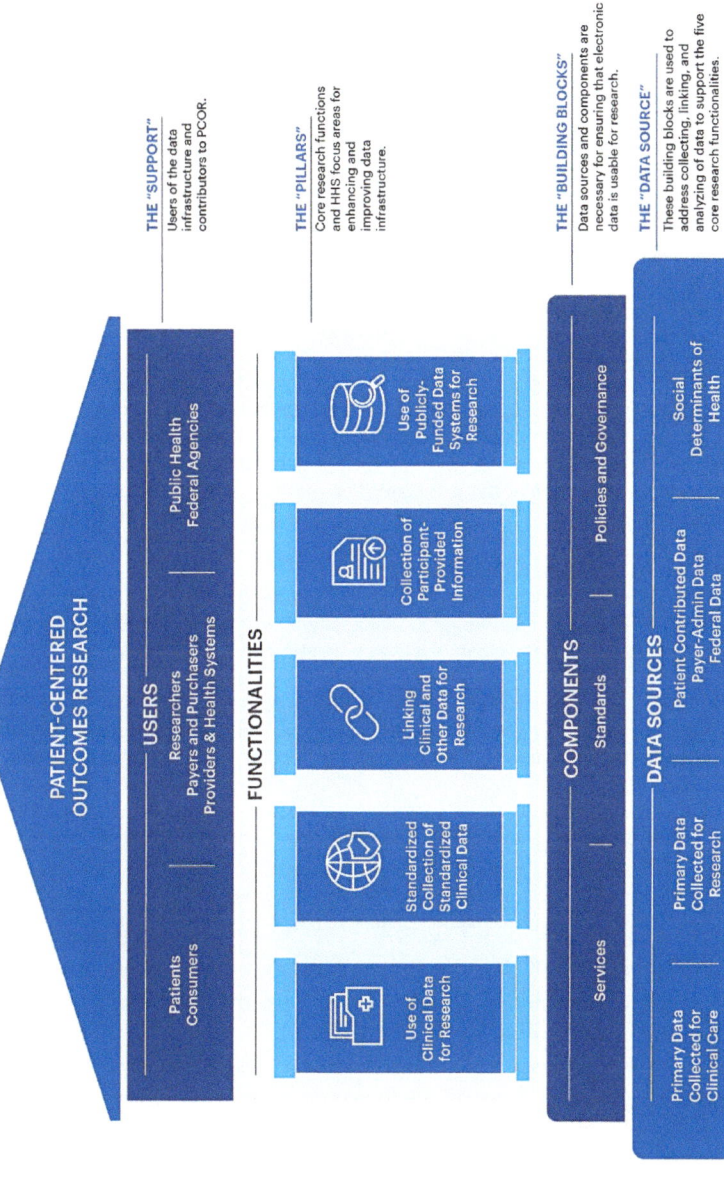

FIGURE 2-1 Office of the Secretary PCOR Trust Fund strategic framework for the PCOR data infrastructure.
SOURCE: Workshop Presentation by ASPE, May 3, 2021.

> **BOX 2-1**
> **Key Data Infrastructure Functionalities in the Existing Strategic Framework for PCOR**
>
> **Use of clinical data for research**
> Researchers will be able to utilize and analyze routinely collected clinical data for implementation of clinical studies (observational and interventional), including data relevant to assessing safety, efficacy, and adherence, as well as genetic data and patient-reported outcomes.
>
> **Standardized collection of standardized clinical data**
> Researchers will be able to use standardized clinical data based on common data element standards across research projects and networks, thereby facilitating linkage and aggregation of data across data sources.
>
> **Linking of clinical and other data for research**
> Researchers will be able to follow patients across the care continuum over time, including those enrolled in clinical trials. Researchers will be able to capture the range of variables influencing health outcomes and link clinical and other types of data (e.g., other clinical data, claims data, participant-provided information, and environmental data) required for research regardless of where the participant goes.
>
> **Collection of participant-provided information**
> Participants, including those in safety net organizations, will be able to participate more fully in clinical research by directly providing information (i.e., data points provided by the participant such as patient-reported outcomes).
>
> **Use of enhanced publicly funded data systems for research**
> Researchers will be able to readily use, retrieve, link, and aggregate publicly funded data for research due to enhancements in publicly funded data systems.
>
> SOURCE: https://aspe.hhs.gov/collaborations-committees-advisory-groups/os-pcortf/about-os-pcortf/building-data-capacity-patient-centered-outcomes-research.

prioritization activity."[4] The findings from that study were among the materials reviewed by the committee as background for its work. The prioritization activity involved stakeholders with a variety of backgrounds, such as health care providers, researchers, and health policy experts, who were asked to generate lists of challenges and needed improvements for the five functionalities included in ASPE's framework for the PCOR data infrastructure. Participants were then asked to vote on the challenges and

---

[4] https://aspe.hhs.gov/sites/default/files/migrated_legacy_files//197426/PCOR-Data-Infrastructure.pdf.

> **BOX 2-2**
> **Building Blocks of the PCOR Data Infrastructure**
>
> *Standards* represent information and meaning to patient-centered data to ensure that health-specific information can be accurately (and securely) exchanged and used. In most cases standards should be nationally accepted, widely approved, or broadly adopted through either market forces, community approval, or regulatory requirements. These include such items as data standards for capturing, storing, representing, and exchanging data in a secure manner such that accurate information is conveyed to the recipient of the data.
>
> *Policies* are standards of behavior that participants can rely on consistently to build patient-centered data for research. Policies may include federal policies, as well as models for standardized state and local policies, that will lead to a trusted framework within the PCOR data infrastructure that ensures productivity, protects the patient and the patient's data, ensures that evidence generation remains in the center of PCOR, and ensures the use of agreed upon standards and services.
>
> *Services* refer to resources that entities can employ on demand to capture, store, or exchange either PCOR data or evidence through a centrally hosted model provided remotely (such as through the Internet) rather than provided locally or on-site. Services make it easy for the research data to interoperate among different systems without having to start from scratch for every connection.
>
> *Governance structures* refer to entities that are needed to develop and apply the rules and policies needed for building an interoperable and sustainable research network. Governance structures support the efficient use of the data infrastructure for research across individual and organizational boundaries of control and ownership. Governance structures are distinguished from "governance," which is what a governing body or governance structure does.
>
> SOURCE: https://aspe.hhs.gov/collaborations-committees-advisory-groups/os-pcortf/about-os-pcortf/building-data-capacity-patient-centered-outcomes-research.

improvements in order to generate prioritized lists. The activity resulted in 87 items described as challenges and 76 items described as needed improvements for the data infrastructure. Box 2-3 summarizes the needs that emerged as priorities from this activity.

BOX 2-3
Key Themes That Emerged from the Stakeholder Prioritization Activity Commissioned by ASPE in 2020

Enhancing consistency in data standardization

The need to enhance consistency in data standardization included a desire for consistent processes for collecting, cleaning, and presenting data. Participants also highlighted the need to encourage the adoption of standards and adherence to standards across health systems.

Improving access to data on the social determinants of health (SDOH) that are not routinely collected during care delivery

Participants highlighted the need for supporting the standardized collection of data of this type and expanded access to federal datasets that contain SDOH data. An example of the data that would be useful for research on this topic is ZIP-code-level data on neighborhood characteristics.

Improving the ability to access, integrate, and use protected personal information, particularly the data generated from medical devices and wearables

Stakeholders underscored the need for facilitating access to protected personal information, including patient-reported outcomes and patient-generated health data, especially from medical devices and wearables. The specific needs described in this area included standards for the collection and use of protected personal information, their integration into electronic health records, and mechanisms to promote the collection of patient-reported outcomes among patients and clinicians.

Increasing access to federal datasets, with an emphasis on access to de-identified datasets

Participants highlighted the need for simplifying access to federal datasets for research, particularly de-identified federal datasets and surveillance data.

Expanding collaboration across organizations at the local, state, and federal levels

Participants highlighted the potential benefits of collaboration to leverage and enhance existing data sources and infrastructure. Among the needed collaborations highlighted were those in the areas of data sharing, enhanced federal datasets, standards, and the regulatory framework.

SOURCE: https://aspe.hhs.gov/sites/default/files/migrated_legacy_files//197426/PCOR-Data-Infrastructure.pdf.

OVERVIEW OF THE DATA INFRASTRUCTURE PROJECTS AND PRODUCTS

This section describes the data infrastructure project and products funded through the OS-PCORTF, in order to provide some additional context about the ongoing work. As of 2021, the OS-PCORTF had funded 61 data infrastructure projects, which included 33 active and 28 completed projects. Appendix E shows the full list of projects, with additional details about each. The 53 projects funded during the first 10 years (from 2010 to 2019) translated to 76 agency awards, totaling approximately $131 million. Many of the projects are conducted as collaborations that involve two or more HHS agencies or with the involvement of additional agencies in an advisory capacity.

As discussed earlier, each project addresses one or more of the five functionalities in the data infrastructure framework. Table 2-1 shows a count of the projects by the infrastructure functionalities they address. Table 2-2 summarizes the number of products that resulted from OS-PCORTF data infrastructure projects by product category, and Table 2-3 provides examples of the types of products that are produced.

"Use cases" based on the priorities of the HHS Secretary play an important role in the way priorities are set for the OS-PCORTF. Table 2-4 shows examples of HHS priorities and PCOR projects. ASPE evaluates these projects in the context of their fit with the current strategic plan and the projects' potential contributions to building a data infrastructure that will support PCOR. Figure 2-2 shows how some of the thematic areas that have been funded over the years map onto the five functionalities in the current conceptual framework.

TABLE 2-1 Number of Office of the Secretary PCOR Trust Fund Projects by Data Infrastructure Functionality Addressed

Data Infrastructure Functionality Addressed	Number of Projects
Standardized collection of standardized clinical data	27
Collection of participant-provided information	12
Linking of clinical and other data for research	38
Use of clinical data for research	35
Use of enhanced publicly funded data systems for research	19

NOTE: Some projects address multiple functionalities.
SOURCE: https://aspe.hhs.gov/collaborations-committees-advisory-groups/os-pcortf/explore-portfolio.

TABLE 2-2 Products Produced by Office of the Secretary PCOR Trust Fund Projects

Product Category	Number of Products
Datasets, databases, and linked data	5
Data elements and information models	3
Health information technology standards	6
Tools and guides	8
Software and analytic services	8
Data governance products	3
Publications	8
Project reports and briefs	20
Vignettes, project spotlights, and portfolio reports	15
Annual reports	6
Evaluation reports	2
Total	84

SOURCE: https://aspe.hhs.gov/collaborations-committees-advisory-groups/os-pcortf/os-pcortf-product-library.

TABLE 2-3 Examples of Products Produced by Office of the Secretary PCOR Trust Fund Projects

TECHNICAL PRODUCTS			
Dataset	**Data Element & Information Model**	**HIT Standards**	**Tools and Guides**
– Research dataset with PII (available only through a repository)	– Common data element (CDE)	– HL7 Implementation guide	– Toolkit
– Research dataset without PII (available through a repository and/or can be downloaded)	– Data element and standards set (DESS)	– Terminology standard guides	– Algorithmic tools
– Linked dataset with PII (available only through a repository)	– Data/Clinical information models	– Data classes for United States Core Data for Interoperability (USCDI)	– Methods documentation
– Linked dataset without PII (available through a repository and/or can be downloaded)	– Metadata/Dataset documentation (schema, semantics, and syntax)	– Other documentations related to HIT standards	– Analytic guidance
			– Manual/user guide
			– Implementation/roll-out guidelines
			– System documentation
Software	**Software and Analytic Services**	**Data Governance**	**Stakeholder Engagement**
– Mobile Application	– Application programming interface (API)	– Data quality guide	– User, TEP, or workgroup engagement documentation
– Web-based Application	– Middleware application	– Privacy and security guidelines	– Training
– Application Module	– Data management platform	– Policy-related output	
– Algorithmic codes	– Development environment	– Data sharing framework	
– Analytic codes	– Analytic service platform		
– Data processing codes			

COMMUNICATION AND DISSEMINATION PRODUCTS		ADMINISTRATIVE DELIVERABLES	
Publications	**Presentations**	**Project implementation plans**	**Contract/grant deliverables**
– Journal publication about the project (Journal-ready, Submitted, Published)	– Conference/meeting Presentation (online and in-person)	– Project work plan	– Contracts
– Journal publication using the dataset produced (Journal-ready, Submitted, Published)	– Conference/meeting Presentation (OSPCORTF-led) (online and in-person)	– Design plan	– RFPs and RFIs
– Journal publications produced/led by OS-PCORTF team (including contractors)	– Conference/meeting presentation by OSPCORTF	– Dissemination/communication plan	– Grant-related output
Web & Social Media	**Project Reports and Briefs**	– Evaluation plan	
– OS-PCORTF web page	– Project final report (Under aspe.hhs.gov, Under agency website)	– Sustainability plan	
– Project web pages (under aspe.hhs.gov)	– Project briefs (by the project, by the portfolio		
– Project Web page/s (under agency website)	– Product briefs		
– Blog post about the project or deliverable	– Data and Issue brief		
Webinar	– Other reports produced by the project		
– Webinar presentation	**Portfolio-related reports**		
– Webinar Sessions (OSPCORTF-led)	– Portfolio vignettes (OSPCORTF-led)		
	– Portfolio annual report		
	– Evaluation reports		

NOTE: HIT = health information technology; PII = personally identifiable information; RFI = request for information; RFP = request for proposals; TEP = technical expert panel.
SOURCE: Presentation by ASPE, January 29, 2021, public meeting.

TABLE 2-4 Examples of HHS Secretarial Priorities and Office of the Secretary PCOR Trust Fund Projects

HHS Secretarial Priority	Example Projects	Lead Agency
Opioids and mental health	An Addiction Medicine Network to Address the United States' Opioid Crisis	NIH
Value-based care	Validating and Expanding Claims-based Algorithms of Frailty and Functional Disability for Value-based Care and Payment	ASPE
Maternal mortality	Surveillance Network: Maternal, Infant, and Child Health Outcomes Associated with Treatment of Opioid Use Disorder during Pregnancy	CDC
Social determinants of health	Creating a National Small-Area Social Determinants of Health Data Platform	AHRQ
Emergency preparedness	Assessing and Predicting Medical Needs in a Disaster	ASPR
Patient empowerment and interoperability	Technologies for Donating Medicare Beneficiary Claims Data to Research Studies	CMS/NIH
Data and innovation	Training Data for Machine Learning to Enhance Patient-Centered Outcomes Research Data Infrastructure	ONC

NOTE: NIH = National Institutes of Health; CDC = Centers for Disease Control and Prevention; AHRQ = Agency for Healthcare Research and Quality; ASPR = Office of the Assistant Secretary for Preparedness and Response; CMS = Centers for Medicare & Medicaid Services; ONS = Office of the National Coordinator for Health Information Technology.
SOURCE: Presentation by ASPE, January 29, 2021, public meeting.

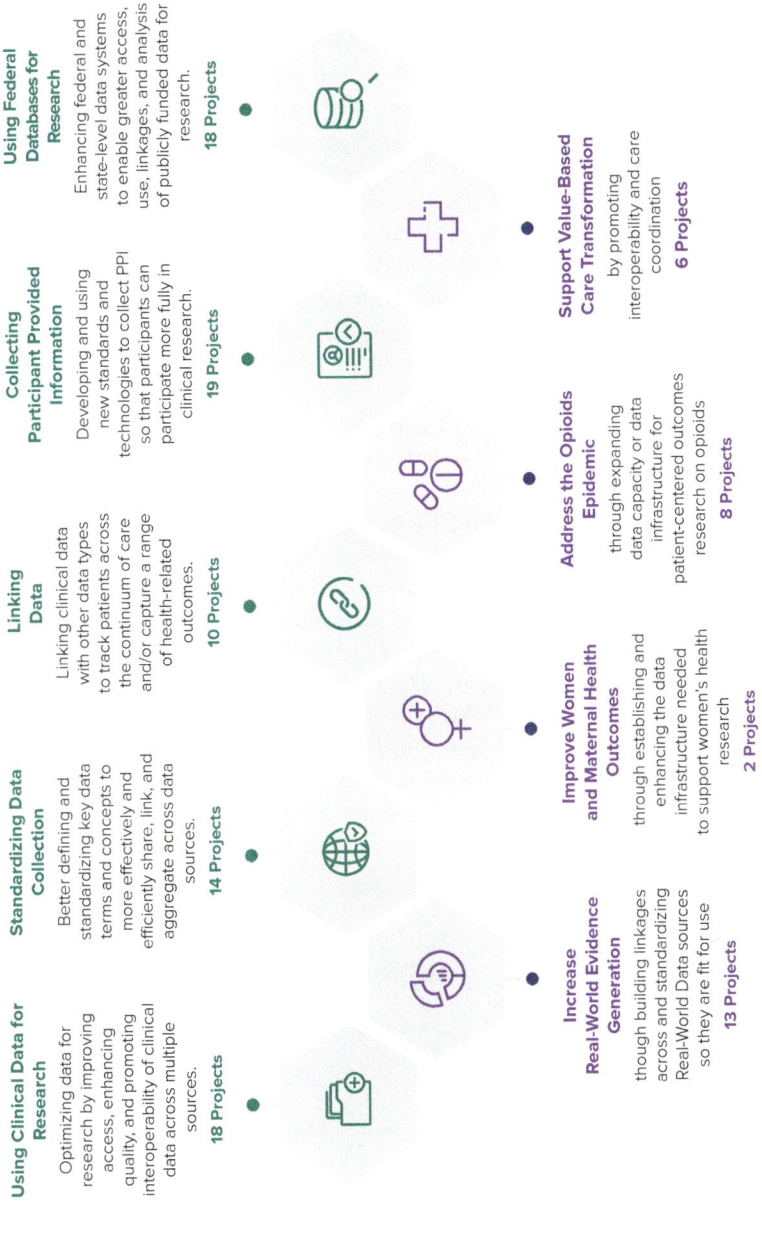

FIGURE 2-2 Relationship between thematic areas funded and the five PCOR data infrastructure functionalities.
SOURCE: Presentation by ASPE, January 29, 2021, public meeting.

2020 Annual Report

The most recent (2020) annual report issued by ASPE for the PCOR data infrastructure work provides a synopsis of the 31 projects that were active in Fiscal Year 2020.[5] As discussed, HHS priorities play an important role in the priorities for the PCOR data infrastructure projects. As such, along with addressing stakeholder priorities for the data infrastructure, the annual report places special emphasis on work that supports women's health and improving maternal health outcomes, as well as COVID-19 pandemic response. Box 2-4 lists the active projects in these key areas. More detailed information about the projects is available on ASPE's website.[6]

The annual report also highlighted three completed projects that enhanced functionalities likely to be useful to researchers:

1. **Adding Cause-Specific Mortality to National Center for Health Statistics' National Hospital Care Survey by Linking to the National Death Index and CMS Master Beneficiary Summary File:** These linkages allow researchers to conduct more robust studies of cause-specific mortality.
2. **Assessing and Predicting Medical Needs in a Disaster:** Increased access to local, state, and federal datasets can improve data availability in a disaster, help analyze and improve response strategies, identify needs and trends for long-term recovery, and track the long-term health outcomes and consequences of a disaster.
3. **Emergency Medicine Opioid Data Infrastructure: Key Venue to Address Opioid Morbidity and Mortality (Project CODE PRO – Capturing Opioid Use Disorder Electronically and Patient Reported Outcomes):** Use of standardized common data elements and patient-reported outcome measures captured in emergency department electronic health records can improve the opioid-use disorder data available in clinical registries for PCOR.

---

[5] https://aspe.hhs.gov/sites/default/files/private/pdf/259016/2020-os-pcortf-portfolio-report.pdf.

[6] https://aspe.hhs.gov/index.php/collaborations-committees-advisory-groups/os-pcortf/explore-portfolio.

> **BOX 2-4**
> **2020 Office of the Secretary PCOR Trust Fund Projects in Three HHS Priority Areas**
>
> **Women's health and improving maternal health outcomes**
> - Developing a Strategically Coordinated Registry Network for Women's Health Technology
> - Bridging the PCOR Infrastructure and Technology Innovation through Coordinated Registry Networks Community of Practice
> - MAT-LINK: MATernaL and Infant NetworK to Understand Outcomes Associated with Treatment for Opioid Use Disorder During Pregnancy
> - Developing a Multi-State Network of Linked Pregnancy Risk Assessment Monitoring System and Clinical Outcomes Data for Patient-Centered Outcomes Research
>
> **COVID-19 pandemic response**
> - SHIELD (Systematic Harmonization and Interoperability Enhancement for Laboratory Data) Collaborative – Standardization of Lab Data to Enhance Patient-Centered Outcomes Research and Value-based Care
> - Harmonization of Various Common Data Models and Open Standards for Evidence Generation
> - Source Data Capture from Electronic Health Records: Using Standardized Clinical Research Data (OneSource)
> - Collection of Patient-Provided Information through a Mobile Device Application for Use in Comparative Effectiveness and Drug Safety Research
> - Capstone for the Outcome Measures Harmonization
> - Enhancing Data Resources for Researching Patterns of Mortality in Patient-Centered Outcomes Research: Project 1 – Adding Cause-Specific Mortality to NCHS's National Hospital Care Survey by Linking to the National Death Index Stakeholder Data Infrastructure Priorities
> - Emergency Medicine Opioid Data Infrastructure – Key Venue to Address Opioid Morbidity and Mortality (Project CODE PRO – Capturing Opioid Use Disorder Electronically and Patient Reported Outcomes)
> - Assessing and Predicting Medical Needs in a Disaster
>
> **Stakeholder data infrastructure priorities**
> - Harmonization of Various Common Data Models and Open Standards for Evidence Generation
> - Enhancing Patient-Centered Outcomes Research: Creating a National Small-Area Social Determinants of Health Data Platform
> - Data Capacity for Patient-Centered Outcomes Research through Creation of an Electronic Care Plan for People with Multiple Chronic Conditions
> - Advancing the Collection and Use of Patient-Reported Outcomes through Health Information Technology
> - A Synthetic Health Data Generation Engine to Accelerate Patient-Centered Outcomes Research
>
> *continued*

> **BOX 2-4 Continued**
>
> - Training Data for Machine Learning to Enhance Patient-Centered Outcomes Research Data Infrastructure
> - Data Linkage: Evaluating Preserving Privacy Methodology and Augmenting the National Hospital Care Survey with Medicaid Administrative Records
> - Childhood Obesity Data Initiative (CODI): Integrated Data for Patient-Centered Outcomes Research Project
> - Assessing and Predicting Medical Needs in a Disaster
>
> SOURCE: https://aspe.hhs.gov/sites/default/files/private/pdf/259016/2020-os-pcortf-portfolio-report.pdf.

2016–2019 Portfolio Review

ASPE periodically commissions in-depth reviews of its portfolio of data infrastructure projects. The most recent review focused on 43 projects that were funded between 2016 and 2019 in the form of individual agency awards (the review did not include multiagency awards).[7] It looked at the extent to which the portfolio of projects advanced the strategic framework, and concluded that approximately three out of four awards included a focus on optimizing the use of clinical data for research. About half of the awards fell into one or more of these categories: enhancing the use of federal datasets for research, standardizing data collections, and (or) developing tools to collect participant-provided information. One out of four projects focused on linking data.

The evaluation also assessed the extent to which the portfolio addressed gaps that had been identified by the previous evaluation, conducted in 2017.[8] The 2019 evaluation concluded that the gap most frequently addressed by the awards was to disseminate research findings, and it noted progress in the areas of implementing standards and improving data quality. Concerning whether the portfolio changed in response to changes in the health policy landscape, the recent evaluation noted that the portfolio expanded to include projects on enhancing the interoperability of health information, improving patient access to health information, and supporting advanced data science methods.

---

[7] https://aspe.hhs.gov/sites/default/files/migrated_legacy_files//194781/OS-PCORTFImpactReport508.pdf.
[8] https://aspe.hhs.gov/sites/default/files/migrated_legacy_files//180436/ASPEPCORTFEvaluation.pdf.

The 2019 assessment also included input from an expert panel on the future direction of the data infrastructure portfolio in several areas. In the area of refinements to the strategic framework, the panel identified the following opportunities for additional progress:[9]

- Integrating external factors such as financial and policy drivers that influence provider documentation and the social determinants that impact health outcomes;
- Identifying and incorporating cross-cutting barriers;
- Highlighting the role of data provenance in the usability of data for research; and
- Forming working groups that can provide input on each of the five functionalities.

The 2019 expert panel further identified the following as priorities for the data infrastructure:

- Addressing nontechnical challenges to the use and sharing of data, including challenges associated with data governance, data privacy, and data security;
- Providing targeted support to products that may be of broad interest and ready for adoption; and
- Engaging end users during the planning phases of project awards.

Finally, the 2019 expert panel identified the need for better metrics to assess the portfolio's impact, including the following:

- Award-specific metrics to assess whether each individual project achieved its objectives;
- Metrics that track how products from projects are being used by other projects within the portfolio;
- A more prescriptive strategic roadmap and metrics that assess progress along the roadmap; and
- Use of website analytics and dissemination and translation metrics that track the number and type of dissemination products, and the ways in which other research initiatives leverage award outputs.

---

[9] https://aspe.hhs.gov/sites/default/files/migrated_legacy_files//194781/OS-PCORTFImpactReport508.pdf.

3

Priority Areas for the PCOR Data Infrastructure

In this chapter we discuss the conclusions reached by the committee based on the information-gathering activities carried out over the course of the study and on the committee's subsequent deliberations and integrated judgment. Key information-gathering activities included (1) reviewing background documentation about the Assistant Secretary for Planning and Evaluation's (ASPE's) work, such as the reports discussed in Chapter 2; (2) public meetings with the U.S. Department of Health and Human Services (HHS) staff; and (3) three public workshops focused on gathering input from stakeholders. Appendixes B through D provide detailed summaries of the workshops, including the input received from the participants and the conclusions reached by the committee on the topics that were discussed.

This chapter focuses on aspects of the patient-centered outcomes research (PCOR) data infrastructure that ultimately emerged as areas that could benefit if prioritized as part of ASPE's work over the next decade. The topics highlighted touch on many of the key elements of the framework currently used by ASPE to manage work related to the PCOR data infrastructure (see Figure 2-1). The chapter also offers additional input on strengthening the overall framework for building the data infrastructure over the coming years.

The committee's charge was to identify issues critical to building data capacity for PCOR and for generating new evidence to inform health care decisions. In its deliberations, the committee noted the limitations of focusing solely on patients and concluded that broadening the focus to *persons* would increase the likelihood that ASPE could develop an infrastructure for research that addresses the priorities identified in the authorizing legislation, by those who participated in workshops, and from the committee members' own experiences in answering questions of interest to people. This distinction between people and patients is not intended to imply that these roles are necessarily separate but rather to underscore the broader context that might be missed when the focus is exclusively on the patient. Furthermore, a desire to broaden the focus does not imply that the challenges associated with the data infrastructure for PCOR have been addressed. As the remainder of this chapter will illustrate, many of the continuing challenges are best addressed in the broader context.

The committee uses the following definitions:

- *People* refers to individuals throughout their life course, whether or not they are interacting with the health services system or have had a clinical diagnosis. A focus on people would enable ASPE to identify the rich set of attributes by which people define themselves and would provide the larger context within which people seek medical intervention for health care problems. The broader context includes people's communities, in other words the health impacts of where individuals live, work, and play. Focusing on people would also be useful for identifying challenges and opportunities in optimizing health.
- *Patients* refers to people who are interacting with the health services system to obtain a diagnosis or treatment for acute or chronic conditions, to manage symptoms that affect their quality of life, or for advice and interventions aimed at preventing disease or enhancing health. In the committee's definitions, patients are people first, but their priorities and preferences may change in response to a new diagnosis or other change in health status.

The committee also offers a first conclusion, which resulted from a recurring theme that emerged from the workshops organized by the committee and from the committee's subsequent deliberations integrating all the input. This conclusion, which serves as the basis of the new approach described above and represents a shift in perspective, could be transformative for both research and health care.

CONCLUSION 3-1: Broadening the focus from the patient to the person more generally and from populations to communities would enable a more comprehensive approach to the data infrastructure and a better understanding of the outcomes that matter to people.

INCLUDING HIGH-PRIORITY TYPES OF DATA IN THE DATA INFRASTRUCTURE

As Figure 2-1 shows, the data serve as the foundation of the PCOR data infrastructure. Data needs and priorities have evolved over the years on the basis of advances in science and policy considerations. The most recent reauthorization of the PCOR Trust Fund highlighted several new areas as priorities, including intellectual and developmental disabilities, maternal mortality, and health care cost as a consideration among the full range of outcomes data.

The committee's first workshop focused on gathering input on emerging data needs and priorities from stakeholders, including researchers and representatives of patient organizations. Among the goals of the workshop were to identify key questions that stakeholders are most likely to want answered going forward and to identify gaps between what stakeholders need and what the data infrastructure allows.

A theme that emerged from the workshop was the magnitude of the gaps in the data on health disparities. Health disparities represent an evolving and expanding area of research, with corresponding data needs and data limitations that affect the ability to identify, understand, and address these disparities. Limitations exist for a variety of social determinants of health data and for a range of populations and communities. Data for specific populations are sometimes unavailable or are not representative. In other cases, the data might not be timely or might have other gaps that make it difficult to understand the impact of changes over long periods of time. The committee's first interim report (see especially Appendix B, Chapter 2) discusses these limitations in further detail and highlights a variety of examples, ranging from gaps in the data available on disabilities to those concerning sexual and gender minorities and racial and ethnic groups. Improving the data available for understanding and addressing these disparities would require data strategies that prioritize these data needs.

The cost of care emerged as another topic area where there are substantial gaps in the information available. Both patient groups and researchers highlighted the clear need for more data on the total cost of care and a better understanding of cost considerations and their impact on the quality and length of life (see Appendix B, Chapters 3 and 4, as well as Appendix D, Chapter 2). Given the limitations on accessing health care delivery and the high cost of health care relative to the financial resources available to families in the United States, the ability to access care and to pay for that care can face barriers that impact the length and quality of people's lives.

The committee's third workshop, focused on identifying ways of enhancing collaborations, data linkages, and the interoperability of electronic databases, highlighted the particular need for and the underutilized potential in performing linkages to mortality data (see Appendix D, Chapter 2). Death records from the Social Security Administration are often challenging to access, and the Centers for Disease Control and Prevention's National Death Index database only makes data available with a substantial time lag and at a high cost. This means that researchers have limited ability to use mortality as an outcome measure in studies. The delayed access to, limited reliability of, and high costs of accessing mortality data impede PCOR and decrease the reliability of the findings related to this important outcome. Given that these data already exist, this might be an area where enhancements to the data infrastructure could yield an impact.

The committee's review of the Office of the Secretary PCOR Trust Fund (OS-PCORTF) data infrastructure projects, summarized in Chapter 2 and Appendix E, shows that ongoing work related to the areas identified are particularly important to stakeholders. However, the examination of whether the PCOR data infrastructure currently contains the data elements needed to study and draw conclusions about optimizing outcomes for people and patients revealed that it does not. Existing data do not capture the richness of people's characteristics and experiences, and some specific areas require more attention. Data types that have more recently been authorized through legislation and other priority-setting activities (e.g., social determinants of health, disability, and cost of care) are less likely to be available in the PCOR data infrastructure.

While such limitations are to be expected, opportunities exist for capturing data that are better able to characterize these complexities. A robust data infrastructure builds on the strengths of what is available today and has the flexibility to adapt, both as measures and terminologies become obsolete and as new technologies emerge. The input received as part of the workshops organized by the committee underscored topics that would be particularly worthwhile to prioritize in the near future. This input echoed findings from the stakeholder prioritization activity[1] and the most recent assessment of the portfolio of PCOR data infrastructure projects.[2]

> **CONCLUSION 3-2:** A variety of data types were identified that are less likely to be available or easily accessible in the PCOR data infrastructure, including data on mortality, cost of care, social determinants of health, and disability status, as well as other characteristics of people associated with disparities in health outcomes. Increased attention to filling gaps in the availability of these data will enhance the utility of

---

[1] https://aspe.hhs.gov/sites/default/files/migrated_legacy_files//197426/PCOR-Data-Infrastructure.pdf.

[2] https://aspe.hhs.gov/sites/default/files/migrated_legacy_files//194781/OS-PCORTFImpactReport508.pdf.

the infrastructure for answering questions that matter to people and will enable research on potential intervention targets.

A fundamental reason for the data limitations that make it difficult to answer questions important for PCOR is that most of the data available for research are not primarily collected for research purposes. While research questions require a relational or integrative perspective, the data collected tend to be transactional, that is, collected for payment or treatment purposes. This has several implications for the data available. First, the data collected are typically limited to or organized within subpopulations (e.g., those insured by Medicaid or Medicare). People who are uninsured, including those who have limited access or interactions with health care services, are likely to be underrepresented in many databases. Second, the information collected (and what is not collected) often makes the datasets poorly suited to answer a variety of research questions. Third, those who collect the data do not have an incentive to collect information in a way that is useful for secondary purposes, such as research. These realities present a challenge to answering critical questions, but the workshops also made it clear that opportunities exist to make the data infrastructure more suitable for answering questions of interest, so long as the potential uses of the data are carefully considered.

Much of the focus of the PCOR data infrastructure to date has been on data generated in the course of patient care or in federally funded research studies. The increasing use of person-generated data from various sources was a recurring theme throughout the workshops (see Appendixes C and D in particular). A focus on person-centered outcomes will enable an expansion of opportunities to incorporate person-generated data in the PCOR infrastructure. Integrating these types of data into PCOR will enhance learning about aspects of people's lives that affect health but do not involve direct engagement with the health services system, including relevant measures of how well people are doing. The fact that this is an emerging area also means that in many domains, research on the validity and reliability of these types of measures is still in its early stages. Additional work and scientific testing are needed to ensure that the measures are useful for their intended purposes.

CONCLUSION 3-3: An area with opportunities for additional expansion is the collection of patient- and person-generated data and the routine integration of these data into data platforms that can be used both for research and for other purposes, including regulatory decision making and to inform shared decision making.

One source of additional data that might not otherwise be available to researchers is disease registries directed by patient groups. Disease registries are compilations of data from a variety of other sources and are typically focused on a specific condition or diagnosis. Collaborations with patient organizations can help facilitate access to these types of databases, build patient engagement, and address patient concerns about participating in research studies, all important aspects of achieving a person-centered approach. For additional details on the input received by the committee on this topic, see in particular the discussion on patient data needs in Appendix B, Chapter 3, and on collaborations with patient groups in Appendix D, Chapter 6.

CONCLUSION 3-4: Patient-directed disease registries can be a source of in-depth, longitudinal, prospective clinical and patient-reported data that are not available from other data sources.

One topic that emerged from the committee's second workshop, which included discussions on approaches and methods that could move PCOR forward, was the potential usefulness of adopting a longitudinal perspective on a person's journey through the health care system and, more broadly, through life events that have a relevance to health (see Appendix C, Chapter 3). The fact that the data available for PCOR are typically not collected primarily for research poses challenges in this area as well, but these challenges could gradually be overcome by addressing the broader limitations of the data infrastructure discussed throughout this chapter, including: the lack of integration of data across the research data ecosystem; the lack of unique health identifiers; and the underutilization of certain sources of data, such as person-generated data and real-world clinical data.

CONCLUSION 3-5: Assembling a comprehensive longitudinal record of individuals' health journeys, which also includes the social context of their lives to the extent possible, would facilitate more far-reaching outcomes research.

ADDRESSING FRAGMENTATION

The health care system in the United States is fragmented, resulting in fragmented data, and the PCOR data infrastructure aspires to overcome some of this fragmentation. The data that exist for PCOR are collected and curated in a variety of databases across the health system. These databases are typically constructed to serve their primary purposes and do not prioritize the ability to link with other databases. Other relevant data, such as data on social determinants of health, sometimes exist only outside of these databases or do not exist at all. The workshops identified these data silos as a major barrier both to research and to increasing the usefulness of the information available for decision making more broadly.

A prolific area of work aimed at facilitating data linkages has been focused on developing technical approaches to address data privacy concerns. Tokenization solutions, for example, assign unique keys to the records that are being linked, enabling the linkage to happen without the sharing of patient identifiers. Competition in this area encourages innovation, but the workshops also revealed the resulting challenges for the PCOR data infrastructure (see Appendix C, Chapters 2 and 4, and Appendix D, Chapter 2). Each approach has unique characteristics, and researchers might favor one over others. Furthermore, the approaches that exist are constantly evolving and cannot always be relied on to work in the future. Some solutions are proprietary, and data that use one method cannot be linked to data that use another method.

CONCLUSION 3-6: The data available for PCOR are fragmented across a variety of databases. Expanding data linkages could greatly increase the usefulness of these data for research.

The workshops highlighted the importance of collaborations among federal agencies and other partners (such as states, patient groups, and others) to continue to build a comprehensive data infrastructure based on fragmented data (see especially Appendix D). These collaborations can be particularly useful in addressing barriers that hinder data linkages, such as the limitations associated with person-level unique health identifiers and patient matching. Other areas identified where collaborations could further mitigate the challenges associated with data fragmentation include increasing consistency in the use of standards for data interoperability and element definitions and working with stakeholders and patients to promote data sharing.

State data collection systems are an especially rich source of detailed data that can be useful to state and local policy makers (see Appendix D, Chapter 3). State-generated data are also valuable at the national level, including for answering broader questions about issues that may be influenced by local policy, such as health care access and disparities. While many states have robust data collection systems, the data collected, their quality, and ease of access to the data all vary by state. Challenges associated with access make the use of state-generated data for research at the national level particularly difficult.

CONCLUSION 3-7: Collaboration among federal agencies and between federal agencies and other partners to address barriers that hinder data linkages, such as the limitations associated with the lack of unique health identifiers and patient or person matching, will improve the PCOR data infrastructure. The usefulness of data available for

PCOR could further be increased by sharing and adopting best practices among the states concerning the collection of data, data quality, and ease of access.

DATA NOT DESIGNED TO ADVANCE KNOWLEDGE

As discussed above, the PCOR data infrastructure relies primarily on data that were not collected primarily for research purposes, and in particular for patient- or person-centered research. Much of the work aimed to facilitate the use of these data for research is focused on the development of standards for clinical data and on enhancing the interoperability of data systems. ASPE has focused on "data standards" as one of the building blocks, and the "standardized collection of standardized clinical data" as one of the pillars in the PCOR data infrastructure framework to improve the data infrastructure (Figure 2-1). As a result, many of the projects funded by the PCOR Trust Fund have been centered on these topics. The previous stakeholder prioritization activity also concluded that additional work on standards should be a priority.

The workshops organized by the committee demonstrated that, within the context of PCOR, standardization is increasingly being applied to collecting, storing, analyzing, and exchanging data. Improvements in clinical data standards, in particular, and the adoption of interoperable systems are improving the availability and usefulness of these data for research.

One of the themes that emerged from the workshops is that standards are most useful when they address a specific problem or are driven by a specific use case (see Appendix C, Chapter 2). Because needs and norms evolve over time, standards need to evolve too. The work on standards that is happening across the globe holds lessons for PCOR in general, and lessons might also be learned from best practices that emerge for the development of standards.

The workshops also made it clear that in some areas there is a fair amount of agreement around what standards are needed and what useful standards look like. In other areas, such as for data on the social determinants of health, the work is just beginning, so wide agreement on standards may not yet be possible. In all cases, extensive testing of the potential standards is necessary.

> **CONCLUSION 3-8:** Standards are most useful when their development is driven by their potential uses and a clear concept of the value they can contribute.
>
> **CONCLUSION 3-9:** Taking an international perspective is important for the development of a PCOR data infrastructure; in particular, the

infrastructure focused on standards would benefit from building on work that happens internationally.

Workshop participants did not see a large role for ASPE in selecting areas for or developing standards (see Appendix C, Chapter 2). ASPE's most valuable contributions in this area could be in developing an architecture and an implementation strategy that facilitate common language and interoperability across datasets as well as accessibility of the data. Other areas where ASPE could play an important role include convening stakeholder meetings to discuss and develop standards and taking the lead in cataloging existing standards.

CONCLUSION 3-10: ASPE, in collaboration with other partners and stakeholders, could add significant value in the area of standards for PCOR by:
- continuing to promote the development of a data infrastructure and an implementation strategy that facilitate the use of standards and access to the data;
- convening stakeholder meetings to enhance communication and work toward developing a common language for standards;
- facilitating access to the data and collaborations with existing organizations working in this area;
- leading efforts to catalogue and exemplify data standards and analytic standards for a holistic view of individuals' health; and
- increasing consistency in the use of standards for data interoperability and element definitions.

CONCLUSION 3-11: Prioritizing projects that address fidelity or use of standards may convey greater value for the PCOR infrastructure than developing new standards.

GOVERNING DATA ACCESS

The way data are accessed, used, and shared for research is governed by privacy laws. The most relevant of these laws are the following four:

1. The Health Insurance Portability and Accountability Act of 1996 (HIPAA);
2. "Part 2", which relates to regulations on substance-abuse data confidentiality;
3. The Family Educational Rights and Privacy Act (FERPA), which covers educational institutions; and
4. The Privacy Act, which covers federal government data resources.

The law that has the most impact on PCOR data is HIPAA, which does not cover all health data but does cover identifiable data from most doctors, hospitals, health plans, and contractors. While identifiable data can be used for research under certain conditions, HIPAA was primarily designed to enable data flows within a health care system rather than to address research considerations. New "information blocking" rules that were set forth by the 21st Century Cures Act[3] and went into effect in April 2021 shift the default to the sharing of electronic health information for any lawful purpose, including research. Information blocking is defined as

> a practice by a health IT developer of certified health IT, health information network, health information exchange, or health care provider that, except as required by law or specified by the Secretary of Health and Human Services as a reasonable and necessary activity, is likely to interfere with access, exchange, or use of electronic health information.[4]

While there are penalties for information blocking, the rules around enforcement were still under discussion during the writing of this report. A more detailed discussion of the privacy laws applicable to PCOR data is included in Chapter 4 of Appendix C (see in particular the overview presented by Deven McGraw).

As discussed above, some of the work in this area focuses on technical and methodological solutions to improve data access while preserving privacy. The Blue Button initiative is an additional effort that facilitates data sharing, primarily by providing a mechanism that enables people to download their own health records and then potentially share them with others for a variety of purposes, including research.[5]

Data access and privacy considerations were a recurring theme during the committee's information-gathering activities (see especially Appendix C, Chapter 4, and Appendix D, Chapter 2). Challenges associated with various approaches to obtaining consent were also discussed as an area that needs more work, in light of secondary uses of data that may not be clear to patients. At the same time, it appears that relatively few OS-PCORTF projects have been funded in this area. The workshops made it clear that there are concerns about the laws and rules governing data access and data sharing.

HIPAA, in particular, was developed several decades ago, and its approach to setting thresholds for data disclosures makes it outdated. Moreover, interpretations of how HIPAA applies to particular situations are

---

[3] https://www.healthit.gov/curesrule/.
[4] https://www.healthit.gov/topic/information-blocking.
[5] https://www.healthit.gov/topic/health-it-initiatives/blue-button.

often inconsistent. There is a need for a new framework with guardrails that balance the risk of disclosure with the need for research that improves people's health. This includes a need for a critical review of current privacy legislation, an understanding of public perspectives, and the development of recommendations for revisions or reform that would be applicable to the protection of health data in the Internet-enabled world, with a focus on preventing misuses of the data.

> **CONCLUSION 3-12:** This is an opportune time to revisit and update the legislation and rules governing data privacy and the sharing of data for research.

> **CONCLUSION 3-13:** Governance challenges that create barriers to developing the PCOR infrastructure can be found at all levels of the system. Data availability could be increased by exploring challenges at the local level, including variable interpretations of federal laws and regulations, and by identifying approaches to address those challenges.

DATA ACCESS OPTIONS

Although it is not unique to PCOR, there is an ongoing challenge in finding the right balance between protecting privacy and enabling increased use of data for research. The workshops touched on a variety of mechanisms for accessing PCOR-relevant data that endeavor to navigate this challenge (see Appendix C, Chapter 4, and Appendix D, Chapter 2). Some examples include Special Sworn Status for individuals; Centers for Medicare & Medicaid Services enclave; network participation; group access (for researchers, patients/people, clinicians, policy makers); and Master Data Use agreements. There was also discussion of the benefits possible when mature projects share with others how they have managed access. These processes could all benefit from additional streamlining to facilitate data use.

> **CONCLUSION 3-14:** Investments in identifying mechanisms for facilitating the ability of researchers, patients, and other people to access data will contribute to increased use of the PCOR infrastructure.

While improving data access is essential, another theme raised by stakeholders was the importance of being transparent about how the data will be used (see especially Appendix B, Chapters 3 and 4). Workshop participants emphasized the need to involve the people whose data are being used, as well as their communities, in decisions at each stage of the process. Building and maintaining trust with those whose data are being sought is essential to ensure that the data obtained are representative, complete, and reliable. This is especially important when the data could be perceived as sensitive, as is the case with some of the data on the social determinants of health. Collaborations with patient organizations can help in addressing patient concerns about participating in research studies and in building patient engagement, which are both important for achieving a patient-centered approach.

Researchers echoed the need to make PCOR data more widely available to empower patients and communities to use this information. Efforts to reduce disparities, in particular, cannot be accomplished by research alone. Clinicians are a key stakeholder group that generates a large portion of the data and also uses the data. Ensuring that relevant and easy-to-use PCOR data are available to clinicians is essential for obtaining their cooperation in producing high-quality data.

> **CONCLUSION 3-15:** Building and maintaining trust among the people and communities whose data are being sought for research is essential for producing high-quality data, and patient groups can be helpful partners in these efforts. Including representatives of patients and other people in the research process to understand how to measure health impacts that matter to individuals is an important component in building trust. Providing value back to data donors, such as through the sharing of research results, could help underscore the importance and benefits of the information to stakeholders, including individuals, families, clinicians, and communities, in addition to enabling them to use the information in ways they find relevant. These uses could play a particularly important role in reducing health disparities, complementing research efforts in this area.

While the benefits of data sharing are clear, the workshops also highlighted some of the reasons behind reluctance to share and underscored the risks involved for the organizations providing the data (see the discussion in Appendix D, Chapter 5). Successful data sharing agreements can be established when these factors are taken into consideration.

> **CONCLUSION 3-16:** Successful data sharing partnerships across health care systems and government agencies require participant trust, clear evidence of mutual benefit, and the ability to control risk.

ADVANCING RESEARCH PRACTICES AND ANALYTIC METHODS

Some of the committee's input-gathering activities focused on advances in the methods used for PCOR and on identifying areas that could benefit from additional attention in the coming years to facilitate research (see

Appendix C, Chapter 3). Workshop participants emphasized the need for transparency and for consideration of related scientific principles, such as reproducibility of the data and methods used for PCOR. These considerations are important for all types of data and analysis, but the increasing use of tools such as machine learning and natural language processing raises the question of whether best practices can ensure that these tools do not introduce biases that hardwire current disparities in care delivery (e.g., algorithmic bias).

The workshops also illustrated the importance of highlighting best practices, not only for how results are shared but also for the sharing of other resources and components associated with the research process, such as the software developed for analyses. Sharing all these resources ensures that the data can be widely used and that the research can be replicated. Ultimately the goal of PCOR is to benefit people, so the questions of what happens to the research after it is completed and how the information is shared with those whose data are being used also deserve further attention.

CONCLUSION 3-17: PCOR products would be enhanced by investing in methods that are essential for the conduct of PCOR, such as including persons throughout the research continuum, addressing problems of missing data, improving study designs, ensuring appropriate inference from methods utilizing observational data, and addressing structural bias in data systems and studies.

CONCLUSION 3-18: Applying best practices to the analytic methods used in PCOR is important to facilitate the reliability and reproducibility of study results.

CONCLUSION 3-19: The results of PCOR are only replicable and most useful when the underlying data and comprehensive research documentation (such as analytic code) are made available for use by others.

PROJECT SELECTION TO SUPPORT THE DATA INFRASTRUCTURE FRAMEWORK

While previous sections discussed specific aspects of the PCOR data infrastructure that could benefit from additional work in the years ahead, this section offers a few general, big-picture observations on project selection. ASPE sets priorities for the OS-PCORTF with assistance primarily from a Leadership Council that consists of HHS agency heads and their designees. The Leadership Council also provides input on the selection of projects to fund. While ASPE regularly obtains additional input from others, such as researchers and patient advocates, the question arises whether their lack of representation on the OS-PCORTF Leadership Council limits critical input on data infrastructure needs.

Although it is clear that the projects funded through the OS-PCORTF are well targeted toward further developing and enhancing key aspects of the data infrastructure, the PCOR data infrastructure has not reached its full potential to provide data that can answer questions that matter to people and enable them to make informed decisions. The committee's work identified several areas that could benefit from additional attention. The emergence of new technologies and approaches (e.g., wearable devices, artificial intelligence, and privacy-preserving record-linkage solutions) are also continuing to present new opportunities for enhancing the data infrastructure.

Leaders from patient organizations that participated in the workshops noted that PCOR data are often not focused on the types of issues that are truly important to people and that would enable them to find answers to the questions they tend to have about their treatment options and potential outcomes (see Appendix B, Chapter 3). The lack of information on the costs of care was highlighted as an example, which is also in line with the goals of the recently broadened scope of PCOR, namely to take into consideration "the potential burdens and economic impacts of the utilization of medical treatments, items, and services."

The workshops also made it clear that the data available do not capture complexities that need to be measured to understand how people's characteristics and experiences influence health outcomes (see Appendix B, Chapter 2). There was an emphasis on the need to build flexibility into the data collection systems to allow them to adapt to evolving terminologies and technologies for capturing and processing data. This is particularly important for social determinants of health, an area that may be rapidly changing.

The workshops also revealed that the policy and regulatory aspects of data sharing and privacy protection need updating (see Appendix C, Chapter 4). To date, these issues have received less direct attention in the context of the PCOR data infrastructure work. Arguably, these questions need to be addressed at a broader level, but ASPE may have a role in facilitating some of the discussions by proactively initiating work focused on these topics.

Previous sections in this chapter touched on some aspects of the issues mentioned above, particularly in the context of emerging priorities for health data. These topics are also highlighted here because the ability to address them has implications for the overall approach to the data infrastructure framework. Beyond the emerging data needs identified, the broader context for the data infrastructure is continuously evolving, due to larger societal shifts, emerging public health concerns (e.g., infectious diseases), new medical treatments (e.g., gene immunotherapy), and other developments. Nimbleness, mechanisms built in for stakeholder engagement, and transparent decision making are the key characteristics necessary for data infrastructure development.

> **CONCLUSION 3-20:** The development of the data infrastructure might be enhanced and critical gaps could be filled by proactively identifying necessary projects in areas that examine the overall framework for the PCOR data infrastructure, particularly in the context of broader issues such as the balance between privacy and increased data use.

The discussions with stakeholders and the review of prior evaluations led the committee to identify two general categories of projects that may be particularly worthwhile to pursue because of a high expected return on the investment. One such category consists of projects focused on topics or aspects of the infrastructure that are unlikely to be funded by other entities, such as other agencies or the private market. HHS is uniquely well positioned to address needs related to the data infrastructure that would otherwise be unmet. The other category covers projects that could result in findings that have application beyond a single condition or disease. These types of projects are most likely to lead to reuse of the data and broader use of the data infrastructure in general.

> **CONCLUSION 3-21:** Investments in areas unlikely to be funded or developed by other entities may have a particularly high value.

> **CONCLUSION 3-22:** Investments in projects that have potential use and application beyond the condition or disease for which they are proposed will accelerate the use of the infrastructure.

DISSEMINATION OF RESULTS AND USE OF THE DATA INFRASTRUCTURE

Over the years, efforts to disseminate information about the PCOR data infrastructure and PCOR studies have increased. The discussions with stakeholders, however, revealed that awareness of the work could be increased by additional attention to this area. Dissemination efforts focused on external stakeholders, in particular, could increase the usefulness of the investments made in the projects by encouraging additional engagement and reuse of the data and methods (see Appendix B, Chapter 3, and Appendix D, Chapter 2).

> **CONCLUSION 3-23:** There is a need to increase awareness among all stakeholders about new data infrastructure developments funded

by the Office of the Secretary PCOR Trust Fund. Increased awareness will enhance the efficiency and effectiveness of research, which in turn will increase the impact of the investments made in infrastructure development.

CONCLUSION 3-24: Investments in implementing and disseminating infrastructure tools and products will accelerate the achievement of overall PCOR infrastructure goals.

Input from patient advocacy groups highlighted the need for additional dissemination focused on diverse stakeholders outside the research community (see Appendix B, Chapter 3). While data on patient-centered outcomes are available in many areas that are important to patients, the information is rarely available in ways that would make it truly accessible to them. More widespread dissemination of information that is easy to use could also increase engagement.

CONCLUSION 3-25: Dissemination and translation of the research findings could be greatly enhanced by using forms of communication that are relevant to those outside the research community.

UPDATING THE DATA INFRASTRUCTURE FRAMEWORK

Building on what was learned from the workshop, and on the basis of the committee's further deliberations, this section offers a few additional observations focused on strengthening the overall framework for building the data infrastructure in the coming years. As discussed in Chapter 2, Figure 2-1 is a visual representation of the framework ASPE has been using for the PCOR data infrastructure to operationalize the mandate for the OS-PCORTF and guide decision making. This representation of the key elements of the data infrastructure allows ASPE to keep track of how funds are invested and which aspects of the infrastructure are enhanced.

ASPE's framework provides a description of the components, but it may not be fully actionable. A fragmented health care system and the resulting fragmented nature of the data available for research continue to be a barrier to developing insights that could ultimately improve health, which is the fundamental motivation for PCOR. The recent experience of the COVID-19 pandemic illustrates how this fragmentation has hindered the development of policies and solutions to address challenges.

Figure 3-1 provides an illustration of the committee's perspective on the data infrastructure framework. This is not intended to replace the existing framework but rather to present an additional view that is explicitly focused on improved health as the goal. Improving health is the North Star

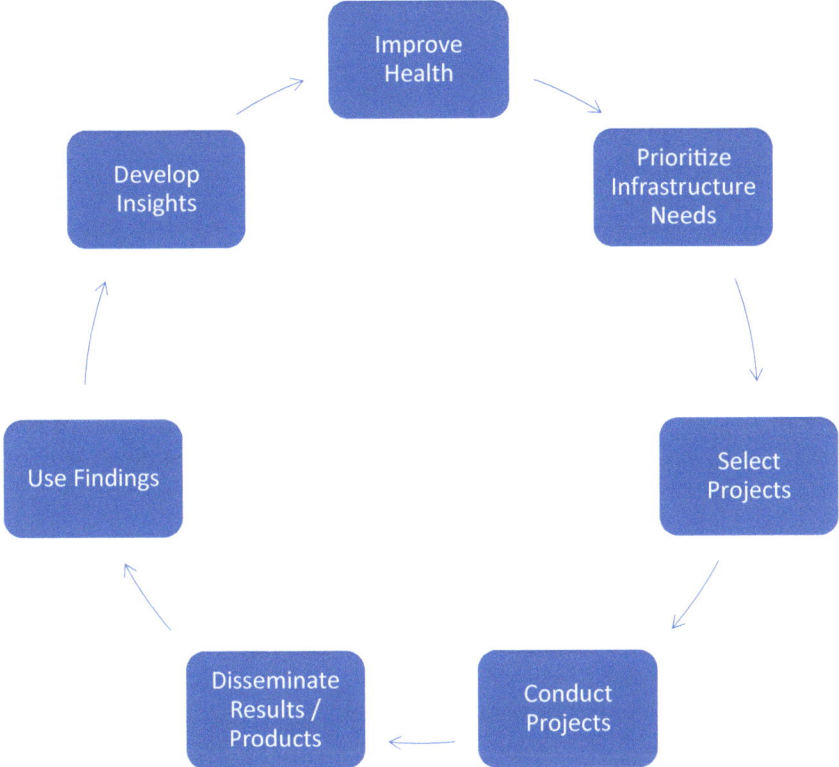

FIGURE 3-1 Framework for the role of enhanced data infrastructure and effective project management in improving health.

that guides the selection of projects and affects every decision. Reducing "voltage drops" at each step in the framework can contribute to realizing the potential of the PCOR data infrastructure. The most challenging need to address is likely between the development of insights and improving health, as shown on the left-hand side of the figure, which can be interpreted broadly to include informing policies, regulations, laws, and other mechanisms that drive improvements.

As discussed earlier, stakeholder input is important at each step. It is also important to note that the steps on the left-hand side of the figure go well beyond what can be accomplished through a solid data infrastructure alone, and therefore might not be directly achievable by ASPE or even by HHS. However, it is important to keep this broader context in mind to the extent that decisions about the data infrastructure are able to have an impact on progress toward the overall goal.

CONCLUSION 3-26: Explicitly focusing on improved health as the goal of the PCOR infrastructure may be a useful way to prioritize projects and target infrastructure investments.

Finally, the committee's deliberations echo the findings of the most recent portfolio assessment concerning the need for additional feedback and metrics that would enable ASPE to assess the impact of the investments in the data infrastructure. ASPE tracks information about what has been produced by each project, showing publications, presentations, and other public resources, as well as narrative summaries of accomplishments, as part of the description of completed projects on its website. Measuring impact (what happened as a result of the work) is always a challenging task, but obtaining additional feedback from stakeholders and building a strong feedback loop that attempts to ascertain what types of evidence have been generated as a result of the work could provide additional insights and strengthen the overall framework for the data capacity infrastructure.

CONCLUSION 3-27: A tighter feedback loop with the external end users and developers of evidence would enhance the value of data infrastructure investments. Examining what evidence was generated due to ASPE interventions and identifying what impact it had on policy and knowledge would also help close the gaps observed in realizing the potential of the PCOR data infrastructure.

Appendix A

Biographical Sketches of Committee Members

GEORGE ISHAM (NAM) (*Chair*) is a senior fellow at the HealthPartners Institute and a senior advisor for the Alliance of Community Health Plans. Previously, he served as a senior advisor to the board of directors and the senior management team of HealthPartners, and prior to that, he was HealthPartners' medical director and chief health officer, responsible for quality of care and health and health care improvement. He has been active in health policy, serving as a member of the Centers for Disease Control and Prevention's Task Force on Community Preventive Services and of the Agency for Healthcare Research and Quality's United States Preventive Services Task Force, as well as a founding co-chair of the National Committee for Quality Assurance's committee on performance measurement and of the National Quality Forum's Measurement Application Partnership. He has an M.D. from the University of Illinois at Chicago and an M.S. in preventive medicine and administrative medicine from the University of Wisconsin–Madison.

JOHN F.P. BRIDGES is professor and vice chair of academic affairs in the Department of Biomedical Informatics at The Ohio State University (OSU) College of Medicine. He is also a professor in the Department of Surgery and an adjunct professor in both the Division of Epidemiology at the OSU College of Public Health and Department of Health Behavior and Society at the Johns Hopkins Bloomberg School of Public Health. Prior to joining OSU he was on the faculty of the Johns Hopkins Bloomberg School of Public Health, the Department of Tropical Hygiene and Public Health within University of Heidelberg School of Medicine, and the Department of

Epidemiology and Biostatistics within the Case Western Reserve University School of Medicine. He has previously held positions in the Department of Economics at the Weatherhead School of Management at Case Western Reserve University, the National Bureau of Economic Research, Center for Medicine in the Public Interest, and the Centre for Health Economics Research and Evaluation in Australia. He has a Ph.D. in economics from the City University of New York.

JULIE BYNUM is the Margaret Terpenning Professor of Medicine in the Division of Geriatric Medicine and vice chair for Faculty Affairs in the Department of Internal Medicine at the University of Michigan. She is also a research professor in the Institute of Gerontology, Geriatric Center Associate Director for Health Policy and Research, and a member of the Institute for Healthcare Policy and Innovation. She currently leads a portfolio of National Institutes of Health–funded research that examines the quality of care, diagnosis, and treatment of people with Alzheimer's disease and related dementia in the community, nursing homes, and assisted living and is the director of the Center to Accelerate Population Research in Alzhiemer's. She is currently a member of the National Academies of Sciences, Engineering, and Medicine's Forum on Aging, Disability, and Independence and was a member of a National Academies committee that authored *Vital Signs: Core Metrics for Health and Health Care Progress*. She has an M.P.H. from the Johns Hopkins University School of Hygiene & Public Health and an M.D. from the Johns Hopkins University School of Medicine.

ANGELA DOBES is vice president of the Crohn's & Colitis Foundation's IBD Plexus Program, a research-information exchange platform designed to centralize data and biosamples from diverse research initiatives to advance science, accelerate precision medicine, and transform the care of inflammatory bowel disease (IBD) patients. She has previously worked for clinical technology and pharmaceutical organizations, where she has led implementation of various technology solutions focused on business optimization and accelerating the delivery of new therapies to patients safely. She is currently serving as principal investigator on a study to enhance engagement, research participation, and collaboration through the IBD Partners Patient Powered Research Network. She has an M.A. in public health from the Icahn School of Medicine at Mount Sinai.

DEBORAH ESTRIN (NAE/NAM) is a professor of computer science at Cornell Tech where she holds the Robert V. Tishman founder's chair, serves as the associate dean for impact, and is an affiliate faculty at Weill Cornell Medicine. Her research activities include technologies for caregiving, immersive health, small data, participatory sensing, and public interest technology.

Estrin was an Amazon Scholar, and before joining Cornell University she was founding director of the National Science Foundation's Center for Embedded Networked Sensing at the University of California, Los Angeles, pioneering the development of mobile and wireless systems to collect and analyze real-time data about the physical world. Estrin cofounded the nonprofit startup Open mHealth and has served on several scientific advisory boards for early-stage mobile health startups. She has a Ph.D. in electrical engineering and computer science from the Massachusetts Institute of Technology.

OLUWADAMILOLA FAYANJU is the Helen O. Dickens Presidential Associate Professor of Surgery at the Perelman School of Medicine at the University of Pennsylvania. She is also chief of breast surgery at Penn Medicine. Previously, she was associate professor of surgery and population health sciences in the Duke University School of Medicine and director of the Durham VA Breast Clinic. She was also associate director for Disparities & Value in Healthcare with Duke Forge, Duke University's center for actionable data science. In 2019, she was recognized by the National Academy of Medicine as an Emerging Leader in Health and Medicine Scholar. She received an M.A. in comparative literature from Harvard University and her M.D. and M.P.H.S. from the Washington University in St. Louis.

CONSTANTINE GATSONIS is the Henry Ledyard Goddard University Professor of Statistical Sciences, director of statistical sciences, and professor of biostatistics at Brown University. He was founding director of the Center for Statistical Sciences and founding chair of the Department of Biostatistics at Brown University. He is a leading authority on the evaluation of diagnostic and screening tests and has made major contributions to the development of methods for medical technology assessment and health services and outcomes research. He is a world leader in methods for applying and synthesizing evidence on diagnostic tests in medicine and is currently developing methods for comparative effectiveness research in diagnosis and prediction and radiomics. Since 2016 he has served as a statistical consultant for the *New England Journal of Medicine*, and was the founding editor-in-chief of *Health Services and Outcomes Research Methods*. He has a Ph.D. in mathematical statistics from Cornell University.

ROBERT GOERGE is a senior research fellow at Chapin Hall at the University of Chicago. He is also a senior fellow and founder of the Master's Degree in Computational Analysis in Public Policy at the University of Chicago Harris School of Public Policy. His research is focused on improving the available data and information on children and families, particularly those who require specialized services related to maltreatment, disability, poverty, or violence. At Chapin Hall, he is principal investigator for the

Family Self-Sufficiency Data Center, the Linking Federal Data to Local Data project, and the National Survey for Early Care and Education. He currently serves on the National Academies of Sciences, Engineering, and Medicine's Committee on National Statistics. He has a Ph.D. in social policy from the University of Chicago.

GEORGE HRIPCSAK (NAM) is the Vivian Beaumont Allen Professor and chair of the Department of Biomedical Informatics at Columbia University. He is also the director of medical informatics services for New York Presbyterian Hospital. He is also a board-certified internist. He led the effort to create the Arden Syntax, a language for representing health knowledge that has become a national standard. As chair of the American Medical Informatics Association Standards Committee, he coordinated the medical informatics community response to the Department of Health and Human Services for the health informatics standards rules under the Health Insurance Portability and Accountability Act of 1996. His current research is on the clinical information stored in electronic health records. Using data mining techniques, he is developing the methods necessary to support clinical research and patient safety initiatives. He has an M.D. and an M.S. in biostatistics from Columbia University.

LISA IEZZONI (NAM) is professor of medicine at Harvard Medical School and the Health Policy Research Center at Massachusetts General Hospital, where she served as director in the past. She was previously co-director of research in the Division of General Medicine and Primary Care at Beth Israel Deaconess Medical Center in Boston. Her research focuses on risk adjustment methods for predicting cost and clinical outcomes of care, and on health care experiences and outcomes of persons with disabilities. She has served on the editorial boards of the *Annals of Internal Medicine*, the *Journal of General Internal Medicine*, *Health Affairs*, *Medical Care*, *Health Services Research*, and the *Disability and Health Journal*, among others. She has an M.D. from Harvard Medical School and an M.Sc. from the Harvard T.H. Chan School of Public Health.

S. CLAIBORNE JOHNSTON (NAM) is the inaugural dean of Dell Medical School, vice president for medical affairs, and the Frank and Charmaine Denius Distinguished Dean's Chair in medical leadership at The University of Texas at Austin. Previously, Johnston was associate vice chancellor for research at the University of California, San Francisco (UCSF). He also directed the Clinical and Translational Science Institute and founded the UCSF Center for Healthcare Value. His research is focused on clinical trials and health services research in stroke. He is also an expert in medical education, research administration, health care value, and population health. He has led several large-cohort studies of cerebrovascular disease and three international multicenter randomized trials. He has an M.D. from Harvard Medical School and a Ph.D. in epidemiology from the University of California, Berkeley.

MIGUEL MARINO is an associate professor with joint appointments in the School of Public Health Division of Biostatistics and the Department of Family Medicine at Oregon Health & Science University. His research focuses on the development and implementation of novel statistical methodology to address complexities associated with the use of electronic health records (EHRs) to study changes in policy, using EHRs to study health disparities, validation of EHRs as a reliable source for observational studies, pragmatic randomized trials, and preventive health maintenance. He was selected by the National Academy of Medicine as an Emerging Leader in Health and Medicine Scholar. He has a Ph.D. in biostatistics from Harvard University.

ELIZABETH McGLYNN (NAM) is vice president for Kaiser Permanente Research and executive director for the Center for Effectiveness & Safety Research at Kaiser Permanente. She is also interim senior associate dean for research and scholarships at the Kaiser Permanente Bernard J. Tyson School of Medicine. She is an internationally known expert on methods for evaluating the appropriateness and quality of health care delivery. She has led major initiatives to evaluate health reform options under consideration at the federal and state levels. She is the lead of Kaiser Permanente & Strategic Partners Patient Outcomes Research To Advance Learning (PORTAL) Network. She was a member of the Strategic Framework Board, which provided a blueprint for the National Quality Forum on the development of a national quality measurement and reporting system. She chaired the board of AcademyHealth, served on the board of the American Board of Internal Medicine Foundation, and served on the Board of Providence-Little Company of Mary Hospital Service Area in Southern California. She has a Ph.D. in public policy from RAND Graduate School.

DAVID MELTZER (NAM) is the Fanny L. Pritzker Professor in the Department of Medicine, chief of the section of Hospital Medicine, and faculty in the Department of Economics and Harris School of Public Policy at the University of Chicago. He is also director of the Center for Health and the Social Sciences and of the Urban Health Lab at the University of Chicago. His research explores problems in health economics and public policy with a focus on the theoretical foundations of medical cost-effectiveness analysis and the cost and quality of hospital care. Since 1997, he has developed the inpatient general medicine services at the University of Chicago as a

Learning Health Care System to produce knowledge on how to improve the care of hospitalized patients, mobilizing the clinical care process to generate and learn from diverse data from electronic health records, claims data, patient interviews, and bio-specimens on more than 100,000 patients. He is the lead of the University of Chicago network site as part of the Chicago Area Patient-Centered Outcomes Research Network. He has an M.D. and a Ph.D. in economics from the University of Chicago.

PAUL TANG (NAM) is an adjunct professor in the Clinical Excellence Research Center at Stanford University and an internist at the Palo Alto Medical Foundation. He was formerly chief innovation and technology officer at the Palo Alto Medical Foundation and vice president, chief health transformation officer at IBM Watson Health. He has more than 25 years of executive leadership experience in health information technology within medical groups, health systems, and corporate settings. He has directed innovation and technology teams in provider organizations, academic institutions, corporate research organizations, and product development organizations. Most recently, he led the creation, development, deployment, and evaluation of the application of artificial intelligence to physician point-of-care solutions integrated within an electronic health record system. He also led a corporate enterprise-wide design team. He has chaired numerous federal and private sector advisory and professional association groups related to health information technology and policy. He received an M.S. in electrical engineering from Stanford University and his M.D. from the University of California, San Francisco.

Appendix B

Building Data Capacity for Patient-Centered Outcomes Research: Interim Report 1– Looking Ahead at Data Needs

(Full text of the committee's first interim report released on September 10, 2021.)[1]

---

[1] https://www.nap.edu/catalog/26297/building-data-capacity-for-patient-centered-outcomes-research-interim-report.

Building Data Capacity for Patient-Centered Outcomes Research

INTERIM REPORT 1 – Looking Ahead at Data Needs

Committee on Building Data Capacity for
Patient-Centered Outcomes Research:
An Agenda for 2021 to 2030

Committee on National Statistics
Division of Behavioral and Social Sciences and Education

Board on Health Care Services
Health and Medicine Division

Computer Science and Telecommunications Board
Division on Engineering and Physical Sciences

A Consensus Study Report of

The National Academies of
SCIENCES · ENGINEERING · MEDICINE

THE NATIONAL ACADEMIES PRESS
Washington, DC
www.nap.edu

THE NATIONAL ACADEMIES PRESS 500 Fifth Street, NW Washington, DC 20001

This activity was supported by a contract between the National Academy of Sciences and the U.S. Department of Health and Human Services (award #HHSP23 3201400020B/75P00120F37102). Any opinions, findings, conclusions, or recommendations expressed in this publication do not necessarily reflect the views of any organization or agency that provided support for the project.

International Standard Book Number-13: 978-0-309-26824-0
International Standard Book Number-10: 0-309-26824-9
Digital Object Identifier: https://doi.org/10.17226/26297

Additional copies of this publication are available from the National Academies Press, 500 Fifth Street, NW, Keck 360, Washington, DC 20001; (800) 624-6242 or (202) 334-3313; http://www.nap.edu.

Copyright 2021 by the National Academy of Sciences. All rights reserved.

Printed in the United States of America

Suggested citation: National Academies of Sciences, Engineering, and Medicine. (2021). *Building Data Capacity for Patient-Centered Outcomes Research: Interim Report 1—Looking Ahead at Data Needs*. Washington, DC: The National Academies Press. https://doi.org/10.17226/26297.

The National Academies of
SCIENCES · ENGINEERING · MEDICINE

The **National Academy of Sciences** was established in 1863 by an Act of Congress, signed by President Lincoln, as a private, nongovernmental institution to advise the nation on issues related to science and technology. Members are elected by their peers for outstanding contributions to research. Dr. Marcia McNutt is president.

The **National Academy of Engineering** was established in 1964 under the charter of the National Academy of Sciences to bring the practices of engineering to advising the nation. Members are elected by their peers for extraordinary contributions to engineering. Dr. John L. Anderson is president.

The **National Academy of Medicine** (formerly the Institute of Medicine) was established in 1970 under the charter of the National Academy of Sciences to advise the nation on medical and health issues. Members are elected by their peers for distinguished contributions to medicine and health. Dr. Victor J. Dzau is president.

The three Academies work together as the **National Academies of Sciences, Engineering, and Medicine** to provide independent, objective analysis and advice to the nation and conduct other activities to solve complex problems and inform public policy decisions. The National Academies also encourage education and research, recognize outstanding contributions to knowledge, and increase public understanding in matters of science, engineering, and medicine.

Learn more about the National Academies of Sciences, Engineering, and Medicine at **www.nationalacademies.org**.

The National Academies of
SCIENCES • ENGINEERING • MEDICINE

Consensus Study Reports published by the National Academies of Sciences, Engineering, and Medicine document the evidence-based consensus on the study's statement of task by an authoring committee of experts. Reports typically include findings, conclusions, and recommendations based on information gathered by the committee and the committee's deliberations. Each report has been subjected to a rigorous and independent peer-review process and it represents the position of the National Academies on the statement of task.

Proceedings published by the National Academies of Sciences, Engineering, and Medicine chronicle the presentations and discussions at a workshop, symposium, or other event convened by the National Academies. The statements and opinions contained in proceedings are those of the participants and are not endorsed by other participants, the planning committee, or the National Academies.

For information about other products and activities of the National Academies, please visit www.nationalacademies.org/about/whatwedo.

COMMITTEE ON BUILDING DATA CAPACITY FOR PATIENT-CENTERED OUTCOMES RESEARCH: AN AGENDA FOR 2021 TO 2030

GEORGE ISHAM (*Chair*), HealthPartners Institute
JOHN F.P. BRIDGES, The Ohio State University
JULIE BYNUM, University of Michigan
ANGELA DOBES, IBD Plexus, Crohn's & Colitis Foundation
OLUWADAMILOLA FAYANJU, The University of Pennsylvania
DEBORAH ESTRIN, Cornell Tech
CONSTANTINE GATSONIS, Brown University
ROBERT GOERGE, Chapin Hall, University of Chicago
GEORGE HRIPCSAK, Columbia University
LISA IEZZONI, Massachusetts General Hospital
S. CLAIBORNE JOHNSTON, The University of Texas at Austin
MIGUEL MARINO, Oregon Health & Science University
ELIZABETH McGLYNN, Kaiser Permanente
DAVID MELTZER, University of Chicago
PAUL TANG, Stanford University and Palo Alto Medical Foundation

KRISZTINA MARTON, *Study Director*
MEGAN KEARNEY, *Associate Program Officer* (until June 2021)
RUTH COOPER, *Associate Program Officer* (from June 2021)
MARY GHITELMAN, *Senior Program Assistant*
BRIAN HARRIS-KOJETIN, *Director, Committee on National Statistics*
SHARYL NASS, *Director, Board on Health Care Services*
JON EISENBERG, *Director, Computer Science and Telecommunications Board*

SAUL RIVAS (*National Academy of Medicine Fellow*), University of Texas Rio Grande Valley

COMMITTEE ON NATIONAL STATISTICS

ROBERT M. GROVES (*Chair*), Georgetown University
ANNE C. CASE, Princeton University
MICK P. COUPER, University of Michigan
JANET M. CURRIE, Princeton University
DIANA FARRELL, JPMorgan Chase Institute
ROBERT GOERGE, Chapin Hall at the University of Chicago
ERICA L. GROSHEN, Cornell University
HILARY HOYNES, University of California, Berkeley
DANIEL KIFER, Pennsylvania State University
SHARON LOHR, Arizona State University (emerita)
JEROME P. REITER, Duke University
JUDITH A. SELTZER, University of California, Los Angeles
C. MATTHEW SNIPP, Stanford University
ELIZABETH A. STUART, Johns Hopkins University
JEANNETTE WING, Columbia University

BRIAN A. HARRIS-KOJETIN, *Director*
CONSTANCE F. CITRO, *Senior Scholar*

BOARD ON HEALTH CARE SERVICES

DAVID BLUMENTHAL (*Chair*), The Commonwealth Fund
ANDREW BINDMAN, Kaiser Foundation Health Plan, Inc.
NIRANJAN BOSE, Gates Ventures
MELINDA J. BEEUWKES BUNTIN, Vanderbilt University School of Medicine
NEIL S. CALMAN, The Institute for Family Health
PAUL CHUNG, Kaiser Permanente School of Medicine
PATRICIA M. DAVIDSON, Johns Hopkins University School of Nursing
MARTHA DAVIGLUS, University of Illinois at Chicago
JENNIFER E. DEVOE, Oregon Health & Science University
R. ADAMS DUDLEY, University of Minnesota
RICHARD G. FRANK, Harvard Medical School
TERRY FULMER, John A. Hartford Foundation
CINDY GILLESPIE, Arkansas Department of Human Services
ELMER HUERTA, The George Washington University Cancer Center
SHARON INOUYE, Harvard Medical School
JOHN LUMPKIN, Blue Cross Blue Shield of North Carolina Foundation
FAITH MITCHELL, The Urban Institute
DAVID B. PRYOR, Ascension Health
TRISH RILEY, National Academy for State Health Policy
WILLIAM SAGE, The University of Texas at Austin
HARDEEP SINGH, Baylor College of Medicine

SHARYL NASS, *Director*

COMPUTER SCIENCE AND TELECOMMUNICATIONS BOARD

LAURA HAAS (*Chair*), University of Massachusetts, Amherst
DAVID CULLER, University of California, Berkeley
ERIC HORVITZ, Microsoft Corporation
CHARLES ISBELL, Georgia Institute of Technology
BETH MYNATT, Georgia Institute of Technology
CRAIG PARTRIDGE, Colorado State University
DANIELA RUS, Massachusetts Institute of Technology
FRED B. SCHNEIDER, Cornell University
NAMBIRAJAN SESHADRI, University of California, San Diego
MARGO SELTZER, University of British Columbia
MOSHE VARDI, Rice University

JON EISENBERG, *Director*

Acknowledgments

This Consensus Study Report was reviewed in draft form by individuals chosen for their diverse perspectives and technical expertise. The purpose of this independent review is to provide candid and critical comments that will assist the National Academies of Sciences, Engineering, and Medicine in making each published report as sound as possible and to ensure that it meets the institutional standards for quality, objectivity, evidence, and responsiveness to the study charge. The review comments and draft manuscript remain confidential to protect the integrity of the deliberative process.

We thank the following individuals for their review of this report: Cheryl R. Clark, Health Equity Research & Intervention, Center for Community Health and Health Equity, Brigham and Women's Hospital; Darrell J. Gaskin, Department of Health Policy and Management, Johns Hopkins Bloomberg School of Public Health; Sherry Glied, Robert F. Wagner Graduate School of Public Service, New York University; Elizabeth Patzer, Department of Surgery and Health Services Research Center, Emory University; Robert L. Phillips, Jr., Center for Professionalism and Value in Health Care, American Board of Family Medicine Foundation; Russell Rothman, Institute for Medicine and Public Health, Vanderbilt University Medical Center; and Mariana F. Wolfner, Department of Molecular Biology and Genetics, Cornell University.

Although the reviewers listed above provided many constructive comments and suggestions, they were not asked to endorse the conclusions of this report, nor did they see the final draft before its release. The review of this report was overseen by Andrew B. Bindman, chief medical officer, Kaiser Foundation Health Plan and Hospitals and Alicia L. Carriquiry,

Department of Statistics, Iowa State University. They were responsible for making certain that an independent examination of this report was carried out in accordance with the standards of the National Academies and that all review comments were carefully considered. Responsibility for the final content rests entirely with the authoring committee and the National Academies.

Contents

Summary   1

1   Introduction   7

2   Health Disparities Data Needs   19

3   Patient Perspectives on Data Needs   29

4   Researcher Perspectives on Data Needs   41

Appendixes

A   Biographical Sketches of Committee Members   57
B   Workshop Agenda   63
C   Biographical Sketches of Workshop Speakers   67

Boxes, Figures, and Table

BOXES

1-1 Key Data Infrastructure Functionalities in the Existing Strategic Framework for Patient-Centered Outcomes Research, 12
1-2 Building Blocks of the Patient-Centered Outcomes Research Data Infrastructure, 13
1-3 Statement of Task for the Overall Study, 15

2-1 An Example of How Data Silos Hinder the Ability to Answer Policy Questions: The Impact of Medicaid Expansion on Equity in Hospitalizations for Complex Cancer Surgery, 21
2-2 An Example of How Data Silos Hinder the Ability to Answer Policy Questions: The Impact of Hospital Value-Based Purchasing on Equity in Posthospitalization Functional Status, 22
2-3 Disability Questions for Potential Inclusion in Electronic Health Records, 23

4-1 Case Study: The Use of the Patient-Centered Outcomes Research Infrastructure to Study Whether Vitamin D Can Reduce the Burden of COVID-19, 42
4-2 Person-Centered Primary Care Measures, 46

FIGURES

1-1 Patient-Centered Outcomes Research Trust Fund: Three streams of work and funding, 9
1-2 ASPE's strategic framework for the patient-centered outcomes research data infrastructure, 11

2-1 Example of data available on social determinants of health, 20

3-1 Evidation Health's vision for person-generated health data framework, 36
3-2 Episodic real-world evidence data points versus continuous data using digital technologies, 38

TABLE

3-1 Examples of Patient-Experience Information Related to Chronic Fatigue Syndrome and Myalgic Encephalomyelitis in the Food and Drug Administration's *The Voice of the Patient* Report, 35

Summary

The Office of the Assistant Secretary for Planning and Evaluation (ASPE), in partnership with other agencies and divisions of the U.S. Department of Health and Human Services (HHS), coordinates a portfolio of projects that build data capacity for conducting patient-centered outcomes research (PCOR). PCOR focuses on producing scientific evidence on the effectiveness of prevention and treatment options to inform the health care decisions of patients, families, and health care providers, taking into consideration the preferences, values, and questions patients face when making health care choices. The data infrastructure includes data sources and functionalities that support the research. Major building blocks are the services, standards, policies, and governance that enable the use of the data.

ASPE asked the National Academies of Sciences, Engineering, and Medicine to appoint a consensus study committee to identify issues critical to the continued development of the data infrastructure for PCOR. The committee's work will contribute to ASPE's development of a strategic plan that will guide its work related to PCOR data capacity over the next decade.

As part of its information-gathering activities, the committee organized three workshops to collect input from stakeholders on the PCOR data infrastructure. This report, the first in a series of three interim reports, summarizes the discussion and committee conclusions from the first workshop, focused on looking ahead at data user needs over the next decade. The workshop included representatives of patient groups with a wide reach and researchers with broad research interests as well as an understanding of the

PCOR infrastructure. The high-level conclusions included in this interim report are based primarily on the input collected as part of the workshop, background documentation received from ASPE and other public sources, and the committee members' synthesis and expert judgment regarding the input received. As an interim report based on one in a series of information-gathering activities, the scope of this report is narrowly focused on a subset of key topics relevant to the committee's charge. The conclusions reached by the committee are, at this stage, fairly high level. After completing all of its information-gathering activities, which include but are not limited to the three workshops, the committee will also issue a final report, containing the study's overall findings and conclusions.

FUNDAMENTAL DATA CHALLENGES

Most data that are available for PCOR are collected for clinical care, billing, or other nonresearch purposes. This presents a fundamental challenge to answering critical questions, but the workshop also made it clear that opportunities exist for making the data infrastructure more suitable for answering questions of interest, so long as the potential uses of the data are carefully considered.

> CONCLUSION 2-2: The data available for patient-centered outcomes research are often collected for reasons other than research, which limits their usefulness. Opportunities exist for increasing the utility of the data infrastructure by carefully considering the multiple uses to which the data might be applied.

Researchers experience barriers that limit their ability to access data available in databases, which range from databases that can be considered a part of the PCOR data infrastructure to those owned by private companies. A focus on facilitating and simplifying access could further enhance the usefulness of PCOR data.

> CONCLUSION 4-3: Researchers encounter substantial barriers to accessing existing data for patient-centered outcomes research. Facilitating and simplifying data access could further increase the usefulness of data for research.

DATA FRAGMENTATION

The data that exist for PCOR are collected and curated in a variety of databases across a fragmented health system. These databases are typically constructed as stand-alone entities for particular administrative or other uses, and without factoring in potential linkages with other databases. The workshop identified these data silos as a major barrier, both to understanding the role of social determinants of health and to research more broadly. A focus on facilitating data linkages could greatly increase the usefulness of the information available.

> CONCLUSION 2-3: Existing data on the social determinants of health are found in a variety of databases. Barriers to linking across these data silos represent a major challenge to understanding how social determinants of health affect health outcomes.

> CONCLUSION 4-2: The data available for patient-centered outcomes research are fragmented across a variety of databases. Expanding data linkages could greatly increase the usefulness of these data for research.

HEALTH DISPARITIES

A theme that emerged from the workshop was the magnitude of the gaps in the data that are available to better understand and address health disparities. Health disparities represent an evolving and expanding area of research, with corresponding data needs. Limitations exist for a variety of social determinants of health data and for a range of populations. Improving the data available for understanding and addressing these disparities would require data strategies that prioritize this goal.

> CONCLUSION 2-1: Health disparities can occur across a broad range of characteristics and populations. Data limitations affect the ability to identify and understand these disparities in many areas. Data for specific populations are sometimes unavailable or are not representative. In other cases, the data might not be timely or might have other gaps that make it difficult to understand the impact of changes over long periods of time.

> CONCLUSION 2-5: Prioritizing and improving the collection of data can lead to a better understanding of health disparities and to potential solutions for reducing disparities.

The workshop also made it clear that the data available do not capture complexities that are necessary to understand how people's characteristics and experiences influence health outcomes. Speakers at the workshop identified several potential ways of capturing data that reflect these complexities, emphasizing the need to build flexibility into the data collection systems to allow them to adapt to evolving terminologies and technologies for capturing and processing data. These considerations are particularly important for social determinants of health, an area that may be rapidly changing.

> CONCLUSION 2-4: Existing data do not capture the richness of people's characteristics and experiences. While such limitations are to be expected, opportunities exist for capturing data that are better able to characterize these complexities. A robust data infrastructure builds on the strengths of what is available today and has the flexibility to adapt, both as measures and terminologies become obsolete and as new technologies emerge.

PATIENT DATA NEEDS AND ENGAGEMENT

Too often, the data available for PCOR are not focused on the issues that are truly important to patients and that would enable them to find answers to their questions about treatment options and potential outcomes. Information about the cost implications of medical care is an area in which data are particularly limited, because it has only recently been included in the statutory scope of PCOR.

> CONCLUSION 3-1: The patient-centered outcomes research data infrastructure has not reached its full potential to provide data that can answer questions that matter to patients and enable them to make informed decisions. Information about the cost of care was highlighted among the types of data that would be particularly useful.

Even for the many areas where data on patient-centered outcomes are available, the information is rarely available in ways that would make it truly accessible to patients for decision-making purposes. More widespread dissemination of information that is easy to use could increase the engagement of patients and communities and could complement research efforts to improve health outcomes.

> CONCLUSION 3-2: Dissemination and translation of the research findings could be greatly enhanced by using forms of communication that are relevant to those outside of the research community.

> CONCLUSION 4-4: Making the data more visible and more widely accessible could enable patients and communities to use the information in ways that reduce health disparities, complementing research efforts in this area.

Both patient groups and researchers highlighted the clear need for more data on the total cost of care.

CONCLUSION 4-5: Data needs related to the total cost of care and a better understanding of cost considerations are areas that deserve more attention.

FOCUS ON THE PERSON AS A WHOLE

The input received from workshop participants made it clear that limiting the focus to the patient limits not only thinking about the data but also the outcomes and impacts that matter to people in general.

CONCLUSION 4-1: Broadening the focus from the patient to the person more generally would enable a more comprehensive approach to the data infrastructure and a better understanding of the outcomes and impacts that matter to people.

1

Introduction

The Office of the Assistant Secretary for Planning and Evaluation (ASPE), in partnership with other agencies and divisions of the U.S. Department of Health and Human Services (HHS), coordinates a portfolio of projects that build data capacity for conducting patient-centered outcomes research (PCOR). The PCOR data infrastructure provides decision makers with objective, scientific evidence on the effectiveness of treatments, services, and other interventions used in health care. This research is frequently focused on analyzing existing data to study questions and provide objective information for the purpose of informing real-world health care decisions.

BACKGROUND

The legal framework that established funding for research on the outcomes and effectiveness of treatments and health care interventions dates back to the 2003 Medicare Prescription Drug, Improvement, and Modernization Act. This act provided authorization for the Agency for Healthcare Research and Quality (AHRQ) to support research comparing the outcomes and effectiveness of treatments and clinical approaches and to disseminate the findings from this research. In 2009, the American Recovery and Reinvestment Act provided additional funding to AHRQ, the National Institutes of Health, and HHS for research that compares the effectiveness of medical options. In 2010, the Patient Protection and Affordable Care Act provided further authorization for research that assists patients, clinicians, purchasers, and policy makers in making informed health decisions.

To facilitate PCOR, in 2010 Congress established the Patient-Centered Outcomes Research Trust Fund (PCOR Trust Fund) with the U.S. Department of the Treasury. The goals of the PCOR Trust Fund are to fund PCOR research, disseminate research findings, and develop a data infrastructure for PCOR. The PCOR Trust Fund has been reauthorized through 2029, through H.R. 1865 of the Further Consolidated Appropriations Act of 2020. The most recent statute specified intellectual and developmental disabilities, as well as maternal mortality, as research priorities. The statute also called for PCOR studies to include consideration of the full range of outcomes data. Specifically, the law states that:

> Research shall be designed, as appropriate, to take into account and capture the full range of clinical and patient-centered outcomes relevant to, and that meet the needs of, patients, clinicians, purchasers, and policymakers in making informed health decisions. In addition to the relative health outcomes and clinical effectiveness, clinical and patient-centered outcomes shall include the potential burdens and economic impacts of the utilization of medical treatments, items, and services on different stakeholders and decision-makers respectively. These potential burdens and economic impacts include medical out-of-pocket costs, including health plan benefit and formulary design, non-medical costs to the patient and family, including caregiving, effects on future costs of care, workplace productivity and absenteeism, and healthcare utilization.[1]

The bulk of the PCOR Trust Fund funding (80%) is allocated for research and is made available through the Patient-Centered Outcomes Research Institute, a nongovernmental organization established by Congress for this purpose. Approximately 16 percent of the PCOR Trust Fund funding is set aside for disseminating research findings, incorporating findings into clinical practice, and training researchers in PCOR. The agency overseeing this work is AHRQ.

The remaining funding, which constitutes 4 percent of the PCOR Trust Fund, is allocated for building data capacity for PCOR and is overseen by ASPE. Specifically, Section 937(f) of the Public Health Service Act instructed the Secretary of HHS to:

> … provide for the coordination of relevant Federal health programs to build data capacity for comparative clinical effectiveness research, including the development and use of clinical registries and health outcomes research networks, in order to develop and maintain a comprehensive, interoperable data network to collect, link, and analyze data on outcomes and effectiveness from multiple sources including electronic health records.[2]

---

[1] https://www.ssa.gov/OP_Home/ssact/title11/1181.htm.
[2] https://aspe.hhs.gov/collaborations-committees-advisory-groups/os-pcortf/about-os-pcortf.

Figure 1-1 shows how the PCOR funding and work is allocated across the three entities. This National Academies of Sciences, Engineering, and Medicine study is focused on issues relevant to ASPE's continued work on the PCOR data infrastructure, in other words, on the priorities for the use of the 4 percent of the funding that is allocated for HHS.

As the coordinating agency for the data infrastructure investment portfolio across HHS agencies, ASPE guides the PCOR data infrastructure's strategic framework and vision, sets funding priorities, and coordinates interagency workgroups. ASPE's work is assisted by a Leadership Council for the PCOR Trust Fund, which includes representatives from other HHS agencies, including the Administration for Children and Families, the Administration for Community Living, AHRQ, the Assistant Secretary for Preparedness and Response, the Centers for Disease Control and Prevention (CDC), the Centers for Medicare & Medicaid Services, the Food and Drug Administration, the Health Resources and Services Administration, the Indian Health Service, the National Institutes of Health, the Office of the Chief Technology Officer, the Office of the National Coordinator for Health Information Technology, and the Substance Abuse and Mental Health Services Administration. The Leadership Council provides input on priorities for the portfolio, including projects to fund. During the period 2010 to 2019, the PCOR Trust Fund funded 53 projects, which translated to 76 agency awards, totaling approximately $131 million.

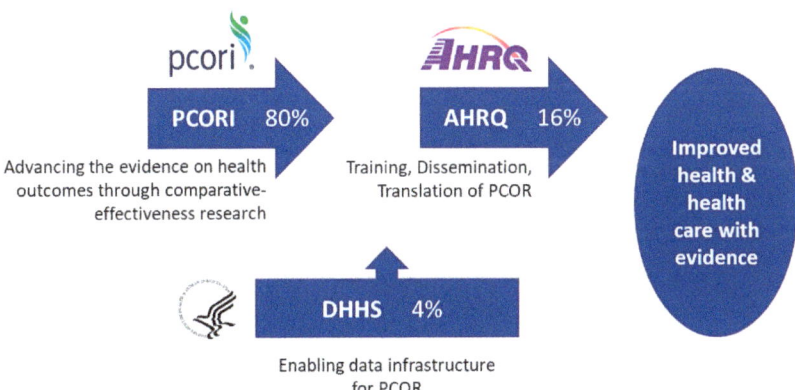

FIGURE 1-1 Patient-Centered Outcomes Research Trust Fund: Three streams of work and funding.
NOTE: AHRQ = Agency for Healthcare Research and Quality; HHS = U.S. Department of Health and Human Services; PCOR = Patient-Centered Outcomes Research; PCORI = Patient-Centered Outcomes Research Institute.
SOURCE: Workshop presentation by ASPE, May 3, 2021.

Figure 1-2 is a visual representation of ASPE's current framework for the PCOR data infrastructure. The bottom row shows the main data sources feeding into the PCOR infrastructure. Data collected as part of clinical care include data collected for health care delivery and for billing purposes. Examples of primary data collected as part of research studies include data from clinical trials and national health surveys. Other examples of data sources include Medicare or Medicaid claims data; quality or outcomes data collected by health care providers for the purposes of improving health care value; Food and Drug Administration data on the safety of medications and medical devices; and CDC data on births and deaths provided by state public health authorities.

The framework describes the relationship between the data sources and the current key functionalities and focus areas (middle row) that support the research. The key functionalities are described in further detail in Box 1-1. Major building blocks are the services, standards, policies, and governance that enable the use of the data for research, described in further detail in Box 1-2. The top row shows the key data users and contributors of data. A more detailed overview of ASPE's work and the projects funded to date will be included in the final report, at the conclusion of the committee's review.

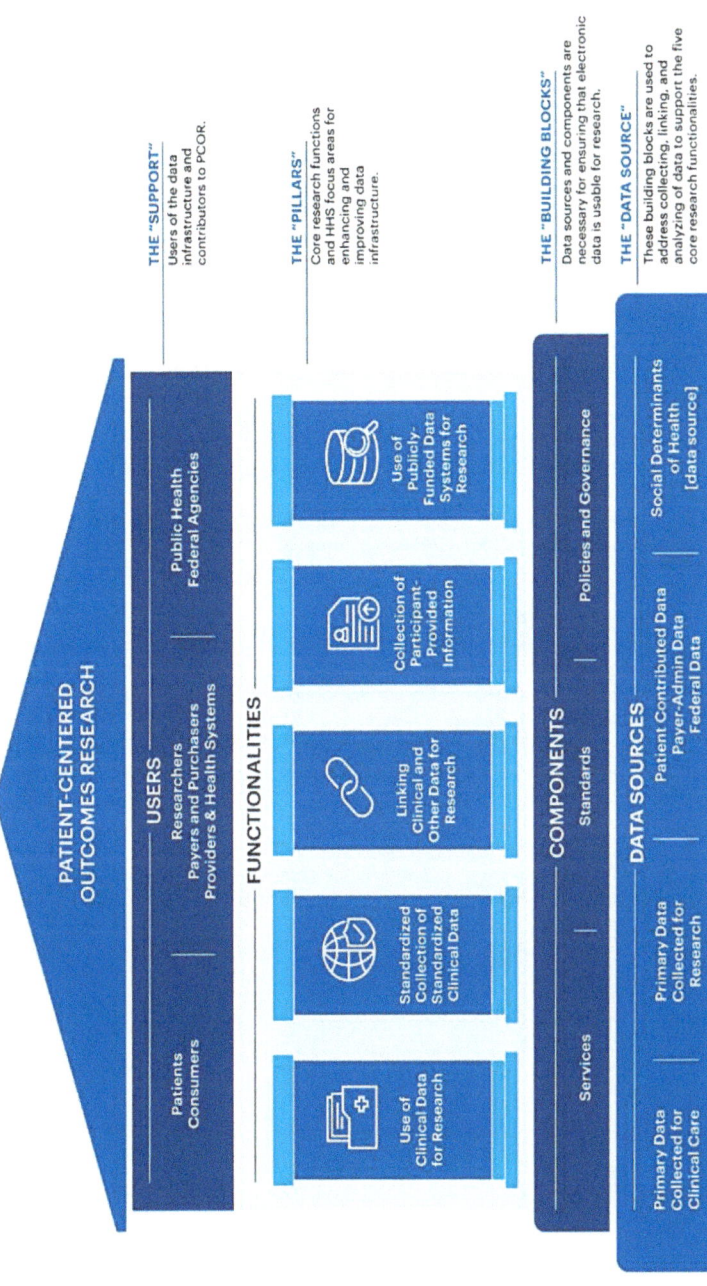

FIGURE 1-2 ASPE's strategic framework for the patient-centered outcomes research data infrastructure.
SOURCE: Workshop presentation by ASPE, May 3, 2021.

> **BOX 1-1**
> **Key Data Infrastructure Functionalities in the
> Existing Strategic Framework for
> Patient-Centered Outcomes Research**
>
> *Standardized Collection of Standardized Clinical Data*
> Researchers will be able to use standardized clinical data based on common data element standards across research projects and networks, thereby facilitating linkage and aggregation of data across data sources.
>
> *Collection of Participant-Provided Information*
> Participants, including those in safety net organizations, will be able to participate more fully in clinical research by directly providing information (i.e., data points provided by the participant such as Patient-Reported Outcomes).
>
> *Linking of Clinical and Other Data for Research*
> Researchers will be able to follow patients across the care continuum over time, including those enrolled in clinical trials. Researchers will be able to capture the range of variables influencing health outcomes and link clinical and other types of data (e.g., other clinical data, claims data, participant-provided information, and environmental data) required for research regardless of where the participant goes.
>
> *Use of Clinical Data for Research*
> Researchers will be able to utilize and analyze routinely collected clinical data for implementation of clinical studies (observational and interventional), including data relevant to assessing safety, efficacy, and adherence, as well as genetic data and Patient-Reported Outcomes.
>
> *Use of Enhanced Publicly Funded Data Systems for Research*
> Researchers will be able to readily use, retrieve, link, and aggregate publicly funded data for research due to enhancements in publicly funded data systems.
>
> SOURCE: https://aspe.hhs.gov/collaborations-committees-advisory-groups/os-pcortf/about-os-pcortf/building-data-capacity-patient-centered-outcomes-research.

> **BOX 1-2**
> **Building Blocks of the**
> **Patient-Centered Outcomes Research Data Infrastructure**
>
> *Standards* represent information and meaning to patient-centered data to ensure that health-specific information can be accurately (and securely) exchanged and used. In most cases standards should be nationally accepted, widely approved, or broadly adopted either through market forces, community approval, or regulatory requirements. These include such items as data standards for capturing, storing, representing, and exchanging data in a secure manner such that accurate information is conveyed to the recipient of the data.
>
> *Policies* are standards of behavior that participants can rely on consistently to build patient-centered data for research. Policies may include federal policies, as well as models for standardized state and local policies, that will lead to a trusted framework within the patient-centered outcomes research (PCOR) data infrastructure that ensures productivity, protects the patient and the patient's data, ensures that evidence generations remains in the center of PCOR, and ensures the use of agreed upon standards and services.
>
> *Services* refer to resources that entities can employ on demand to capture, store, or exchange either PCOR data or evidence through a centrally hosted model provided remotely (such as through the internet) rather that provided locally or onsite. Services make it easy for the research data to interoperate among different systems without having to start from scratch for every connection.
>
> *Governance* structures refer to entities that are needed to develop and apply the rules and policies needed for building an interoperable and sustainable research network. Governance structures support the efficient use of the data infrastructure for research across individual and organizations' boundaries of control and ownership. Governance structures are distinguished from "governance," which is what a governing body or governance structure does.
>
> SOURCE: https://aspe.hhs.gov/collaborations-committees-advisory-groups/os-pcortf/about-os-pcortf/building-data-capacity-patient-centered-outcomes-research.

ISSUES FOR THE COMMITTEE

ASPE asked the National Academies to appoint a consensus study committee and identify issues critical to building data capacity for PCOR and for generating new evidence to inform health care decisions. The input provided by the committee will contribute to ASPE's strategic planning for its work related to the data infrastructure over the next decade. The study is part of a broader initiative by ASPE intended to update the strategic plan in light of the reauthorization of the PCOR Trust Fund and advances in health information technology and interoperability tools in recent years.

The study is a collaboration of three units of the National Academies: the Committee on National Statistics, the Board on Health Care Services, and the Computer Science and Telecommunications Board. The consensus study committee of 15 members had a diverse membership, including experts with decades of experience, as well as emerging leaders, in the broad fields of (1) PCOR; (2) research methods, statistics, and demography; (3) computer science and data infrastructure; and (4) patient engagement and patient perspectives. Appendix A contains the biographical sketches of the committee members.

As part of its information-gathering activities, the committee was asked to organize three workshops to collect input from stakeholders on aspects of the charge developed in consultation with ASPE. The workshops focused on key topics that the committee believed would particularly benefit from broad input from a variety of data users and other stakeholders. The conclusions from each workshop are summarized in interim reports. This first interim report summarizes the discussion and conclusions from the first workshop, which focused on looking ahead at data user needs over the next decade. The second workshop in the series centered on data standards, methods, and policies that could make the PCOR data infrastructure more useful. The third workshop discussed research and data collaborations.

As an interim report focused on one in a series of information-gathering activities, the scope of this report is limited to a subset of the topics relevant to the committee's charge and the conclusions reached by the committee are, at this stage, fairly high level. Some aspects of the topics discussed will be examined in further detail in subsequent workshops. For example, the first workshop focused on the additional data that stakeholders would like to have access to for PCOR. The second workshop will examine ways that the existing data could be better utilized to meet data needs, as well as the challenges associated with data sharing and addressing privacy concerns. After completing all of its information-gathering activities, the committee will issue a final report, which will integrate and examine these topics in further detail.

Box 1-3 shows the committee's Statement of Task for the overall study; the committee will address this charge in its final report, integrating what

> **BOX 1-3**
> **Statement of Task for the Overall Study**
>
> The National Academies will appoint an ad hoc committee to conduct a series of three 1-day public workshops and develop conclusions to help guide the data capacity development for patient-centered research from 2021 through 2030. Each workshop will seek input from key stakeholders on topics relevant to the committee charge, and the specific focus of each workshop will be determined by the committee in consultation with the Assistant Secretary for Planning and Evaluation.
> As part of its activities, the committee will also
>
> - Consider the published review of the history and trajectory of the Office of the Secretary Patient-Centered Outcomes Research Trust Fund (OS-PCORTF) portfolio of investments and the OS-PCORTF roadmap.
> - **Assess anticipated changes to health care priorities and priorities for health data and their impact on building data capacity into the foreseeable future, as identified by the Assistant Secretary for Planning and Evaluation.**
> - Evaluate the feasibility and utility of developing a phased-in approach to building the interoperable data capacity for patient-centered outcomes research with existing databases in the Department of Health and Human Services, other federal departments, and the private sector in a phased approach, such as projects identified in the Cures Act Title III Section 4003 (Interoperability).
> - Consider other existing legislation, regulations, and the like, as deemed relevant.
> - **Receive input from individuals or groups that represent stakeholders including patients and their caregivers or families and their health care providers.**
>
> The committee will issue interim reports after each public workshop with conclusions, and will produce a final written report with findings and conclusions to help guide a future course to continue building the data capacity for patient-centered research. All reports will follow institutional guidelines and be subject to the National Academies review procedures prior to release.

was learned from the workshops, and from all other forms of input, including public meetings with HHS staff and background documentation available on the history and operations of the PCOR Trust Fund. The final report will contain overall findings and conclusions from the study, on the basis of the committee's further deliberations and integrated judgment on the input received and materials reviewed.

Appendix B shows the agenda for the workshop, which was held on May 3, 2021. The committee's goal for this event was to bring together researchers and representatives of patient organizations to understand the needs of these two important data user groups. Specifically, the goals of the workshop were to:

- Provide a high-level overview of the types of data included in the data infrastructure for PCOR.
- Identify key questions that stakeholders are most likely to want answered going forward, including general themes that cut across health conditions and circumstances.
- Discuss the implications of the broadened statutory scope for PCOR.
- Identify gaps in what stakeholders need and what the infrastructure allows. Consider both limitations in the existing data and improvements that could be made to new data collections.
- Discuss what questions cannot be answered and who is not served by the current PCOR data infrastructure.
- Discuss what HHS is best positioned to address and how the agency could maximize resources available for the PCOR data infrastructure (representing 4% of the PCOR Trust Fund), in the context of HHS's public mission, authorities, programs, and data resources.

Invited speakers in each of the sessions were asked to reflect on the general topics above. The specific questions for each session are described in Chapters 2 through 4. An obvious limitation of any activity of this type is that only a small number of stakeholders can be invited to speak. To compensate for this limitation to the extent possible, the committee invited representatives of patient groups with a broad reach, representing a variety of different interests and medical conditions. The researchers included were also individuals with broad research interests and an understanding of the PCOR infrastructure. In addition to sessions focused on the data needs of patient groups and researchers, the workshop also included a session on health disparities research and the data needed to explore this topic in more depth. The workshop also featured a case study on data challenges encountered as part of a study related to COVID-19. Appendix C contains biographical sketches for the speakers. A recording of the workshop and the presentation slides used by the speakers are available on the National Academies' website at www.nationalacademies.org/PCORData.

Information about the workshop was disseminated through National Academies' mailing lists and on the project website. To collect additional stakeholder input, members of the public were invited to provide comments on topics related to the workshop (or any other topic related to the committee's charge), using a public input form available on the National Academies' website.

OVERVIEW OF THE REPORT

This report is organized around the three main sessions of the workshop. Chapter 2 discusses presentations on the data needs related to health disparities, Chapter 3 focuses on patient organization needs, and Chapter 4 describes the input received from researchers. The points conveyed by the workshop participants do not necessarily reflect the views of the committee; instead, in each chapter, a summary of the input received is followed by the committee's conclusions. These conclusions are based primarily on the input collected as part of the workshop, background documentation received from ASPE and other public sources, and the committee members' synthesis and expert judgment. Because this is an interim report, the committee's conclusions at this stage are big-picture conclusions, which will be integrated with additional input over the course of the study.

2

Health Disparities Data Needs

This chapter summarizes presentations and discussion focused on data that could further the understanding of health disparities. Speakers participating in this session were asked to focus on the questions below. The brief overview of the input received from the presenters is followed by the committee's conclusions.

- What are the limitations of the patient-centered outcomes research (PCOR) data infrastructure in terms of
  - disparities in the data, including knowledge about patient outcomes, taking into consideration differences in patient preferences and values?
  - challenges associated with using the data to understand disparities and health equity?
  - lack of data on some populations?
- What are opportunities and priorities for enhancing data capacity in this area?
- What data capacity challenges is the U.S. Department of Health and Human Services (HHS) best positioned to address in the context of its public mission, authorities, programs, and data resources?

The first speaker, Karen Joynt Maddox, Washington University in St. Louis, argued that one of the main reasons why it is challenging to use health data for research in general, and for PCOR in particular, is that the health and personal data that are available are typically not collected for PCOR to begin with. Instead, the reasons for collecting the data tend to be for recordkeeping for clinical care or for payment. As a result, the data available are not centered on the person and do not enable an understanding of the person's context, including his or her medical journey, demographic information, health status, and comorbidities, as well as the social context in which the person lives.

Data that could be useful for studying disparities are collected in a variety of settings and are housed in separate databases. To take full advantage of the information, it is necessary to link these data, something that is often difficult to accomplish. Figure 2-1 is an illustration of these data silos. Joynt Maddox noted that one positive characteristic of the data collected on the social determinants of health is that some of the information available is particularly detailed. This includes, for example, data from hospitals' electronic medical records modules, as well as data from social work and care coordination assessments.

Joynt Maddox highlighted Z-codes, which are a subset of the codes contained in the International Classification of Diseases (Tenth Revision, Clinical Modification, or ICD-10-CM). Z-codes are used to capture information such as the factors that influence a person's health status and the reason for contact with health services. This includes information about employment, family characteristics, housing, psychosocial characteristics, socioeconomic characteristics, and nonadherence (e.g., intentional underdosing of medication due to financial hardship). While these codes are widely available and detailed, they appear at a lower-than-expected rate in records, which suggests that they may be underused.

As an example of how data silos hinder the ability to answer policy questions, Joynt Maddox discussed efforts to answer the question of how

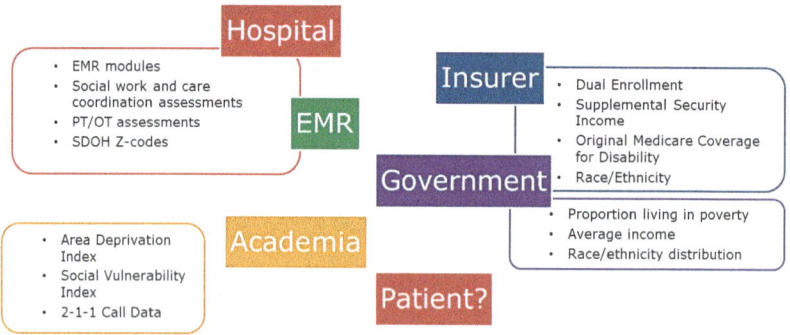

FIGURE 2-1 Example of data available on social determinants of health.
NOTES: EMR = electronic medical records; OT = occupational therapy; PT = physical therapy; SDOH = social determinants of health.
SOURCE: Workshop presentation by Karen Joynt Maddox, May 3, 2021.

potential Medicaid expansion in Missouri could impact equity in hospitalizations for complex cancer surgery. Box 2-1 summarizes the databases that could potentially be considered to examine this question, along with their limitations. None of these datasets has reliable information on social determinants of health.

Box 2-2 summarizes data sources that could be considered to examine another question with policy implications: the impact of the Hospital Value-Based Purchasing Program on equity in posthospitalization functional status.

The ideas shared by Joynt Maddox for improving the data available in this area were to (1) include hospital and state identifiers in national datasets, such as the National Inpatient Sample, and other related datasets from the Healthcare Cost and Utilization Project; (2) create mapping and linkages across data sources; (3) incentivize the collection of Z-codes relevant to social determinants of health and data on functional status through payment policy; and (4) make data available more quickly and more easily accessible for research and policy decisions.

Megan Morris, University of Colorado Anschutz Medical Campus, discussed data needs related to disability status. She noted that there is growing evidence that individuals with disabilities experience significant health

---

BOX 2-1
An Example of How Data Silos Hinder the Ability to Answer Policy Questions: The Impact of Medicaid Expansion on Equity in Hospitalizations for Complex Cancer Surgery

- *National Medicaid data*: Not up to date; do not include the uninsured, so no baseline.
- *National in-patient sample*: Has a 2-year lag at least; does not include state or hospital identifiers, so not possible to know the impact of Medicaid expansion on hospital utilization for cancer surgery.
- *Medicare data*: Has less of a time lag; has geographic information, but no information on young Medicaid patients or the uninsured.
- *State all-payer claims databases*: Not widely available, not standardized, usually do not include the uninsured.
- *Local hospital data*: Not widely available, not generalizable, no easy comparison group.
- *VA and Kaiser*: Not nationally representative, limiting utility for estimating broad policy effects.

SOURCE: Workshop presentation by Karen Joynt Maddox, May 3, 2021.

> **BOX 2-2**
> **An Example of How Data Silos Hinder the
> Ability to Answer Policy Questions:
> The Impact of Hospital Value-Based Purchasing on Equity in
> Posthospitalization Functional Status**
>
> - *National Medicare data*: Updated, but includes no data on functional status; race and ethnicity data are highly aggregated.
> - *Medicare skilled nursing facility data*: Has a 1- to 2-year lag; only includes fee-for-service patients in skilled nursing facilities.
> - *Medicare home health aide services, long-term care, and inpatient rehabilitation facility data:* Same as above (Medicare skilled nursing facility data); not necessarily comparable across settings.
> - *Medicare outpatient data*: No patient-reported outcomes.
> - *Medicare Current Beneficiary Survey data*: Has a small sample of patients; not useful for small subgroups including racial/ethnic minoritized groups.
>
> SOURCE: Workshop presentation by Karen Joynt Maddox, May 3, 2021.

and health care disparities. She discussed recent work she conducted with support from the Patient Centered Outcome Research Institute (PCORI) to identify research priorities for advancing equitable health care for individuals with disabilities. As part of the study, she collected input from a range of stakeholders, including researchers, patient advocacy organizations, health systems, payers, policy makers, and agencies within the HHS. The key finding from this work was the need to improve data on people with disabilities.

Morris said that data on disabilities are rarely collected or documented in common data sources, such as electronic health records, patient experience surveys, or in big data sources, such as claims data. ICD-9-CM or ICD-10-CM codes are often insufficient for identifying who has a disability. For example, for a study of individuals who had total laryngectomies and were nonverbal, Morris reviewed medical charts and found that less than 30 percent of patients with this condition had an ICD-9-CM code for their communication disability in their medical record (likely because this code does not affect payment for the service).

Morris argued that the priority need in this area is for data that make it possible to (1) identify the quality of health and health care of individuals with disabilities; (2) develop, implement, and measure the effects of interventions; and (3) provide accommodations to individuals with disabilities.

In 2011, HHS released data collection standards that included standards for data on disability status. The HHS guidelines included six questions, and Morris suggested that these six could be integrated into electronic health records, along with an additional question on communication disabilities. The question of communication disabilities has already been tested for potential inclusion in several national surveys. Box 2-3 reproduces these seven disability questions. Morris said her research indicates that these questions would be well received by patients.

To reduce disability disparities, Morris suggested (1) recognizing persons with disabilities as a population at high risk for experiencing health disparities; (2) supporting initiatives and infrastructure for documenting disability status at the point of care; (3) ensuring that disability demographics and accessibility quality measures are included in surveys; and (4) developing methods to identify persons with disabilities in claims data.

Mitchell Lunn, Stanford University, discussed health disparities among and the lack of data for sexual- and gender-minority populations. Lunn said that data collected by the Gallup organization indicate that sexual and gender minorities represent about 5.6 percent of the U.S. population. However, the lesbian, gay, bisexual, transgender, queer (LGBTQ+) population is a heterogeneous group, and the umbrella term encompasses people with differing health needs. Further, high-quality, detailed data on the breakdown of sexual and gender minorities by race and ethnicity are not available.

Lunn emphasized the differences among the concepts of sexual orientation, gender identity, and sex assigned at birth, and argued that data on sexual orientation and gender identity are inadequately collected in most clinical and research settings. As an example, the sexual orientation item

---

BOX 2-3
Disability Questions for Potential Inclusion in Electronic Health Records

1. Are you deaf or do you have serious difficulty hearing?
2. Are you blind or do you have difficulty seeing, even when wearing glasses?
3. Do you have serious difficulty walking or climbing stairs?
4. Do you have difficulty concentrating, remembering, or making decisions?
5. Do you have difficulty dressing or bathing?
6. Do you have difficulty doing errands alone such as visiting a doctor's office or shopping?
7. Using your usual language, do you have difficulty communicating (for example, understanding or being understood)?

SOURCES: Workshop presentation by Megan Morris, May 3, 2021. Questions 1–6, U.S. Department of Health and Human Services (2011). https://aspe.hhs.gov/reports/hhs-implementation-guidance-data-collection-standards-race-ethnicity-sex-primary-language-disability-0.

in the electronic health records used by Stanford Medicine collects information only on the identity construct, not on sexual attraction or sexual behavior. The options available to describe sexual orientation are more limited than the range of terms used by the community (for example, "pansexual" and "queer" are not available) and only one option can be selected, although a write-in option is available. In terms of gender identity, Stanford Medicine's electronic health records also limit the answer to one option, with a narrower range of options than the terms used by the community.

To illustrate limitations in a research setting, Lunn discussed the *All of Us* program, a National Institutes of Health (NIH) research program that aims to enroll and collect data from more than one million participants. The sexual orientation and gender identity questions used by *All of Us* also measure the identity construct. The items were developed with input from subject matter experts and the community, and contain terms that are more commonly used by the community. It is also possible to select more than one answer for both sexual orientation and gender identity. Some of the options become available in the form of a submenu, and Lunn argued that it would be preferable to include more items on the initial list, since that would give respondents more options to consider that might be applicable to them. He added that some of the terms used in the NIH program are antiquated and are being revised.

Lunn also discussed the PRIDE study, a large-scale national health study of people who identify as LGBTQ+ or as another sexual or gender minority. He said that with multiple selections allowed in that study, around 35 percent of participants in the sample select more than one option for sexual orientation and around 18 percent select more than one option for gender identity. The terms used are revised every few years with community engagement.

Lunn argued that current clinical approaches, such as electronic health records systems and data models, do not allow patients to comprehensively report their sexual orientation and gender identity. Not using people's stated identity (e.g., grouping or administratively classifying them instead) could result in the loss of valuable data that may have health implications. Research studies can serve as models for developing sexual orientation and gender identity data standards, because these studies tend to involve researchers who are focused on this field. Lunn also emphasized that sexual and gender minority terms tend to change at a rapid pace, and therefore frequent re-evaluation with community engagement is critical to selecting the optimal terms to use.

Kaleab Abebe, University of Pittsburgh, echoed comments made by other speakers related to some of the key challenges associated with the data infrastructure for PCOR. First, he said, regardless of what data are collected and in what context they are collected, it is important to ask whether or not the data are representative of the population that could benefit from them. Second, data being housed in disparate locations and being owned by different entities leads to a substantial barrier to their use, and it is important to think of ways to curate and harmonize these data.

Abebe noted that the various data sources have varying degrees of completeness and representativeness. When these data sources are linked, the resulting datasets have their own patterns of data gaps and lack of representativeness, particularly in terms of the populations who could benefit from the availability of the data the most. He described this as "disparities on top of disparities." If data are not available or are incomplete, it is difficult to act on the information in a way that could benefit people. Abebe also underscored the importance of efforts to standardize data but, again, without losing sight of the larger underlying question of whether the data have gaps in terms of the populations that are covered.

Thinking about opportunities, Abebe mentioned the example of the clinical trial infrastructure in the United Kingdom, which not only facilitates the carrying out of trials, but also aggregates the data that have been accumulated as part of trials. In the United States, it may be possible to build on what already exists to link more of the data. Abebe also highlighted opportunities to build on work already started that puts patient preferences in the center, including the development of an interoperable electronic care (eCare) plan. He also emphasized the need to develop metrics for the data infrastructure portfolio to enable researchers to better understand successes and failures and potentially utilize this information when considering future work.

Abebe noted that the social determinants of health can change over time, so measures need to be developed with the understanding that they need to be flexible. He also argued that there should be more of a spotlight on disparities, not only on measuring them but also on capturing metrics for ways of addressing disparities, whether in the form of interventions, therapeutics, or other potential solutions.

Thomas Sequist, Harvard University and Brigham and Women's Hospital, discussed data needs with a particular focus on Native Americans. He said that during the COVID-19 pandemic it took a long time to recognize the impact of the pandemic on Native American communities, in part because of an inability to generate data at a level that would make it possible to understand the health issues specific to American Indians. One reason for this is that small sample sizes often result in data on American Indian populations being combined with data on other populations. Another challenge is that many studies on American Indians draw on data available from the Indian Health Service, but only about half of this population receives health care through that agency. The American Indian population that is left out of research that relies on that agency's data is heavily skewed toward an urban population.

Sequist said that an important step toward addressing these challenges would be to develop more robust ways to identify American Indians in all existing datasets, which would make it possible to better characterize their experiences. Information about people's tribal affiliations would further help in understanding their culture and the experiences they may have related to their health.

Sequist pointed out that social determinants of health come into play not only at an interpersonal level, but also at a geographic level, so better data are needed to understand these risk factors at that level. He discussed how geography can be relevant in addressing inequities, arguing that the use of geography needs to be carefully considered and standardized to better understand the interplay between it and race, ethnicity, and language.

Concerning language, Sequist highlighted the need for accurate and reliable data, noting that lack of standardization in the way language information is collected has been a challenge both for research and for improving health care. For example, he underscored the need to differentiate among someone's preferred language, their primary language, the languages in which they are fluent, and the languages in which they have achieved health literacy. The COVID-19 pandemic, which affected non-English-speaking patients in a particularly severe way, has illustrated the need for language-appropriate care.

Sequist said that the array of information that exists on patient-reported outcomes does not always reflect the types of outcomes that patients themselves value or the experiences that they are having with the system, particularly concerning race-specific issues, ethnicity-specific issues, and language-specific issues. The relative value people place on various outcomes is likely to depend on their background, and substantial investments would be needed in patient-reported outcomes projects to begin to really understand those variations.

CONCLUSIONS

In this section we summarize the committee's conclusions based on the presentations and discussion. The research of those experts who presented at the workshop focuses on health disparities in a variety of areas, affecting various populations. The underlying theme that emerged from the presentations was that there are data limitations for a variety of populations, and that these limitations hinder the ability to understand health disparities.

> **CONCLUSION 2-1:** Health disparities can occur across a broad range of characteristics and populations. Data limitations affect the ability to identify and understand these disparities in many areas. Data for specific populations are sometimes unavailable or are not representa-

tive. In other cases, the data might not be timely or might have other gaps that make it difficult to understand the impact of changes over long periods of time.

A fundamental reason for the data limitations that make it difficult to answer questions important for PCOR is that most of the data available for research are not primarily collected for research purposes. While research questions require a relational or integrative perspective, the data collected tend to be transactional, that is, collected for payment or treatment purposes, and therefore do not vary according to most personal characteristics. This has several implications for the data available. First, the data collected are typically limited to or organized within subpopulations (for example, those insured by Medicaid or Medicare). People who are uninsured, including those who have limited access or interactions with health care services, are likely to be underrepresented in many databases. Second, the information collected (and the absence of what is not collected) often makes the data poorly suited to answer a variety of research questions. Third, those who collect the data do not necessarily have an obvious incentive to collect information in a way that is useful for secondary purposes, such as research. The workshop identified a variety of data needs and potential opportunities for enhancing the data infrastructure, and these deserve further attention.

CONCLUSION 2-2: The data available for patient-centered outcomes research are often collected for reasons other than research, which limits their usefulness. Opportunities exist for increasing the utility of the data infrastructure by carefully considering the multiple uses to which the data might be applied.

The data that do exist are stored in a variety of databases across a fragmented health care system. The workshop identified data silos (e.g., within settings, at a point in time, or for a specific payer) as a major barrier to the efficient use of the information that is available.

CONCLUSION 2-3: Existing data on the social determinants of health are found in a variety of databases. Barriers to linking across these data silos represent a major challenge to understanding how social determinants of health affect health outcomes.

The workshop made it clear that the data available do not capture the complexities that are necessary to understand in order to determine how people's characteristics and experiences influence outcomes. The speakers identified several potential ways of capturing more of these complexities, and they emphasized the need to build flexibility into the data collection systems to allow them to adapt as both the terminologies and the available technologies for capturing and processing data evolve.

CONCLUSION 2-4: Existing data do not capture the richness of people's characteristics and experiences. While such limitations are to be expected, opportunities exist for capturing data that are better able to characterize these complexities. A robust data infrastructure builds on the strengths of what is available today and has the flexibility to adapt, both as measures and terminologies become obsolete and as new technologies emerge.

The workshop underscored the magnitude of the data gaps in the area of health disparities. Improving the data available for understanding and addressing disparities would require an effort concentrated on this goal.

CONCLUSION 2-5: Prioritizing and improving the collection of data can lead to a better understanding of health disparities and to potential solutions for reducing disparities.

3

Patient Perspectives on Data Needs

This chapter summarizes data needs conveyed by patient organizations. Speakers in this session were asked to focus on the questions below. The brief overview of the input received from the presenters is followed by the committee's conclusions.

- Looking ahead, what are the main data needs?
- What are the implications of the (recently broadened) statutory scope for patient-centered outcomes research (PCOR)?
- What questions cannot be answered and who is not served by the current PCOR data infrastructure?
- What new data sources could be incorporated into the PCOR data infrastructure?
- What data capacity challenges is the U.S. Department of Health and Human Services (HHS) best positioned to address in the context of its public mission, authorities, programs, and data resources?

Rebekah Angove shared her perspective based on her role as vice president for patient experience and program evaluation at the Patient Advocate Foundation (PAF), a nonprofit organization that provides case management services and financial aid to those with chronic, life-threatening, and debilitating illnesses. Angove also previously served as engagement director of REACHnet, a clinical research network that is part of the National Patient-Centered Clinical Research Network.

As part of its work focused on assisting patients, PAF also collects data from patients with the goal of translating evidence into research and policy work focused on improving health care and the patient experience. Angove said that because PAF works with patients who experience access and affordability challenges, its patient and caregiver network represents populations that are often underrepresented in research initiatives because they are underinsured or uninsured and, consequently, are less likely to be represented in large health care systems that have robust data collections and clinical trials.

Angove discussed challenges associated with obtaining patient agreements for participating in data collection as well as broader engagement in research. PAF's experience and the research it has done on this topic indicate that most patients have a very limited understanding of research, and especially of terminology such as "comparative effectiveness" research and "patient-centered outcomes" research. Patients are also often confused or uninformed about how research data are used and the implications of giving their consent for the use of their data. She argued that confusion in these areas leads to mistrust or distrust.

Angove highlighted several characteristics of meaningful patient engagement. First, she noted that engagement requires careful thinking about the range of experiences that are included in order to achieve representativeness. Beyond the dimensions of diversity discussed in Chapter 1, diversity along additional dimensions such as treatment experiences, life experiences, urban vs. rural, and ability to pay for and access health care also need to be represented. If the patients engaged in and contributing to research are not representative of a broad range of experiences, the findings could exacerbate disparities. Angove also underscored the role transparency plays in meaningful patient engagement. This means being clear about who owns the data and how the data are being used, as well as better communication about how patients are involved in the process.

Angove argued that meaningful patient involvement means involvement in all activities that are part of PCOR, and not just involvement in an activity that is specifically carved out for patient involvement (for example, recruitment and patient committees). For example, patients could be more involved in conversations about methodology, about how the results are interpreted, or about how information about the research is communicated. Angove emphasized that the fact that the data are patient reported does not necessarily mean they are patient centered. Validated measures for patient-reported outcomes (PROs) have historically been developed without patient involvement. For example, when patients are involved in projects, they often point out issues related to the PRO measurement scales that are used, but ultimately their input is not incorporated because researchers are reluctant to deviate from PRO measures that have been validated.

Another aspect of meaningful patient engagement discussed by Angove is training in how research is done, not only for patients but also for the researchers themselves, as well as policy makers and health care workers. This is particularly important given the sensitive nature of the health information that patients are being asked to share. Angove also emphasized the importance of communicating to patients the value of their contributions.

Gary Epstein-Lubow, Brown University, discussed his experiences as team leader for the stakeholder engagement team for the National Institute on Aging's Imbedded Pragmatic Alzheimer's Disease and AD-related Dementias Clinical Trials Collaboratory (IMPACT Collaboratory). The IMPACT Collaboratory's goal is to build the nation's capacity to conduct pragmatic clinical trials of interventions imbedded within health care systems for people at risk of dementia, people living with dementia, and their family members and care partners.

While there are no disease-modifying treatments available for dementia, nonpharmacologic interventions show promise, although they have had limited adoption. Epstein-Lubow said that to address this, embedded pragmatic clinical trials (ePCTs) need improved patient-centered outcomes data that are systematically available. Patients and caregivers are important stakeholders who provide input to the trial implementation, and the interventions need to be integrated into the routine clinical flow and not add a reporting burden. To do this, it is essential for electronic health records to capture patient-centered outcomes in a systematic way, with special attention paid to confirming that data are collected from underrepresented groups and groups disproportionately harmed by dementia. Finally, outcomes of ePCTs must be relevant and usable by decision makers, including health care systems.

Epstein-Lubow said that there are special considerations for ePCTs when it comes to dementia research. From the perspective of patients, applicable ethical considerations and regulations deserve particular attention, because people living with dementia are a vulnerable population and there are questions about their capacity to provide informed consent and to self-report their preferences. Another area that deserves attention is the role of care partners and family members, including the potential for linking caregiver data with patient data.

Concerning data needs in the area of dementia, Epstein-Lubow highlighted five needs, namely the need for:

1. information that can lead to improvements in person-centered care;
2. improved reporting on functional status, including physical, social, occupational, and emotional functioning, in addition to cognitive functioning;
3. data linkages between information provided by people living with dementia and their caregivers;
4. strategies for capturing information about lived experiences; and

5. methods for standardizing proxy reporting for people who have partial capacity or who lack capacity to report directly.

Epstein-Lubow argued that the broadened statutory scope for PCOR increases opportunities for learning about patient-centered outcomes but also involves some risks. For example, if inadequate attention is paid to underrepresented groups, including members of groups at higher risks of negative health effects of dementia, this could lead to underrepresented patient-centered outcomes data in these areas. There is also the risk of potential added burden for family members and caregivers in their roles as proxy respondents and missed opportunities for data linkage in the case of missing data from caregivers.

Additional data challenges exist for research on dementia, according to Epstein-Lubow, including the following:

- There is no standard measure set for people living with dementia.
- There is no standard measure set for family caregivers.
- Quality measures for dementia care are optional in most reporting systems.
- There are challenges regarding the collection of patient-centered outcomes from people living with moderate or severe dementia.
- Accommodations for data collection may be required for people with limited health literacy.
- There are methodological challenges associated with linking data from people living with dementia and their caregivers.

Epstein-Lubow highlighted several dementia measures that are part of the Merit-Based Incentive Payment System (MIPS), which is a Centers for Medicare & Medicaid Services (CMS) program that eligible health care clinicians can participate in to report data to better connect care quality with Medicare payments. These dementia measures are optional, but Epstein-Lubow argued that they could be required. The measures highlighted include

- dementia-associated behavioral and psychiatric symptom screening and management;
- dementia: cognitive assessment;
- dementia: education and support of caregivers for patients with dementia;
- dementia: functional status assessment; and
- dementia: safety concern screening and follow-up for patients with dementia.

In addition, Epstein-Lubow suggested that the Consumer Assessment of Healthcare Providers and Systems questions on patient and caregiver experience of care could be expanded to include proxy reports of dementia.

To strengthen the PCOR data infrastructure in ways that could benefit people living with dementia, Epstein-Lubow said that HHS would be particularly well positioned to address one of the recommendations made by the public members of the HHS Advisory Council on Alzheimer's Research, Care and Services, which urged HHS to "Encourage further development, evaluation, and use of health care models for AD/ADRD that align performance measures, the experience of care by persons living with AD/ADRD and their caregivers, and payment."[1]

Epstein-Lubow further suggested using the definitions of care "value" used by CMS and studying models that enhance value. One way to do this would be to rely on the CMS "Meaningful Measures" initiative, including use of new care planning codes, the annual wellness visit, and the MIPS dementia measures discussed earlier.

Elisabeth Oehrlein discussed insights from her work at the National Health Council (NHC), a nonprofit association of more than 140 health-related organizations, including leading patient advocacy groups. She identified a list of key data needs based on what the NHC's patient groups are hearing from the patients these organizations serve, and based on NHC's work in the areas of regulations, real-world evidence, and value assessment:

- patient-centered outcomes and impacts that really matter to patients, collected consistently;
- burden, including costs incurred by patients and their families;
- social determinants of health (for example, transportation, housing);
- evidence based on representative populations;
- quality and satisfaction with care, defined from the perspective of patients;
- accessibility of the research results to patients; and
- interoperability.

Oehrlein said that in addition to measuring the outcomes and impacts that patients truly care about, it is also important to use language that patients will use. For example, in the case of alopecia areata (an autoimmune disease that causes hair loss), the patient-reported outcome measure has traditionally been the percentage of the skin that is covered in hair, but talking to patients made it clear that what they care about is not

---

[1] https://aspe.hhs.gov/public-members-advisory-council-alzheimers-research-care-and-services-2020-recommendations#clinical, see recommendation 5.

necessarily the difference between a 20 percent or 40 percent improvement in skin covered, but rather whether or not they need to wear a wig.

In terms of increasing patient accessibility of the research results and evidence, Oehrlein mentioned the expansion of dashboards that patients can use to enter certain criteria and find out what treatments might work better for them or what the outcomes experienced by others with similar conditions have been. These types of communication vehicles could be a model going forward.

To further illustrate the types of outcomes that matter to patients, Oehrlein discussed findings from a Food and Drug Administration report focused on chronic fatigue syndrome and myalgic encephalomyelitis (Table 3-1).[2] The table shows that many aspects of a patient's experience that are traditionally considered important to measure are indeed important to patients. These aspects include disease-related impacts, feelings, and functions. However, patients also care about and want more information on treatment-related impacts, financial impacts, and caregiver impacts. This type of patient input can help narrow the scope of the data that are collected in order to better focus resources and reduce the burden on patients.

Oehrlein said that the broadened statutory scope for PCOR presents opportunities to more effectively assess treatment alternatives and value from the patients' perspective. In particular, she finds that patient advocates and patients are often surprised to discover that data on out-of-pocket costs and other costs important to patients have not been systematically collected. Having these types of data available would lead to more holistic evidence relevant to patient decision-making and more informed decisions as patients navigate their options and understand what the treatment impacts might be, beyond clinical outcomes. These types of decisions increasingly have an impact on patients' access to care.

As an illustration of a model for moving forward, Oehrlein discussed the work of the EveryLife Foundation for Rare Diseases. Its report assessing the total economic burden of rare diseases was born out of the realization that the data that have been collected to date on direct medical costs really do not reflect the full patient experience, especially when it comes to rare diseases.[3] EveryLife Foundation researchers have thought carefully about which costs are important to patients and how those data might be collected.

In terms of data needs that HHS would be best positioned to address, Oehrlein highlighted the need for better data for underserved populations and communities. Supporting dashboard-type solutions to make more of the data available to inform individual patient decisions would also be

---

[2] https://www.fda.gov/media/86879/download.
[3] https://everylifefoundation.org/wp-content/uploads/2021/02/The_National_Economic_Burden_of_Rare_Disease_Study_Summary_Report_February_2021.pdf.

TABLE 3-1 Examples of Patient-Experience Information Related to Chronic Fatigue Syndrome and Myalgic Encephalomyelitis in the Food and Drug Administration's *The Voice of the Patient* Report

Disease-Related Impact on Feelings and Function	Treatment-Related Impacts	Financial-Related Impacts	Caregiver-Related Impacts
• Postexertional malaise • Weakness • Muscle and joint pain • Unrefreshing sleep • Decreased quality of family life • Social isolation • Feelings of hopelessness	• Willing to accept significant risk from new treatment to alleviate or cure condition	• Loss of career • Harsh financial difficulties as a result of decreased or lost employment income • High cost of treatment, often because unapproved treatments are not covered by insurance	• Stress on family and family members

SOURCE: U.S. Food and Drug Administration (2013). https://www.fda.gov/media/86879/download. Workshop presentation by Elisabeth Oehrlein, May 3, 2021.

useful. The COVID-19 dashboard operated by the National Center for Advancing Translational Sciences is an example of a government initiative along those lines.

Bray Patrick-Lake, Evidation Health, shared her insights in part based on her career working in patient advocacy, leading a patient foundation, and working on national research programs, such as *All of Us* and PCORnet. Her current work is focused on measuring what matters most to patients in everyday life. Evidation Health is a digital research and health engagement company whose members participate in research studies. Members provide person-generated health data, which enable continuous monitoring of health outcomes at the individual level. The platform collects 750 million data points daily. The data include individually generated, individually permissioned data, such as data from wearables and environment data, as well as system-generated individually permissioned data, such as data from electronic health records. Figure 3-1 illustrates the range of data sources considered by Evidation.

Patrick-Lake argued that the traditional sources of data (shown on the left side of Figure 3-1) provide episodic snapshots of the experiences of patients living with disease over time. Most of what constitutes people's lives, and therefore the richest data about patients' experiences with disease,

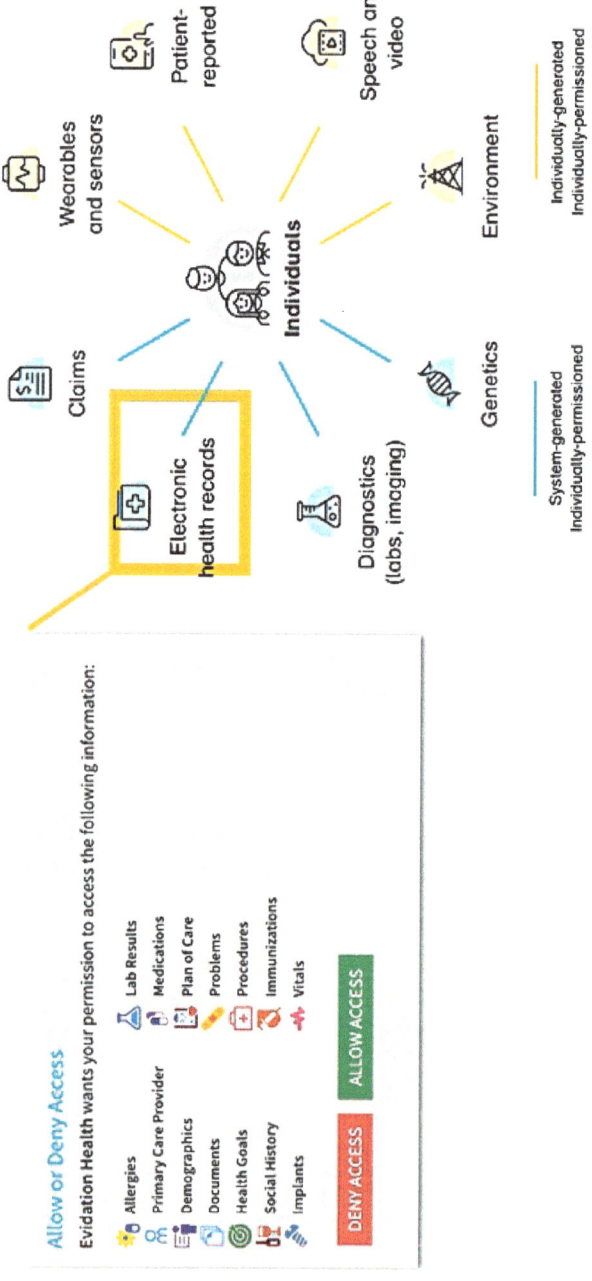

FIGURE 3-1 Evidation Health's vision for person-generated health data framework.
SOURCE: Workshop presentation by Bray Patrick-Lake, May 3, 2021. Evidation Health (2021).

is currently invisible to the health care system. Figure 3-2 illustrates how real-world evidence data points (i.e., evidence obtained from real-world data, such as data generated during routine clinical practice) contrast with data from digital technologies that have the potential to continuously and passively collect data, without substantial burden to patients.

Patrick-Lake argued that digital technologies that continuously collect data have the potential to result in:

- better characterization and understanding of living with the disease;
- better understanding of disease progression;
- earlier identification of at-risk individuals;
- real-world, objective Quality of Life and Activities of Daily Living measures; and
- pattern detection for public health.

Patrick-Lake echoed a point made by other speakers, namely that traditional sources of real-world data might not capture what is truly important to patients. For example, a measure used in the context of cardiac care is mortality, but a patient living with cardiac disease would more likely want information on how to improve his or her quality of life, what the progression of the disease might be like, and how the disease might impact activities of daily living over time.

As an illustration of how data from wearable devices can greatly enhance real-world data, Patrick-Lake suggested considering two asthma patients who seem to be nearly identical based on traditional sources of real-world data: they both have moderate or severe asthma; they are both nonsmokers; they are on the same inhaled medications; and they are both adhering to their physician-prescribed treatments. In terms of symptom control, one person might report waking up often (every night or almost every night) due to asthma symptoms, while the other reports waking up 2 or fewer days a month due to asthma symptoms. When data from (the same brand of) wearable device are added, it becomes clear that the first person is asleep 49 percent of the time, while the second person is asleep 90 percent of the time, while in bed.

Patrick-Lake argued that digital technologies can result in data that accelerate and enhance clinical care, accelerate clinical research, and improve public health. Examples discussed included predicting flare events in an autoimmune condition using wearable and survey data; enhancing recovery modeling for limb surgeries with personalized predictions of outcome tailored to individual characteristics; and early detection, monitoring, and management of COVID-19 in everyday life.

For a potential roadmap of how to achieve the full potential of person-generated health data and digital clinical measures, Patrick-Lake referenced

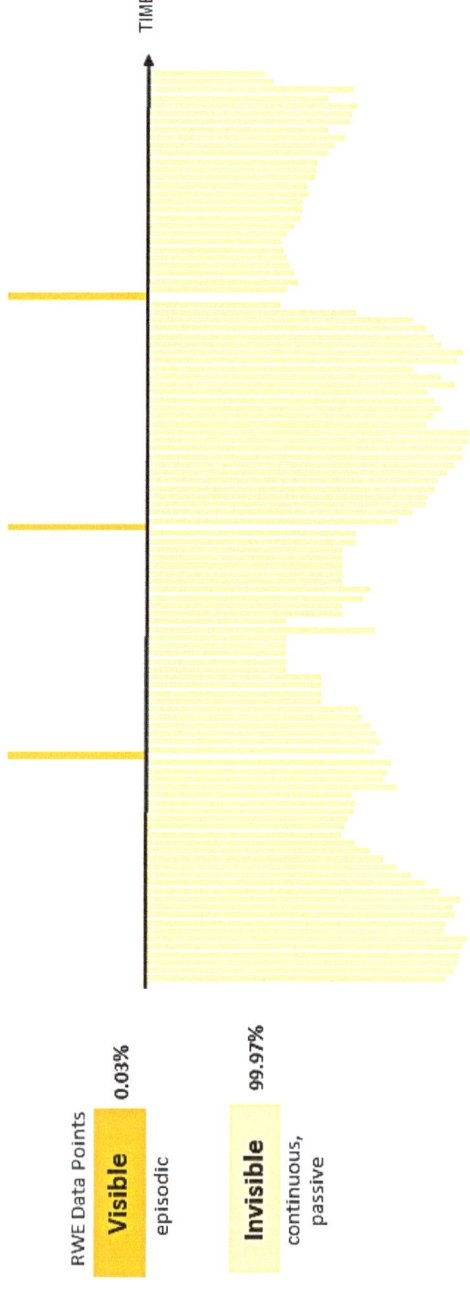

FIGURE 3-2 Episodic real-world evidence data points versus continuous data using digital technologies.
SOURCE: Workshop presentation by Bray Patrick-Lake, 2021. Evidation Health (2021).

The Playbook, a document released by the Digital Medicine Society.[4] She highlighted the need for standards for organizing and analyzing digital data and to serve as a foundation for further developing methodologies for their use. There is also a need to develop an evidentiary framework, which would make this type of data more broadly accepted in health care, research, and public health settings.

Patrick-Lake argued that HHS could have a role in developing incentives and rewards that could reduce barriers to collaboration and promote the use and reuse of innovations. She said that there is also need for policy leadership to advance data rights and the work of the National Human Genome Research Institute's Ethical, Legal and Social Implications Research Program, which supports the appropriate balance between individual protections and public benefit, ensuring that individuals are well informed and protected against discrimination based on their digital specimens.

CONCLUSIONS

Representatives of patient organizations argued that PCOR data are often not focused on the types of issues that are truly important to people and that would enable them to find answers to the questions they tend to have about their treatment options and potential outcomes. Information on costs was highlighted as particularly important, which is in line with the goals of the recently broadened scope of PCOR to take into consideration "the potential burdens and economic impacts of the utilization of medical treatments, items, and services."

> **CONCLUSION 3-1: The patient-centered outcomes research data infrastructure has not reached its full potential to provide data that can answer questions that matter to patients and enable them to make informed decisions. Information about the cost of care was highlighted among the types of data that would be particularly useful.**

While data on patient-centered outcomes are available in many areas that are important to patients, the information is rarely available in ways that would make it truly accessible to them for decision-making purposes. More widespread dissemination of information that is easy to use could also increase engagement.

> **CONCLUSION 3-2: Dissemination and translation of the research findings could be greatly enhanced by using forms of communication that are relevant to those outside of the research community.**

---

[4] https://playbook.dimesociety.org.

4

Researcher Perspectives on Data Needs

This chapter summarizes data needs conveyed by researchers. Speakers in this session were asked to focus on the questions below. The chapter also discusses a case study on the use of the patient-centered outcomes research (PCOR) infrastructure to study whether vitamin D can reduce the burden of COVID-19. The chapter concludes with the committee's conclusions.

- Looking ahead, what are the main data needs?
- What are the implications of the (recently broadened) statutory scope for PCOR?
- What questions cannot be answered and who is not served by the current PCOR data infrastructure?
- What new data sources could be incorporated into the PCOR data infrastructure?
- What data capacity challenges is the U.S. Department of Health and Human Services (HHS) best positioned to address in the context of its public mission, authorities, programs, and data resources?

David Meltzer, University of Chicago, discussed the use of existing data, including PCOR datasets, to conduct research on whether vitamin D could reduce the burden of COVID-19. Box 4-1 summarizes some of the key studies to date, including the studies initiated by Meltzer at the beginning of the pandemic, using University of Chicago data. This case study was intended to illustrate a specific application of how the data infrastructure can be used to study an emerging health question, and how research projects can build on each other. Box 4-1 illustrates limitations and sum-

> **BOX 4-1**
> **Case Study:**
> **The Use of the Patient-Centered Outcomes Research Infrastructure to Study Whether Vitamin D Can Reduce the Burden of COVID-19**
>
> Observational Analysis at University of Chicago Medicine
> - 489 patients with vitamin D level, 14-365 days before
> - COVID-19 test (March 3–April 10, 2020)[a]
> - March 3 to April 10 (4,314 pts ->489 pts in analytic sample)[b]
>
> Other Epidemiological Studies
> - Merzon et al.:
>   - N = 7,807, Israeli health system cohort
> - Kaufman et al.:
>   - N = 190,000 U.S. cases tested by Quest Diagnostics
>   - Race imputed by zipcode
> - Hastie et al.:
>   - N = 348,958, UK Biobank study cohort
> - Ma et al.:
>   - N = 8,297, UK Biobank study cohort
>
> Randomized Controlled Trials of Vitamin D and COVID-19 Severity
> - Castillo et al.: RCT of calcifediol vs. usual care
> - Murai et al.: RCT D3 200,000 IU vitamin D x 1 vs. placebo
> - Rastogi et al.: RCT D3 60,000 IU/d x 7d vs. placebo
>
> Additional Observational Analyses in Progress
> - National COVID Cohort Collaborative (N3C)
>   - Funded by NCATS, ~ 50 sites, >1 million COVID patients plus controls
>   - Data continuously added; some paring of controls vs. COVID cases
>   - Secure computing environment, collaborative ecosystem
>   - Sample size/coverage to allow analysis of levels, seasonality, location, racial subgroups

marizes Meltzer's observations related to the usefulness of the PCOR data based on this work.

Andrew Bazemore, American Board of Family Medicine, noted that although we live in a time of unprecedented health-data availability, there are also some structural blind spots in the U.S. health care system. He cited Kerr White's research on the ecology of medical care and the notion that out of 1,000 people in a community in a given month, 750 might experience illness or injury, 250 will seek primary care, and 10 will be hospitalized, of which just one will be hospitalized in an academic health center,

- Epic Cosmos
  - Several times larger than N3C
  - Only Epic personnel can access data
- VA data (with Robert Gibbons and others)
  - Includes Rx of vitamin D
  - Examine hazard of COVID diagnosis after new vitamin D prescription
- PCORNet/CAPriCORN
  - Multicenter EHR data with deep Chicago-area coverage and ability to extend nationally
  - Linked contextual data, little PRO data, biomarkers only via routine care

Observations Based on the University of Chicago Medicine Study
- PCOR data provided important insights, sometimes rapidly
  - Ease of access, including administrative and technical barriers, cost affected use
  - Relevant data infrastructure diverse and overlapping
  - Multiple public and private sources provided opportunities
  - International data sources also advanced the field
- Data completeness and quality questions evident
- Contextual and patient-reported variables relevant
- Biomarker data valuable, additional biomarker data important (e.g., *All of Us*)
- Initiating RCTs important and complementary with observational studies

---

[a]D.O. Meltzer, T.J. Best, H. Zhang, T. Vokes, V. Arora, and J. Solway. (2020). Association of vitamin D status and other clinical characteristics with COVID-19 test results, *JAMA Network Open* 3(9), e2019722 (doi:10.1001/jamanetworkopen.2020.19722).
[b]D.O. Meltzer, T.J. Best, H. Zhang, T. Vokes, V. Arora, and J. Solway. (2021). Association of vitamin D levels, race/ethnicity, and clinical characteristics with COVID-19 test results, *JAMA Network Open* 4(3), e214117 (doi:10.1001/jamanetworkopen.2021.4117).
NOTE: COVID = coronavirus disease 2019; EHR = electronic health records; NCATS = National Center for Advancing Translational Sciences; PCOR = patient-centered outcomes research; PRO = patient-reported outcome; RCT = randomized controlled trial; Rx = prescription; VA = U.S. Department of Veterans Affairs.
SOURCE: Workshop presentation by David Meltzer, May 3, 2021.

---

in other words in the type of place where most of the research is being conducted.[1] While Kerr White's original study was published in the early 1960s, this "ecology" has not changed. Bazemore said that it is important to understand where people land within the broader health care setting, and where the borders are between wellness and illness, between illness and care-seeking, and between primary care and the hospital, in order to

---

[1]K.L. White, T.F. Williams, and B.G. Greenberg. (1996). The ecology of medical care. *Bulletin of the New York Academy of Medicine* 73(1), 187–212.

better understand how to provide access to high-quality care that is truly patient-centered.

Bazemore noted that primary care, which is the largest platform for health care delivery, is not well represented in the data available. For example, about 0.3 percent of National Institutes of Health (NIH) research funding ends up in family medicine research settings. A study that looked at the first six cycles and then the subsequent six cycles of funding from PCORI found that between 18 and 30 percent involved primary care sites, even though about half of U.S. health care delivery happens in those settings. Even in the case of studies that involved primary care sites, typically their role was focused on patient recruitment. Places where patients with the highest risk of poor patient-centered outcomes are receiving care, including safety net clinics, federally qualified health centers, small health clinics, and rural health clinics, would be even less likely to be included.

Bazemore said that it would be useful to better understand patients' experiences in primary care settings, including how they differ from the experiences of those who receive care from a specialist, in an emergency room, or in other places. It would also be important to understand how the characteristics of primary care influence patient outcomes. Patients often report that what is important to them is that their primary care doctor involve them as much as they want to be involved in their health care. Information about community health risk factors facing patients would provide further context.

Among the data sources that are missing from the current PCOR data infrastructure, according to Bazemore, are not only primary care practices themselves but also two other data sources: primary care registries and health information exchanges focused on primary care and the safety net. On the analytical side, Bazemore noted that a major concern is that new technologies such as artificial intelligence and machine learning do not typically involve primary care patients in their algorithm development. This has implications for the data that are being generated for PCOR.

Bazemore also underscored the need to incorporate social determinants of health data into the data environments being built. This includes geo-coded secondary ecological data, ranging from individual variables to indices, such as the social deprivation index, the area deprivation index, and the social vulnerability index. Patient-reported data on social determinants of health are also needed, in combination with the ecological proxies. This information together can enable researchers to really understand the patient experience and the dynamic neighborhood features that inform and complement the patient perspective.

Kurt Stange, Case Western Reserve University, began by saying that as a family and public health physician, he has spent his career doing "stealth" research, trying to understand how to advance health and health care for whole people in a system that is designed to fragment them into their parts. The problem for PCOR is not only fragmented and siloed data but also a system that is designed for fragmentation in data use.

Stange raised the question of whether it would be possible to shift the model from trying to use data to drive quality from the top down to using data to support the local agency of those on the front lines who are trying to integrate, personalize, and prioritize care for all people. In the effort to solve the puzzle of health and patient-centered health care, the current approach tends to divide things up into parts: diseases, risk factors, risk groups. The parts are valued, but efforts to integrate the whole are not sufficiently supported.

Regarding specific needs, Stange highlighted data that would support the functions of integrating, personalizing, and prioritizing care for whole people. There is also a need to support care for people whose health needs cannot be addressed by relying on a single disease label, or a risk label, or a group label. Linking different sectors affecting health is also necessary.

As a starting point for addressing the prioritizing function, Stange cited a 2015 National Academies of Sciences, Engineering, and Medicine *Vital Signs* report that provided a useful framework for identifying core metrics for assessing health and progress in health care.[2] The report proposed the following criteria for core measures:

- importance for health,
- strength of linkage to progress,
- understandability of the measure,
- technical integrity,
- potential for broader system impact, and
- utility at multiple levels.

Stange argued that this is an efficient and effective way of thinking about data. He noted that the report also provides guidance on measuring performance for useful PCOR domains. Stange said that the broadened statutory scope of PCOR provides an opportunity to focus on the whole as well as the parts. It also provides opportunities to support those on the front lines trying to contextualize care, as well as to support relationship-centered care.

Concerning the question of who is poorly served by the current PCOR data infrastructure, Stange underscored previous points about the limitations of the data on people living with multiple chronic conditions and various disadvantaged groups. He added that the data also have limitations

---

[2]Institute of Medicine. (2015). *Vital Signs: Core Metrics for Health and Health Care Progress*. Washington, DC: The National Academies Press.

> **BOX 4-2**
> **Person-Centered Primary Care Measures**
>
> - My practice makes it easy for me to get care.
> - My practice is able to provide most of my care.
> - In caring for me, my doctor considers all of the factors that affect my health.
> - My practice coordinates the care I get from multiple places.
> - My doctor or practice know me as a person.
> - My doctor and I have been through a lot together.
> - My doctor or practice stand up for me.
> - The care I get takes into account knowledge of my family.
> - The care I get in this practice is informed by knowledge of my community.
> - Over time, my practice helps me stay healthy.
> - Over time, my practice helps me to meet my goals.
>
> SOURCE: Workshop presentation by Kurt Stange, May 3, 2021.

for those who are not "helpfully defined by their disease" or are defined by other data collected for another purpose. The health care system tends to offer people a disease label, but that is not necessarily the label or the data most helpful to them in terms of what is important in their lives.

For additional data that could be incorporated into the PCOR data infrastructure, Stange suggested the Person-Centered Primary Care Measures, which he and his coauthors developed based on what patients, clinicians, and (to a lesser extent) payors said was important to them in health care.[3] Box 4-2 shows these measures, which Stange said are widely used and are also pending endorsement by the National Quality Forum and the Centers for Medicare & Medicaid Services (CMS) for use in the CMS Quality Payment Program.

Stange also discussed specific data challenges that he believes HHS could be particularly well positioned to address. These include

- reframing data use to support *primary care* as a force for integration and equity for individuals and families;
- reframing data use to support *public health* as a force for integration and equity for communities and populations;
- supporting the integration of primary care and public health;
- supporting primary care research about the *care of whole people*;

---

[3] R.S. Etz, S.J. Zyzanski, M.M. Gonzalez, S.R. Reves, J.P. O'Neal, and K.C. Stange. (2019). A new comprehensive measure of high-value aspects of primary care, *The Annals of Family Medicine*, 17(3), 221–230. http://www.annfammed.org/content/17/3/221.

- bringing together the Office of the Assistant Secretary for Planning and Evaluation, the Centers for Disease Control and Prevention, and the National Committee on Vital and Health Statistics in their congressionally mandated role to update the Health Insurance Portability and Accountability Act of 1996 to make data sharing safe and less onerous; and
- raising the budget cap for NIH research project grants.

Robert Califf, Verily Life Sciences and Google Health, started by saying that in his experience the key question people want answered in most health care scenarios is this: *Out of the options at my disposal, which diagnostic strategy and treatment is best for me?* While this is at the core of the terminology *comparative effectiveness*, the data available and associated context are not enabling researchers to design and conduct crisp, reliable comparative effectiveness studies.

Califf pointed out the important role the pragmatic randomized trial played in providing answers related to the COVID-19 pandemic. He said that a priority going forward should be to identify a core set of data that would provide reliable information that, when coupled with appropriate study design, could enable multiple pragmatic clinical trials to be conducted to answer the many questions that people have about the options they have, and about the option that would ultimately be best for them. These trials could include not only drugs and devices but also behavioral and health service interventions and systems of care as well. He noted that more data is not necessarily better, and that time invested in identifying the essential data that are needed would be time well spent.

Califf also pointed out that computing has changed since the early days of PCOR and that some questions that were not feasible to be examined before are within scope now. This includes questions related to the roles of deep molecular, behavioral, and social determinants of health, given that it has long been recognized that social, cultural, behavioral, and biological determinants not only interact to combine in complex ways to impact individual outcomes, but also have common dimensions across groups of people. Going forward, it will be important to look at opportunities afforded by different ways to integrate information using a different approach to computing. He cited the example of COVID-19 trackers, which constantly scrape information off the Internet, integrate the data, and present them at a variety of levels, ranging from countries to states, counties, and even individual hospitals. This information has been useful for optimizing clinical trial recruitment and for deploying interventions. In theory, this approach could now be used for all diseases, starting with a substrate of real-time information about the status of health from a geospatial and temporal reference point.

Califf also argued that "de-identified data" is somewhat of a myth, because re-identification is usually possible if someone is determined to accomplish that. Furthermore, in many cases identifiable data are going to be the most useful for research and the most valuable for translating research into practice. He argued that the current rules that exist are not fit for purpose, because they make research very difficult. What is needed, Califf said, is a system that enables researchers to use identifiable data more easily, while at the same time imposing extreme penalties on people who take advantage of this access and misuse the data. He added that health systems already use fully identified data for operations purposes, and if that is done, then the data should perhaps also be available to produce generalizable knowledge that could be spread across health systems and could benefit people beyond those involved in a specific health care operation.

Califf echoed the arguments made by others about the importance of integrating research and care. He noted that PCOR has already made a big difference in this area, but it would make a bigger difference yet to continue this work.

Califf also brought up the challenges associated with patient-reported outcome data collected through cell phones. The use of cell phones is widespread and access to broadband internet is also growing, but these types of data collections do not reach everyone equally. In the case of digital technologies, older people are one group that is likely to be underrepresented, not only because of challenges related to access to cell phones, but also due to more limited skills at using the technology effectively. Califf also echoed challenges associated with the lack of data for a variety of populations more broadly, as discussed in Chapter 2. He highlighted two additional groups that receive relatively little attention: people living in rural areas and those struggling with addictions. There are rising health concerns specific to both of these populations, and therefore there is a need to develop approaches that would address the data limitations associated with these groups.

David Cella, Northwestern University, summarized key data needs as a common data model for patient-reported outcomes; common data elements for patient-reported outcomes; comparative effectiveness metrics across conditions; and medical and nonmedical cost data. He said that despite advances in artificial intelligence and natural language processing, structured data are still useful, in part because they enable comparative effectiveness research not only within conditions, but also across conditions, and they enable a look at overall value for cost. Cella listed insurance deductibles, copayments, caregiver expenses, and work productivity (for example, absenteeism) as the key components of medical and nonmedical cost data needed.

Cella argued that the broadened statutory scope for PCOR opens a major opportunity to examine costs in the context of effectiveness, which has not previously been possible. It also opens the potential for interagency collaboration around cost-effectiveness research and application. These collaborations could include Agency for Healthcare Research and Quality, NIH, CMS, and possibly the U.S. Food and Drug Administration. The broadened statutory scope of PCOR also provides ingredients for a learning health systems approach across provider organizations.

Concerning the questions that cannot be answered with the current PCOR infrastructure, Cella said it continues to be difficult to answer crosscutting comparative effectiveness research questions as they relate to patient-reported outcomes. He echoed earlier points about the difficulty of accessing patient-reported outcomes data, particularly through the Chicago Area Patient-Centered Outcomes Research Network, which is 1 of 13 Clinical Data Research Networks.

Cella mentioned that in 2014 he was part of the PCORnet Patient-Reported Outcomes Common Measures Working Group, which recommended a set of common measures for PCORnet. The recommendations included nine core items for adults, focused on general health, quality of life, physical function (two questions), depression, fatigue, sleep, social roles and activities, and pain. For children, the core items recommended were focused on: general health, quality of life, pain, fatigue, stress, depression, peer relationships, and family relationships. Most of these items are from the Patient-Reported Outcomes Measurement Information System, which provides deep and wide item banks to cover these domains. From each of the domains, the working group selected a single question that would work best, if one could only ask a single question. Cella said that with large networks such as PCORnet, sometimes one question is sufficient to obtain a good estimate for a cohort. The working group's recommendations were not implemented, however, because of technology limitations, such as electronic health records that could not adequately speak to one another and share a common data model overall.

Cella cited a 2019 paper that found that among member organizations of the New England Journal of Medicine Catalyst Insights Council, around 38 percent used the Patient-Reported Outcome Measures System (PROMS) and an additional 17 percent had plans to start using it within 3 years. Cella added that even those who use PROMS capture information on less than 50 percent of patients, often excluding underrepresented minorities and patients with lower educational levels. Most who collect these data do so primarily for operational reasons, to improve their metrics, or to improve their own patients' experience or engagement. And there is still not much outward-facing incentive for doing patient-reported outcome assessments in clinical settings.

Cella listed the following as data-capacity activities that he considers HHS to be best positioned to address:

- promoting technologies to capture patient-provided data, including patient-reported outcome measures;
- promoting patient activation and engagement;
- endorsing health care quality initiatives and patient-reported outcome performance measures; and
- "funding the mandate" or finding other ways of encouraging clinical providers and provider organizations to collect the data.

Giselle Corbie-Smith, University of North Carolina, argued that having incomplete data on race, ethnicity, and other social identities leads to erasures of the experiences of some populations. This lack of data and these erasures diminish the potential of PCOR to advance health equity. The data infrastructure needs to be robust enough to allow data to be disaggregated in ways that can detect differences among small populations. For example, an inability to disaggregate data to compare Filipino health care workers to other Asians and Pacific Islanders could mean missing a disproportionate impact of the COVID-19 pandemic on Filipino nurses and nurses of Filipino descent.

Corbie-Smith said there has been growing momentum to understand the social determinants of health and that some information of this kind is being captured in electronic medical records. However, she added, below that surface there is a need to better understand the role of structural racism, community context, and social drivers of health. There is a need for data on patients' experiences within the health care systems, as well as outside the walls of hospitals and clinics. Specifically, there are limited data on community health resources outside the health care system: the data are either completely missing or, when available, are often dissociated from the health care system. In the case of the COVID-19 pandemic, it became clear that this information is necessary to be able to provide equitable testing resources and equitable vaccine resources.

Corbie-Smith also discussed the critical role of engagement, particularly engagement of patients, community-based organizations, and faith-based organizations, in the case of disasters such as the COVID-19 pandemic. Borrowing a term used by Ralph Ellison in the *Invisible Man*, Corbie-Smith said that the network of community service providers is "unvisible" to health care and public health systems. There is a tendency to think that health is created within the health care system when, in fact, community service providers are often the ones addressing social determinants of health. She also pointed out that there is a crisis around trust in science, and that misinformation is filling the gap. If researchers made their work more accessible to patients, providers, and communities, trust in the work of scientists would likely also increase.

With regard to opportunities, Corbie-Smith referred to "data democratization," which echoed what other speakers said about the need to make the data more widely visible and accessible beyond the research community, and particularly to patients and communities. Beyond obviously benefiting from the use of the data, patients can also help researchers interpret the meaning of data.

Communities can also benefit from the use of data to think about how to effect change around health equity, because it is unreasonable to expect that achieving health equity could happen within the PCOR context alone. Corbie-Smith noted that data visualizations are a helpful tool for democratizing data.

As also discussed by others, collecting more complete data on race and ethnicity is another area that represents an opportunity. This includes avoiding misclassification and collecting data that allow for disaggregation to understand small populations. The data and research also need to reflect the intersection of social identities.

Corbie-Smith emphasized the need for robust stakeholder engagement in defining strategic areas of research. This includes not only stakeholder input on research questions within a particular study, but also input on the overall strategy for PCOR. Stakeholder engagement needs to include communities not commonly reflected or recognized.

Corbie-Smith also highlighted the opportunities presented by including networks of community service providers in the research. These stakeholders include not only federally qualified community health centers but also community service providers that are providing a matrix of care. Keeping these providers visible will lead to a better understanding of the lived experiences of patients, what is important to them, and how they actually can be healthy.

Corbie-Smith also discussed the use of mobile technologies to collect person- and community-level data. While not all of her patients are technologically savvy enough to use telehealth, many of them have smartphones. Smartphones, wearables, and methodologies such as ecological momentary assessment make it possible to understand what is happening with patients outside of the health care context. Combining person-centered data with community-level data makes it possible to understand the interaction between the community, the physical built environment, and the social environments and how that impacts health. Corbie-Smith said that ecological momentary assessment can help provide answers to questions such as the impact of structural racism and interpersonal racism on the health of individuals, particularly in communities that are over-policed.

In terms of analytical opportunities, Corbie-Smith said that there is a need for analyses that reflect the complexities. She said that traditional approaches assume that factors such as food insecurity, housing insecurity, and intimate partner violence are independent of each other. There is also a tendency to assume linearity, instead of recognizing the complexity of the systems in which patients live, work, grow, play, and age. Corbie-Smith also underscored the need for transparency in research and around data democratization in order to demonstrate the trustworthiness of science, which fundamentally is what is needed to move forward.

Scott Ramsey, Fred Hutchinson Institute for Cancer Outcomes Research (HICOR), began by discussing that institute's mission and its Value in Cancer Care initiative, which engages oncology providers, patient partners, payers, health system representatives, and researchers to improve the value and efficiency of cancer care delivery in Washington State. This initiative was formed based on the realization that the rising costs of cancer care and problems with care coordination threaten society's ability to eliminate cancer as a cause of suffering and death.

HICOR's community engagement program shares data about clinic performance and costs across a common population-based data platform. The network includes all of the 28 oncology practices in Washington State, five of the state's major health insurance providers, representatives from local and state government, and a number of patient advocacy groups and patient advocates, including those who represent typically underrepresented minorities.

The database, which is updated on a regular basis throughout the year, includes insurance claims from major payors in the state and is linked to the two cancer registries. The data are used to produce an annual community cancer care report, which documents several oncology quality metrics and the average cost of care for each clinic for specific services. The database also serves as a platform for the oncology community to share best practices, and for a low-cost way to capture outcomes from prospective studies that have started in response to quality issues that were identified from the database and that were prioritized by the stakeholders.

Based on this work, Ramsey shared the lessons learned about key characteristics of databases that can best serve patients. His list included

- comprehensive capture of the patient experience;
- data elements informed by patients and other stakeholders;
- data relevant to treatment decisions;
- ongoing mechanism for direct feedback on patient-identified priorities;
- information that is relevant and accessible; and
- information that is timely.

He noted that in his experience, inadequate accessibility and timeliness have been problems for cancer data for many years.

Ramsey asked whether databases are built from the perspective of a patient or that of a researcher who is trying to adapt the patient perspective. Thinking about the patient as a data consumer is one way to begin to address this issue. When patients seek medical care, they arrive with a particular medical history and a range of social determinants might influence their perspectives. Their neighborhood and their network influence the care available to them, their interest and ability to understand the health system that serves them, their care plan, and the rationale for that plan. Because a subset of patients wants to interrogate the data themselves to understand what they should do, it is important to think about whether a proposed data infrastructure allows understanding of health systems and interrogation in a way that makes sense to patients. Ramsey said he believes that the technology industry is ahead of government agencies in thinking about these issues.

Thinking specifically about cancer care, Ramsey said that based on the literature and based on his own experience working with cancer patients, measures of patient satisfaction do not correlate well with the process measures of care and key outcomes. To address these disparities, there is a need for more granular and relevant measures of patient experience. According to Ramsey, the factors that influence patients' sense of well-being during cancer care, and that are not always addressed by providers, include feeling that they are supported, dealing with uncertainty, perceived loss of autonomy, and trust in the health system.

Ramsey said that in seeking to understand the relationship between treatment and outcomes, the research community sometimes suffers from the well-known "streetlight effect," using only the data that are available. Those data typically focus on what happens in the health care system, whereas, he believes, in many cases the individual's experiences and environment play a bigger role in their care and outcomes.

The social determinants of health are generally not captured in traditional claims and electronic health records databases. However, it is becoming increasingly clear to the cancer care community that social determinants of health may play a bigger role than any other factor in the observed differences in outcomes among cancer patients. Social determinants of health influence patients over a lifetime, but to date little has been done to understand this at a level of specificity that can address policy. The limited data available certainly limit the ability to do this research.

Ramsey also discussed his research on financial toxicity in cancer care, and the emerging picture of vast and lasting impacts on patients' financial well-being, which translates into impact on their well-being in other domains. He argued that there is a need for a data infrastructure that allows researchers to study this problem in other chronic conditions. This would necessitate linking to existing financial databases, such as credit reporting databases, to understand the scale and scope of this problem. He noted that HICOR has been able to link its cancer registry with credit data from Transunion, although accomplishing this took 2 years.

Ramsey argued that HHS does not necessarily need to create new data. Instead, he said, the agency is best positioned to facilitate access to existing data that currently live in the private sector; create regulations that foster interoperability; establish privacy safeguards; and improve timeliness of databases, particularly in areas such as cancer care, which is quickly evolving.

CONCLUSIONS

The final session of the workshop included researchers working in a variety of areas related to patient-centered outcomes. Their input echoed many of the points made by others throughout the workshop. In particular, it is clear that limiting the focus to the person as the patient, as opposed to the person as a whole, limits not only thinking about the data but also the outcomes and impacts that matter to people, both inside their medical relationships when they are patients and, more generally, outside of medical relationships.

CONCLUSION 4-1: Broadening the focus from the patient to the person more generally would enable a more comprehensive approach to the data infrastructure and a better understanding of the outcomes and impacts that matter to people.

The fragmented nature of the data infrastructure and the data silos represents a particular hurdle for researchers. This hurdle could be overcome by a focus on facilitating data linkages, which in turn could increase the usefulness of the information available for research as well as for decision making more broadly.

CONCLUSION 4-2: The data available for patient-centered outcomes research are fragmented across a variety of databases. Expanding data linkages could greatly increase the usefulness of these data for research.

Researchers described a variety of barriers that limit their ability to access the data available in the many existing databases, ranging from databases that can be considered a part of the PCOR data infrastructure to databases owned by private companies. Focusing on facilitating and simplifying access represents an area that could further enhance the usefulness of PCOR data.

CONCLUSION 4-3: Researchers encounter substantial barriers to accessing existing data for patient-centered outcomes research. Facilitating and simplifying data access could further increase the usefulness of data for research.

Researchers echoed the need to make PCOR data more widely available to empower patients and communities to use this information. Efforts to reduce disparities, in particular, cannot be accomplished by research alone.

CONCLUSION 4-4: Making the data more visible and more widely accessible could enable patients and communities to use the information in ways that reduce health disparities, complementing research efforts in this area.

The need for information on the cost of health care and the ways cost factors into care decisions represented another area where researchers echoed the need expressed by other stakeholders for more data.

CONCLUSION 4-5: Data needs related to the total cost of care and a better understanding of cost considerations is an area that deserves more attention.

Appendix A

Biographical Sketches of Committee Members

GEORGE ISHAM (NAM) (*Chair*) is a senior fellow at the HealthPartners Institute and a senior advisor for the Alliance of Community Health Plans. Previously, he served as a senior advisor to the board of directors and the senior management team of HealthPartners, and prior to that, he was HealthPartners' medical director and chief health officer, responsible for quality of care and health and health care improvement. He has been active in health policy, serving as a member of the Centers for Disease Control and Prevention's Task Force on Community Preventive Services, a member of the Agency for Healthcare Research and Quality's United States Preventive Services Task Force, as a founding co-chair of the National Committee for Quality Assurance's committee on performance measurement, and a founding co-chair of the National Quality Forum's Measurement Application Partnership. He has an M.D. from the University of Illinois at Chicago and an M.S. in preventive medicine and administrative medicine from the University of Wisconsin–Madison.

JOHN F.P. BRIDGES is professor and vice chair of academic affairs in the Department of Biomedical Informatics at the Ohio State University (OSU) College of Medicine. He is also a professor in the Department of Surgery and an adjunct professor in both the Division of Epidemiology at the OSU College of Public Health and Department of Health Behavior and Society at the Johns Hopkins Bloomberg School of Public Health. Prior to joining OSU, he was on the faculty of the Johns Hopkins University Bloomberg School of Public Health, the Department of Tropical Hygiene and Public Health within the University of Heidelberg School of Medicine, and the

Department of Epidemiology and Biostatistics within the Case Western Reserve University School of Medicine. He has previously held positions in the Department of Economics at the Weatherhead School of Management at Case Western Reserve University, the National Bureau of Economic Research, Center for Medicine in the Public Interest, and the Center for Health Economics, Research and Evaluation in Australia. He has a Ph.D. in economics from the City University of New York.

JULIE BYNUM is the Margaret Terpenning Professor of Medicine in the Division of Geriatric Medicine and vice chair for faculty affairs in the Department of Internal Medicine at the University of Michigan. She is also a research professor in the Institute of Gerontology, Geriatric Center Associate Director for Health Policy and Research, and a member of the Institute for Healthcare Policy and Innovation. She currently leads a portfolio of National Institutes of Health–funded research that examines the quality of care, diagnosis, and treatment of people with Alzheimer's disease and related dementia in the community, nursing homes, and assisted living and is the director of the Center to Accelerate Population Research in Alzhiemer's. She is currently a member of the National Academies of Sciences, Engineering, and Medicine's Forum on Aging, Disability, and Independence and was a member of a National Academies' workshop planning committee on adverse consequences of cancer treatment. She has an M.P.H. from the Johns Hopkins University School of Hygiene & Public Health and an M.D. from the Johns Hopkins University School of Medicine.

ANGELA DOBES is vice president of the Crohn's & Colitis Foundation's IBD Plexus Program, a research-information exchange platform designed to centralize data and biosamples from diverse research initiatives to advance science, accelerate precision medicine, and transform the care of inflammatory bowel disease patients. Previously, she has worked for clinical technology and pharmaceutical organizations, where she has led implementation of various technology solutions focused on business optimization and accelerating the delivery of new therapies to patients safely. She is currently serving as principal investigator on a study to enhance engagement, research participation, and collaboration through the IBD Partners Patient Powered Research Network. She has an M.A. in public health from the Icahn School of Medicine at Mount Sinai.

OLUWADAMILOLA FAYANJU is the Helen O. Dickens Presidential Associate Professor of Surgery at the Perelman School of Medicine at the University of Pennsylvania. She is also chief of breast surgery at Penn Medicine. Previously, she was associate professor of surgery and population health sciences in the Duke University School of Medicine and director of the

Durham VA Breast Clinic. She was also associate director for Disparities & Value in Healthcare with Duke Forge, Duke University's center for actionable data science. In 2019, she was recognized by the National Academy of Medicine as an Emerging Leader in Health and Medicine Scholar. She received an M.A. in comparative literature from Harvard University and her M.D. and M.P.H.S. from the Washington University in St. Louis.

DEBORAH ESTRIN (NAE/NAM) is a professor of computer science at Cornell Tech where she holds the Robert V. Tishman founder's chair, serves as the associate dean for impact, and is an affiliate faculty at Weill Cornell Medicine. Her research activities include technologies for caregiving, immersive health, small data, participatory sensing, and public interest technology. Estrin was an Amazon Scholar, and before joining Cornell University she was founding director of the National Science Foundation's Center for Embedded Networked Sensing at the University of California, Los Angeles, pioneering the development of mobile and wireless systems to collect and analyze real-time data about the physical world. Estrin cofounded the nonprofit startup, Open mHealth, and has served on several scientific advisory boards for early-stage mobile health startups. She has a Ph.D. in electrical engineering and computer science from the Massachusetts Institute of Technology.

CONSTANTINE GATSONIS is the Henry Ledyard Goddard University Professor of Statistical Sciences, director of statistical sciences, and professor of biostatistics at Brown University. He was founding director of the Center for Statistical Sciences and founding chair of the Department of Biostatistics at Brown University. He is a leading authority on the evaluation of diagnostic and screening tests and has made major contributions to the development of methods for medical technology assessment and health services and outcomes research. He is a world leader in methods for applying and synthesizing evidence on diagnostic tests in medicine and is currently developing methods for comparative effectiveness research in diagnosis and prediction and radiomics. Since 2016, he has served as a statistical consultant for the *New England Journal of* Medicine and was the Founding Editor-in-Chief of *Health Services and Outcomes Research Methods*. He has a Ph.D. in mathematical statistics from Cornell University.

ROBERT GOERGE is a senior research fellow at Chapin Hall at the University of Chicago. He is also a senior fellow and founder of the Master's Degree in Computational Analysis in Public Policy at the University of Chicago Harris School of Public Policy. His research is focused on improving the available data and information on children and families, particularly those who require specialized services related to maltreatment, disability,

poverty, or violence. At Chapin Hall, he is principal investigator for the Family Self-Sufficiency Data Center, the Linking Federal Data to Local Data project, and the National Survey for Early Care and Education. He currently serves on the National Academies of Sciences, Engineering, and Medicine's Committee on National Statistics. He has a Ph.D. in social policy from the University of Chicago.

GEORGE HRIPCSAK (NAM) is the Vivian Beaumont Allen professor and chair of the Department of Biomedical Informatics at Columbia University. He is also the director of medical informatics services for New York Presbyterian Hospital. He is also a board-certified internist. He led the effort to create the Arden Syntax, a language for representing health knowledge that has become a national standard. As chair of the American Medical Informatics Association Standards Committee, he coordinated the medical informatics community response to the Department of Health and Human Services for the health informatics standards rules under the Health Insurance Portability and Accountability Act of 1996. His current research is on the clinical information stored in electronic health records. Using data mining techniques, he is developing the methods necessary to support clinical research and patient safety initiatives. He has an M.D. and an M.S. in biostatistics from Columbia University.

LISA IEZZONI (NAM) is professor of medicine at Harvard Medical School and the Health Policy Research Center at Massachusetts General Hospital, where she served as director in the past. She was previously co-director of research in the Division of General Medicine and Primary Care at Beth Israel Deaconess Medical Center in Boston. Her research focuses on risk adjustment methods for predicting cost and clinical outcomes of care, and on health care experiences and outcomes of persons with disabilities. She has served on the editorial boards of the *Annals of Internal Medicine*, the *Journal of General Internal Medicine, Health Affairs, Medical Care, Health Services Research*, and the *Disability and Health Journal*, among others. She has an M.D. from Harvard Medical School and an M.Sc. from the Harvard T.H. Chan School of Public Health.

S. CLAIBORNE JOHNSTON (NAM) is the inaugural dean of Dell Medical School, vice president for medical affairs, and the Frank and Charmaine Denius Distinguished Dean's Chair in medical leadership at The University of Texas at Austin. Previously, Johnston was associate vice chancellor for research at the University of California, San Francisco (UCSF). He also directed the Clinical and Translational Science Institute and founded the UCSF Center for Healthcare Value. His research is focused on clinical trials and health services research in stroke. He is also an expert in medical education, research administration, health care value, and population health. He has led several large-cohort studies of cerebrovascular disease and three international multicenter randomized trials. He has an M.D. from Harvard Medical School and a Ph.D. in epidemiology from the University of California, Berkeley.

MIGUEL MARINO is an associate professor with joint appointments in the School of Public Health Division of Biostatistics and the Department of Family Medicine at Oregon Health & Science University. His research focuses on the development and implementation of novel statistical methodology to address complexities associated with the use of electronic health records (EHRs) to study changes in policy; using EHRs to study health disparities; validation of EHRs as a reliable source for observational studies; pragmatic randomized trials; and preventive health maintenance. He was selected by the National Academy of Medicine as an Emerging Leader in Health and Medicine Scholar. He has a Ph.D. in biostatistics from Harvard University.

ELIZABETH McGLYNN (NAM) is vice president for Kaiser Permanente Research and executive director for the Center for Effectiveness & Safety Research at Kaiser Permanente. She is also interim senior associate dean for research and scholarships at the Kaiser Permanente Bernard J. Tyson School of Medicine. She is an internationally known expert on methods for evaluating the appropriateness and quality of health care delivery. She has led major initiatives to evaluate health reform options under consideration at the federal and state levels. She is the lead of Kaiser Permanente & Strategic Partners Patient Outcomes Research To Advance Learning (PORTAL) Network. She was a member of the Strategic Framework Board, which provided a blueprint for the National Quality Forum on the development of a national quality measurement and reporting system. She chaired the board of AcademyHealth, served on the board of the American Board of Internal Medicine Foundation, and served on the Board of Providence-Little Company of Mary Hospital Service Area in Southern California. She has a Ph.D. in public policy from RAND Graduate School.

DAVID MELTZER (NAM) is the Fanny L. Pritzker Professor in the Department of Medicine, chief of the section of Hospital Medicine and faculty in the Department of Economics and Harris School of Public Policy at the University of Chicago. He is also director of the Center for Health and the Social Sciences and of the Urban Health Lab at the University of Chicago. His research explores problems in health economics and public policy with a focus on the theoretical foundations of medical cost-effectiveness analysis and the cost and quality of hospital care. Since 1997, he has developed the inpatient general medicine services at the University of Chicago as a Learning Health Care System to produce knowledge on how to improve the care of hospitalized patients, mobilizing the clinical care process to generate and learn from diverse data from electronic health records, claims data, patient interviews, and bio-specimens on more than 100,000 patients. He is the lead of the University of Chicago network site as part of the Chicago Area Patient Centered Outcomes Research Network. He has an M.D. and a Ph.D. in economics from the University of Chicago.

PAUL C. TANG (NAM) is an adjunct professor in the Clinical Excellence Research Center at Stanford University and an internist at the Palo Alto Medical Foundation. He was formerly chief innovation and technology officer at the Palo Alto Medical Foundation and vice president, chief health transformation officer at IBM Watson Health. He has more than 25 years of executive leadership experience in health information technology within medical groups, health systems, and corporate settings. He has directed innovation and technology teams in provider organizations, academic institutions, corporate research organizations, and product development organizations. Most recently, he led the creation, development, deployment, and evaluation of the application of artificial intelligence to physician point-of-care solutions integrated within an electronic health record system. He also led a corporate enterprise-wide design team. He has chaired numerous federal and private-sector advisory and professional association groups related to health information technology and policy. He received an M.S. in electrical engineering from Stanford University and his M.D. from the University of California, San Francisco.

Appendix B

Workshop Agenda

Building Data Capacity for Patient-Centered Outcomes Research: An Agenda for 2021 to 2030

Virtual Workshop 1: Looking Ahead at Data Needs

MAY 3, 2021, 11 AM–5 PM EDT

OBJECTIVES FOR THE WORKSHOP
- Provide a high-level overview of what kind of data are included in the patient-centered outcomes research data infrastructure.
- Identify key questions that stakeholders are most likely to want answered going forward, including general themes that cut across health conditions and circumstances.
- Discuss implications of the broadened statutory scope for PCOR.
- Identify gaps in what stakeholders need and what the infrastructure allows. Consider both limitations in the existing data and improvements that could be made to new data collections (e.g., at point of care or in prospective studies).
- Discuss what questions cannot be answered and who is not served by the current PCOR data infrastructure.
- Discuss what HHS is best positioned to address and how the agency could maximize resources available for the PCOR data infrastructure (representing 4% of the PCOR trust fund), in the context of the HHS public mission, authorities, programs, and data resources.

11:00-11:05 AM EDT	**Goals for the Workshop** GEORGE ISHAM (Committee Chair) HealthPartners Institute
11:05-11:30 AM EDT	**Overview of the Data Infrastructure for Patient-Centered Outcomes Research** Moderator: GEORGE ISHAM BENJAMIN SOMMERS, Deputy Assistant Secretary for Health Policy, ASPE NANCY DE LEW, Associate Deputy Assistant Secretary for Health Policy, ASPE SCOTT R. SMITH, Director, Division of Healthcare Quality and Outcomes, ASPE

11:30 AM-1:00 PM EDT	**PCOR Data Infrastructure Limitations and Opportunities: Disparities and Health Equity Research**
	
	Discussion questions:
	• What are the limitations of the PCOR data infrastructure in terms of:
	   o disparities in the data, including knowledge about patient outcomes, taking into consideration differences in patient preferences and values
	   o challenges associated with using the data to understand disparities and health equity
	   o lack of data on some populations
	• What are opportunities and priorities for enhancing data capacity in this area?
	• What data capacity challenges is HHS best positioned to address in the context of their public mission, authorities, programs, and data resources?
	
	Moderator: OLUWADAMILOLA (LOLA) FAYANJU, Duke University
	
	Speakers:
	
	KAREN JOYNT MADDOX, Washington University in St. Louis

	MEGAN MORRIS, University of Colorado MITCHELL LUNN, Stanford University KALEAB ABEBE, University of Pittsburgh THOMAS SEQUIST, Harvard University and Brigham & Women's Hospital
1:00-1:10 PM EDT	**Break**
1:10-1:30 PM EDT	**PCOR Data Infrastructure Limitations and Opportunities: COVID-19 as Use Case** **Moderator:** PAUL TANG, Palo Alto Medical Foundation and Stanford Clinical Excellence Research Center **Speaker:** DAVID MELTZER, University of Chicago
1:30-2:45 PM EDT	**Patient Perspectives on Data Needs** Discussion questions: • Looking ahead, what are the main data needs? • What are the implications of the (recently broadened) statutory scope for PCOR? • What questions cannot be answered and who is not served by the current PCOR data infrastructure? • What new data sources could be incorporated into the PCOR data infrastructure? • What data capacity challenges is HHS best positioned to address in the context of their public mission, authorities, programs, and data resources? **Moderator:** ANGELA DOBES, Crohn's & Colitis Foundation **Speakers:** REBEKAH ANGOVE, Patient Advocate Foundation GARY EPSTEIN-LUBOW, Brown University ELISABETH OEHRLEIN, National Health Council BRAY PATRICK-LAKE, Evidation Health

2:45-3:05 PM EDT	**Break**
3:05-4:55 PM EDT	**Researcher Perspectives on Data Needs**
	Discussion questions:
	• Looking ahead, what are the main data needs?
	• What are the implications of the (recently broadened) statutory scope for PCOR?
	• What questions cannot be answered and who is not served by the current PCOR data infrastructure?
	• What new data sources could be incorporated into the PCOR data infrastructure?
	• What data capacity challenges is HHS best positioned to address in the context of their public mission, authorities, programs, and data resources?
	Moderator: ELIZABETH MCGLYNN, Kaiser Permanente Research
	Speakers:
	ANDREW BAZEMORE, American Board of Family Medicine
	ROBERT CALIFF, Verily
	DAVID CELLA, Northwestern University
	GISELLE CORBIE-SMITH, University of North Carolina
	SCOTT RAMSEY, Fred Hutch
	KURT STANGE, Case Western Reserve University
4:55-5:00 PM EDT	**Wrap-up**
	GEORGE ISHAM (Committee Chair) HealthPartners Institute

Appendix C

Biographical Sketches of Speakers

KALEAB ABEBE is an associate professor of medicine, biostatistics, and clinical and translational science at the University of Pittsburgh. He also directs the Center for Research on Health Care Data Center as well as the Center for Clinical Trials & Data Coordination. His collaborative research focuses on design, conduct, coordination, and analysis of multicenter randomized controlled trials. Most recently, he led the Data Coordinating Center for the HALT-PKD Network, which comprised two seven-site clinical trials evaluating the impact of hypertensive medications and blood pressure control on the progression of polycystic kidney disease. Additionally, he collaborates with the Adolescent Medicine Division on the design and analysis of cluster randomized trials in sexual violence prevention. In addition to his research collaborations, Abebe is the director of the Clinical Trials Track for the M.S. in Clinical Research at the Institute for Clinical Research Education. He received his B.A. in mathematics from Goshen College and an M.A. and a Ph.D. in statistics from the University of Pittsburgh.

REBEKAH ANGOVE is vice president for patient experience and program evaluation at Patient Advocate Foundation (PAF), where her work is focused on strategically expanding PAF's patient-centered research and program evaluation initiatives. Angove is a health services researcher and leader in patient engagement. She leads efforts to identify patient needs, translate those needs to direct service and policy recommendations, and evaluate the impact of these programs and services on patients and the patient community. In her previous role at the Louisiana Public Health Institute, she served as associate director of health services research and engagement director of

REACHnet, a PCORnet Clinical Data Research Network. Her expertise spans numerous clinical research programs and advisory groups including service on the PCORnet Engagement committee and the Tulane Preventive Medicine Residency Advisory Committee. Angove received her Ph.D. in public and community health from the Medical College of Wisconsin.

ANDREW BAZEMORE (NAM) is the senior vice president of research and policy at the American Board of Family Medicine and also serves as the director of the Robert Graham Center for Policy Studies in Family Medicine. Bazemore helped cultivate the growth and evolution of the Graham Center into an internationally known primary care research center with diverse funding sources. He guided and participated in the Graham Center's research with special interest in access to care for underserved populations, health workforce and training, and spatial analysis. Bazemore also led the Graham Center's emphasis on developing tools that empower primary care providers, leaders, and policy makers. He serves on the faculties of the Departments of Family Medicine at Georgetown University and Virginia Commonwealth University. Bazemore received his M.D. from the University of North Carolina and his M.P.H. from Harvard University School of Public Health.

ROBERT M. CALIFF (NAM) is the head of clinical policy and strategy for Verily and Google Health. Previously, Califf was the vice chancellor for health data science for the Duke University School of Medicine; director of Duke Forge, Duke University's center for health data science; and the Donald F. Fortin, MD, professor of cardiology. He has led major initiatives aimed at improving methods and infrastructure for clinical research, including the Clinical Trials Transformation Initiative, a public-private partnership cofounded by the U.S. Food and Drug Administration (FDA) and Duke University. He also served in the FDA as deputy commissioner for medical products and tobacco from 2015 to 2016 and as commissioner of food and drugs from 2016 to 2017. He is a nationally and internationally recognized leader in cardiovascular medicine, health outcomes research, health care quality, and clinical research, and one of the most frequently cited authors in biomedical science. Califf received his M.D. from the Duke University School of Medicine.

DAVID CELLA (NAM) is Ralph Seal Paffenbarger professor and chair of the Department of Medical Social Sciences, and professor of neurology, pediatrics, preventive medicine (Health and Biomedical Informatics), and psychiatry and behavioral sciences, at Northwestern University. He is also director of the Institute for Public Health and Medicine Center for Patient-Centered Outcomes at Northwestern. Cella plays a leadership role in the development and orchestration of transdisciplinary scientific collaborations and oversees basic and applied social science research to advance the understanding of the mechanisms and measurement of health and disease. Currently he is the multiple principal investigator of the Environmental Children's Health Outcomes Consortium PRO Core grant, and he also leads a health systemwide symptom monitoring and management project under the National Cancer Institute Moonshot Program. A theme of his work has been ensuring that the voice of the patient is reflected in clinical care, research, and policy. A major focus of many of these initiatives has been ensuring that measurement is sensitive and appropriate to diverse populations. Cella received his Ph.D. from Loyola University of Chicago.

GISELLE CORBIE-SMITH (NAM) is a Kenan distinguished professor of the Departments of Social Medicine and Medicine, director of the University of North Carolina (UNC) Center for Health Equity Research in the UNC School of Medicine and associate provost for UNC Rural Initiatives at the UNC at Chapel Hill. She is nationally recognized for her scholarly work on the inclusion of disparity populations in research and is accomplished in drawing communities, faculty, and health care providers into working partnerships in clinical and translational research. Her empirical work, using both qualitative and quantitative methodologies, has focused on the methodological, ethical, and practical issues of research to address racial disparities in health. She is currently the co-principal investigator for the Advancing Change Leadership Clinical Scholars Program. Corbie-Smith currently serves as a multiple principal investigator on the National Institutes of Health/National Institute on Minority Health and Health Disparities–funded RADx-Underserved Populations Coordination and Data Collection Center. Corbie-Smith received her M.Sc. in clinical research from Emory University and her M.D. from the Albert Einstein College of Medicine.

NANCY DE LEW is the associate deputy assistant secretary for health policy in the Office of the Assistant Secretary for Planning and Evaluation at HHS. She leads a team who apply their skills in policy development, strategic planning, research, and evaluation to some of the department's most challenging health policy problems. She provides executive leadership and coordination on a broad range of health care financing, coverage, access, public health, and quality issues. She has worked with Congress on a number of major pieces of legislation over the course of her career including the Affordable Care Act in 2010, the Medicare Modernization Act of 2003, the Balanced Budget Act of 1997, the Health Insurance Portability and Accountability Act of 1996, and the Medicare Catastrophic Coverage Act of 1988. De Lew received her M.A. and M.P.A. in political science and public administration from the University of Illinois at Urbana.

GARY EPSTEIN-LUBOW is an associate professor of psychiatry and human behavior and associate professor of medical science at Alpert Medical School of Brown University. He is also an associate professor of health services, policy and practice at the Brown University School of Public Health. Epstein-Lubow is a geriatric psychiatrist with research, teaching, policy, clinical, and administrative expertise related to geriatric psychiatry patients and family caregiver health, and serves as team leader of the stakeholder engagement team for the National Institute on Aging's Imbedded Pragmatic Alzheimer's Disease and AD-Related Dementias Clinical Trials Collaboratory. He is also an associate director of the Centers for Disease Control and Prevention BOLD Public Health Center of Excellence for Dementia Caregiving. He earned his M.D. from the Ohio State University's College of Medicine and Public Health; he completed his general psychiatry residency, geriatric psychiatry fellowship, and postdoctoral research at Brown University and Butler Hospital.

KAREN E. JOYNT MADDOX is a practicing cardiologist at Barnes-Jewish Hospital and an assistant professor at the Washington University School of Medicine and School of Social Work, as well as a health policy advisor for BJC Healthcare. Her research interests include (1) improving the measurement of the quality and efficiency of physicians, hospitals, and health systems; (2) understanding the impact of policy interventions on health care, with a focus on value-based and alternative payment models; and (3) reducing disparities in care, with a focus on vulnerable populations including racial and ethnic minorities, individuals living in poverty, individuals with disabilities, frail elders, and those in rural areas. Joynt Maddox received her A.B. in public policy from the Woodrow Wilson School at Princeton University and her M.D. from the Duke University School of Medicine. She trained in internal medicine at Duke University Medical Center and in cardiovascular medicine at Brigham and Women's Hospital. She also completed a research fellowship in health policy at the Harvard School of Public Health, from which she received her M.P.H.

MITCHELL (MITCH) R. LUNN is an assistant professor in the Division of Nephrology of the Department of Medicine at the Stanford University School of Medicine. As an internist and nephrologist with a strong interest in technology and sexual and gender minority (SGM) health, his research is designed to characterize the health and well-being of these populations. Through the use of existing and emerging technologies, Lunn focuses on improving understanding of the factors that positively and negatively influence SGM health including research on SGM health disparities, SGM societal experiences (in and out of health care), provider education about SGM health, and institutional climate toward SGM people. He is the codirector of PRIDEnet, a participant-powered research network of SGM people that engages SGM communities at all stages of the biomedical research process: research question generation and prioritization, study design, recruitment, participation, data analysis, and results dissemination. He is also the codirector of The PRIDE Study, a national, online, prospective, longitudinal general health cohort study. He earned his M.D. from the Stanford University School of Medicine and his M.A.S. in clinical research from the University of California, San Francisco (UCSF). He completed internal medicine internship and residency training at Brigham and Women's Hospital and nephrology fellowship at UCSF.

DAVID O. MELTZER (NAM) is the Fanny L. Pritzker Professor in the Department of Medicine, chief of the section of Hospital Medicine and faculty in the Department of Economics and Harris School of Public Policy at the University of Chicago. He is also director of the Center for Health and the Social Sciences and of the Urban Health Lab at the University of Chicago. His research explores problems in health economics and public policy with a focus on the theoretical foundations of medical cost-effectiveness analysis and the cost and quality of hospital care. Since 1997, he has developed the inpatient general medicine services at the University of Chicago as a Learning Health Care System to produce knowledge on how to improve the care of hospitalized patients, mobilizing the clinical care process to generate and learn from diverse data from electronic health records, claims data, patient interviews, and bio-specimens on more than 100,000 patients. He is the lead of the University of Chicago network site as part of the Chicago Area Patient Centered Outcomes Research Network. He has an M.D. and a Ph.D. in economics from the University of Chicago.

MEGAN MORRIS is an associate professor in the Division of General Internal Medicine at the University of Colorado, Anschutz Medical Campus, and she is the founder/director of the Learning Collaborative to Address Disability Equity in Healthcare, a national consortium of health care organizations working toward advancing equitable health care for patients with disabilities. Morris researches disparities in care experienced by persons with disabilities, with a focus on provider and health care organization-level factors that negatively impact the quality of care delivered to patients with disabilities. Using qualitative and mixed methods, she has led multiple studies in the area, including studies examining providers' implicit disability bias and a Patient-Centered Outcomes Research Institute-funded trial comparing methods to improve the quality of communication between patients with disabilities and their health care team. Morris received her M.S. in speech-language pathology, her M.P.H. in health systems and policy, and her Ph.D. in rehabilitation science from the University of Washington.

ELISABETH M. OEHRLEIN is assistant vice president, Research and Programs at the National Health Council (NHC). In this role, she crafts the NHC's annual research and programmatic agenda in service to the organization's mission and leads the NHC's research and programmatic work on value, real-world evidence, and patient engagement. She is a mixed-methods researcher with expertise in epidemiologic, qualitative, and patient-engagement methods, as well as patient-focused medical product development. Her research interests include developing new methods for applying patient-provided information when developing real-world evidence to ensure studies reflect the "real world" as closely as possible, as well as developing new methods for patient-journey mapping. Oehrlein holds an M.S. in epidemiology from the University of Maryland School of Medicine's Department of Epidemiology and Human Genetics, and a Ph.D. in pharmaceutical health services research with a concentration in comparative effectiveness research/patient-centered outcomes research from the University of Maryland School of Pharmacy.

BRAY PATRICK-LAKE is senior director of Strategic Partnerships at Evidation Health, where she develops collaborations to support the design and implementation of participant-centered studies and the regulatory and clinical acceptance of digital measures. She serves on the Digital Medicine Society's Scientific Leadership Board, Reagan Udall Foundation's IMEDS Steering Committee, and American College of Cardiology's National Cardiovascular Data Registry Oversight Board. Previously, she was a member of the *All of Us* National Advisory Panel, member of the National Academies of Sciences, Engineering, and Medicine Health Science Policy Board, and director of Stakeholder Engagement for the Clinical Trials Transformation Initiative (CTTI) at Duke University, where her work involved actively engaging patient advocacy organizations and other stakeholders in the CTTI's efforts to improve clinical trials. She holds a B.S. from the University of Georgia and an M.F.S. from National University.

SCOTT RAMSEY is a physician, cancer researcher, and health economist. He codirects the Hutchinson Institute for Cancer Outcomes Research, or HICOR at Fred Hutch. The institute aims to reduce the economic and human burden of cancer by improving the efficiency and effectiveness of cancer care. Ramsey's research focuses on cancer outcomes, health care delivery, and economic evaluations of new and existing cancer screening and treatment technologies. He also explores methods for engaging a diverse range of stakeholders to help inform how research studies are prioritized and designed. He designs and conducts studies that weigh the costs and benefits of various treatment and screening approaches. Ramsey received his M.D. from the University of Iowa, College of Medicine, and his Ph.D. from the University of Pennsylvania, Wharton School.

THOMAS SEQUIST is the chief patient experience and equity officer at Mass General Brigham. In this role, he leads systemwide strategies for improving patient experience and health care equity, while also overseeing quality and safety. He is a practicing general internist at Brigham and Women's Hospital and is a professor of medicine and professor of health care policy at Harvard Medical School. Sequist's research interests include ambulatory quality measurement and improvement, with a focus on patient and provider education, and the innovative use of health information technology. He is particularly interested in health policy issues affecting care for Native Americans and has worked collaboratively with the Indian Health Service to evaluate the provision of care for this population. He is a member of the Taos Pueblo tribe in New Mexico and is committed to improving Native American health care, serving as director of the Four Directions Summer Research Program at Harvard Medical School and the medical director of the Brigham and Women's Hospital Physician Outreach Program with the Indian Health Service. He graduated from Cornell University with a B.S. in chemical engineering. He received his M.D. from Harvard Medical School and an M.P.H. from the Harvard School of Public Health.

SCOTT R. SMITH is director of the Division of Health Care Quality and Outcomes in the Office of the Assistant Secretary for Planning and Evaluation. His division conducts research on how health policies influence health care quality and outcomes in state and federal programs. In addition, the division is responsible for managing the patient-centered outcomes research data infrastructure portfolio across HHS. His interests are studying quality metrics in Medicare and Medicaid, building national data capacity for conducting patient-centered outcomes research, strengthening research programs, and facilitating support for a learning health care system. He has directed research programs on comparative effectiveness and pharmaceutical outcomes at the Agency for Healthcare Research and Quality and was a member of the tenured faculty at the University of North Carolina at Chapel Hill. He received an M.S.P.H. from the University of Illinois at Urbana-Champaign and a Ph.D. from the University of Michigan.

BENJAMIN SOMMERS (NAM) was appointed the deputy assistant secretary for health policy in the Office of the Assistant Secretary for Planning and Evaluation (ASPE). Before joining ASPE, he was the Huntley Quelch Professor of Health Care Economics at the Harvard School of Public Health and professor of medicine at the Harvard Medical School and Brigham & Women's Hospital. He is a health economist and primary care physician whose main research interests are health policy for vulnerable populations and the health care safety net. He has received numerous awards including the Health Services Research Impact Award and the Article-of-the-Year Award from Academy Health, and the Outstanding Junior Investigator Award from the Society of General Internal Medicine. His research has been published in the *New England Journal of Medicine*, *Journal of the American Medical Association*, *Journal of Health Economics*, and *Health Affairs*, and covered by *The New York Times*, *Wall Street Journal*, and *Washington Post*. He received both his Ph.D. in health policy and his M.D. from Harvard University.

KURT C. STANGE (NAM) is distinguished university professor, Dorothy Jones Weatherhead professor of medicine, and professor in the Departments of Family Medicine and Community Health, Population and Quantitative Health Sciences, and Sociology at the Case Western Reserve University, where he serves as director of the Center for Community Health Integration. He is a family and public health physician, practicing at Neighborhood Family Practice, a federally qualified community health center in Cleveland, Ohio. Stange is active in practice-based, multimethod, participatory research and development that aims to understand and improve primary health care and community health. He uses complexity science to guide and interpret integrated qualitative and quantitative research, and has been working on participatory methods to advance community health and to develop computational models of primary health care and patient-centered, population health and equity outcomes. He has been locally active in the COVID-19 pandemic response and produced a report on the lessons of the pandemic for the National Academies' report *Implementing High-Quality Primary Care: Rebuilding the Foundation of Health Care*. He is an American Cancer Society clinical research professor and a scholar of the Institute for Integrative Health. Stange received his M.D. from Albany Medical College and his Ph.D. from the University of North Carolina School of Public Health.

Appendix C

Building Data Capacity for Patient-Centered Outcomes Research: Interim Report 2– Data Standards, Methods, and Policy

(Full text of the committee's second interim report released on October 27, 2021.)[1]

---

[1] https://www.nap.edu/catalog/26298/building-data-capacity-for-patient-centered-outcomes-research-interim-report.

# Building Data Capacity for Patient-Centered Outcomes Research

INTERIM REPORT 2–
Data Standards, Methods, and Policy

Committee on Building Data Capacity for
Patient-Centered Outcomes Research:
An Agenda for 2021 to 2030

Committee on National Statistics
Division of Behavioral and Social Sciences and Education

Board on Health Care Services
Health and Medicine Division

Computer Science and Telecommunications Board
Division on Engineering and Physical Sciences

A Consensus Study Report of

The National Academies of
SCIENCES · ENGINEERING · MEDICINE

THE NATIONAL ACADEMIES PRESS
Washington, DC
www.nap.edu

THE NATIONAL ACADEMIES PRESS   500 Fifth Street, NW   Washington, DC 20001

This activity was supported by a contract between the National Academy of Sciences and the U.S. Department of Health and Human Services (award #HHSP233201400020B/75P00120F37102). Any opinions, findings, conclusions, or recommendations expressed in this publication do not necessarily reflect the views of any organization or agency that provided support for the project.

International Standard Book Number-13: 978-0-309-27262-9
International Standard Book Number-10: 0-309-27262-9
Digital Object Identifier: https://doi.org/10.17226/26298

Additional copies of this publication are available from the National Academies Press, 500 Fifth Street, NW, Keck 360, Washington, DC 20001; (800) 624-6242 or (202) 334-3313; http://www.nap.edu.

Copyright 2022 by the National Academy of Sciences. All rights reserved.

Printed in the United States of America

Suggested citation: National Academies of Sciences, Engineering, and Medicine. (2022). *Building Data Capacity for Patient-Centered Outcomes Research: Interim Report 2—Data Standards, Methods, and Policy.* Washington, DC: The National Academies Press. https://doi.org/10.17226/26298.

The National Academies of
SCIENCES · ENGINEERING · MEDICINE

The **National Academy of Sciences** was established in 1863 by an Act of Congress, signed by President Lincoln, as a private, nongovernmental institution to advise the nation on issues related to science and technology. Members are elected by their peers for outstanding contributions to research. Dr. Marcia McNutt is president.

The **National Academy of Engineering** was established in 1964 under the charter of the National Academy of Sciences to bring the practices of engineering to advising the nation. Members are elected by their peers for extraordinary contributions to engineering. Dr. John L. Anderson is president.

The **National Academy of Medicine** (formerly the Institute of Medicine) was established in 1970 under the charter of the National Academy of Sciences to advise the nation on medical and health issues. Members are elected by their peers for distinguished contributions to medicine and health. Dr. Victor J. Dzau is president.

The three Academies work together as the **National Academies of Sciences, Engineering, and Medicine** to provide independent, objective analysis and advice to the nation and conduct other activities to solve complex problems and inform public policy decisions. The National Academies also encourage education and research, recognize outstanding contributions to knowledge, and increase public understanding in matters of science, engineering, and medicine.

Learn more about the National Academies of Sciences, Engineering, and Medicine at **www.nationalacademies.org**.

The National Academies of
SCIENCES • ENGINEERING • MEDICINE

Consensus Study Reports published by the National Academies of Sciences, Engineering, and Medicine document the evidence-based consensus on the study's statement of task by an authoring committee of experts. Reports typically include findings, conclusions, and recommendations based on information gathered by the committee and the committee's deliberations. Each report has been subjected to a rigorous and independent peer-review process and it represents the position of the National Academies on the statement of task.

Proceedings published by the National Academies of Sciences, Engineering, and Medicine chronicle the presentations and discussions at a workshop, symposium, or other event convened by the National Academies. The statements and opinions contained in proceedings are those of the participants and are not endorsed by other participants, the planning committee, or the National Academies.

For information about other products and activities of the National Academies, please visit www.nationalacademies.org/about/whatwedo.

COMMITTEE ON BUILDING DATA CAPACITY FOR PATIENT-CENTERED OUTCOMES RESEARCH: AN AGENDA FOR 2021 TO 2030

GEORGE ISHAM (*Chair*), HealthPartners Institute
JOHN F.P. BRIDGES, The Ohio State University
JULIE BYNUM, University of Michigan
ANGELA DOBES, IBD Plexus, Crohn's & Colitis Foundation
DEBORAH ESTRIN, Cornell Tech
OLUWADAMILOLA FAYANJU, University of Pennsylvania
CONSTANTINE GATSONIS, Brown University
ROBERT GOERGE, Chapin Hall, University of Chicago
GEORGE HRIPCSAK, Columbia University
LISA IEZZONI, Massachusetts General Hospital
S. CLAIBORNE JOHNSTON, The University of Texas at Austin
MIGUEL MARINO, Oregon Health & Science University
ELIZABETH McGLYNN, Kaiser Permanente
DAVID MELTZER, University of Chicago
PAUL TANG, Stanford University and Palo Alto Medical Foundation

KRISZTINA MARTON, *Study Director*
CRYSTAL BELL, *Associate Program Officer*
RUTH COOPER, *Associate Program Officer*
MARY GHITELMAN, *Senior Program Assistant*
BRIAN HARRIS-KOJETIN, *Director, Committee on National Statistics*
SHARYL NASS, *Director, Board on Health Care Services*
JON EISENBERG, *Director, Computer Science and Telecommunications Board*

SAUL RIVAS, *National Academy of Medicine Fellow*, University of Texas Rio Grande Valley

COMMITTEE ON NATIONAL STATISTICS

ROBERT M. GROVES (*Chair*), Georgetown University
ANNE C. CASE, Princeton University
MICK P. COUPER, University of Michigan
JANET M. CURRIE, Princeton University
DIANA FARRELL, JPMorgan Chase Institute
ROBERT GOERGE, Chapin Hall at the University of Chicago
ERICA L. GROSHEN, Cornell University
HILARY HOYNES, University of California, Berkeley
DANIEL KIFER, The Pennsylvania State University
SHARON LOHR, Arizona State University, emerita
JEROME P. REITER, Duke University
JUDITH A. SELTZER, University of California, Los Angeles
C. MATTHEW SNIPP, Stanford University
ELIZABETH A. STUART, Johns Hopkins University
JEANETTE WING, Columbia University

BRIAN A. HARRIS-KOJETIN, *Director*
CONSTANCE F. CITRO, *Senior Scholar*

BOARD ON HEALTH CARE SERVICES

DAVID BLUMENTHAL (*Chair*), The Commonwealth Fund
ANDREW BINDMAN, Kaiser Foundation Health Plan, Inc.
NIRANJAN BOSE, Gates Ventures
MELINDA J. BEEUWKES BUNTIN, Vanderbilt University School of Medicine
NEIL S. CALMAN, The Institute for Family Health
PAUL CHUNG, Kaiser Permanente School of Medicine
PATRICIA M. DAVIDSON, Johns Hopkins University School of Nursing
MARTHA DAVIGLUS, University of Illinois at Chicago
JENNIFER E. DeVOE, Oregon Health & Science University
R. ADAMS DUDLEY, University of Minnesota
RICHARD G. FRANK, Harvard Medical School
TERRY FULMER, John A. Hartford Foundation
CINDY GILLESPIE, Arkansas Department of Human Services
ELMER HUERTA, The George Washington University Cancer Center
SHARON INOUYE, Harvard Medical School
JOHN LUMPKIN, BlueCross BlueShield of North Carolina Foundation
FAITH MITCHELL, The Urban Institute
DAVID B. PRYOR, Ascension Health
TRISH RILEY, National Academy for State Health Policy
WILLIAM SAGE, The University of Texas at Austin
HARDEEP SINGH, Baylor College of Medicine

SHARYL NASS, *Director*

COMPUTER SCIENCE AND TELECOMMUNICATIONS BOARD

LAURA HAAS (*Chair*), University of Massachusetts Amherst
DAVID CULLER, University of California, Berkeley
ERIC HORVITZ, Microsoft Corporation
CHARLES ISBELL, Georgia Institute of Technology
BETH MYNATT, Georgia Institute of Technology
CRAIG PARTRIDGE, Colorado State University
DANIELA RUS, Massachusetts Institute of Technology
FRED B. SCHNEIDER, Cornell University
MARGO SELTZER, The University of British Columbia
NAMBIRAJAN SESHADRI, University of California, San Diego
MOSHE VARDI, Rice University

JON EISENBERG, *Senior Board Director*

Acknowledgments

This Consensus Study Report was reviewed in draft form by individuals chosen for their diverse perspectives and technical expertise. The purpose of this independent review is to provide candid and critical comments that will assist the National Academies of Sciences, Engineering, and Medicine in making each published report as sound as possible and to ensure that it meets the institutional standards for quality, objectivity, evidence, and responsiveness to the study charge. The review comments and draft manuscript remain confidential to protect the integrity of the deliberative process.

We thank the following individuals for their review of this report: Rebecca A. Hubbard, Department of Biostatistics, Epidemiology and Informatics, Perelman School of Medicine, University of Pennsylvania; Sue Jinks-Robertson, Department of Molecular Genetics and Microbiology, Duke University; Harold Lehman, Division of General Internal Medicine, Department of Medicine, Johns Hopkins University School of Medicine; Vincent X. Liu, Division of Research, Kaiser Permanente; Keith Marsolo, Population Health Sciences, Duke University School of Medicine; Emily O'Brien, Department of Population Health Sciences, Duke Clinical Research Institute, Duke University School of Medicine; and Jerome Reiter, Department of Statistical Science, Duke University.

Although the reviewers listed above provided many constructive comments and suggestions, they were not asked to endorse the conclusions of this report, nor did they see the final draft before its release. The review of this report was overseen by Andrew B. Bindman, Chief Medical Officer, Kaiser Foundation Health Plan and Hospitals, and Alicia L. Carriquiry, Department of Statistics, Iowa State University. They were responsible for making certain that an independent examination of this report was carried out in accordance with the standards of the National Academies and that all review comments were carefully considered. Responsibility for the final content rests entirely with the authoring committee and the National Academies.

Contents

Summary 1
1 Introduction 7
2 Patient-Centered Outcomes Research Data Standards 17
3 Methods for Patient-Centered Outcomes Research 33
4 Data Policies and Other Data Infrastructure Considerations 45

Appendixes

A Biographical Sketches of Committee Members 55
B Workshop Agenda 61
C Biographical Sketches of Workshop Speakers 65

Boxes and Figures

BOXES

1-1 Key Data Infrastructure Functionalities in the Existing Strategic Framework for Patient-Centered Outcomes Research, 12
1-2 Building Blocks of the Patient-Centered Outcomes Research Data Infrastructure, 13
1-3 Statement of Task for the Overall Study, 15

2-1 A Perspective on Data Required for Patient-Centered Outcomes Research and Standards to Consider, 23

FIGURES

1-1 Patient-Centered Outcomes Research Trust Fund: Three streams of work and funding, 9
1-2 ASPE's strategic framework for the patient-centered outcomes research data infrastructure, 11

2-1 Clinical language engineering workbench: Key functionalities in the natural language processing machine learning process, 27

3-1 A patient timeline view of data, 34

Summary

The Office of the Assistant Secretary for Planning and Evaluation (ASPE), in partnership with other agencies and divisions of the U.S. Department of Health and Human Services (HHS), coordinates a portfolio of projects that build data capacity for conducting patient-centered outcomes research (PCOR). PCOR focuses on producing scientific evidence on the effectiveness of prevention and treatment options to inform the health care decisions of patients, families, and health care providers, taking into consideration the preferences, values, and questions patients face when making health care choices. The data infrastructure includes data sources and functionalities that support the research. Major building blocks are the services, standards, policies, and governance that enable the use of the data.

ASPE asked the National Academies of Sciences, Engineering, and Medicine to appoint a consensus study committee to identify issues critical to the continued development of the data infrastructure for PCOR. The committee's work will contribute to ASPE's development of a strategic plan that will guide their work related to PCOR data capacity over the next decade.

As part of its information-gathering activities, the committee organized three workshops to collect input from stakeholders on the PCOR data infrastructure, which includes a variety of types of data, such as clinical data, research data, administrative data from payer records, and patient-provided data. This report, the second in a series of three interim reports, summarizes the discussion and committee conclusions from the second workshop, which focused on data standards, methods, and policies that could make the PCOR data infrastructure more useful in the years ahead.

Participants in the workshop included researchers and policy experts working in these areas. The first report in the series centered on emerging data needs.[1] The third report will discuss research and data collaborations.

The conclusions included in this interim report are based primarily on the input collected as part of the workshop, background documentation received from ASPE and other public sources, and the committee members' synthesis and expert judgment regarding the input received. As an interim report based on one in a series of information-gathering activities, the scope of this report is narrowly focused on a subset of key topics relevant to the committee's charge. The conclusions reached by the committee are, at this stage, fairly high level. After completing all of its information-gathering activities, which include but are not limited to the three workshops, the committee will also issue a final report, containing the study's overall findings and conclusions.

DATA STANDARDS

Part of the workshop discussed in this report focused on standards for PCOR. Standards are increasingly widely used for a variety of purposes, including collecting, storing, analyzing, and exchanging data. One theme that emerged from the workshop was that these standards are most useful when they are focused on addressing a specific problem or are driven by the specific value they can contribute. The needs and norms evolve over time, and because of this, standards need to evolve too. The workshop also identified some key areas where ASPE's role is particularly important.

> **CONCLUSION 2-1:** Standards are most useful when their development is driven by their potential uses and a clear concept of the value they can contribute.
>
> **CONCLUSION 2-2:** The Office of the Assistant Secretary for Planning and Evaluation could add significant value in the area of standards for patient-centered outcomes research by
>
> - continuing to promote the development of a data infrastructure and an implementation strategy that facilitates the use of standards and access to the data;
> - convening stakeholder meetings to enhance communication and work toward developing a common language for standards;

---

[1] https://www.nap.edu/catalog/26297/building-data-capacity-for-patient-centered-outcomes-research-interim-report.

- facilitating accessibility to the data and collaborations with existing organizations working in this area; and
- leading efforts to catalogue and exemplify data standards and analytic standards.

CONCLUSION 2-3: While data standards are important to conducting patient-centered outcomes research, applying standards to the analytic methods as well is important to facilitate the reliability and reproducibility of study results.

Learning from the work on standards happening across the globe would further advance PCOR.

CONCLUSION 2-4: An international perspective is an important consideration for the patient-centered outcomes research data infrastructure, and the infrastructure focused on standards specifically would benefit from building on work that happens internationally.

METHODS

A promising area of research focuses on better understanding the longitudinal, holistic experiences of people across time and different settings, which requires matching records across databases. To balance these opportunities and concerns, it would be useful to develop a carefully thought-out strategy for linking data from a variety of sources, and to focus on strengthening the data infrastructure in additional ways that would enable longitudinal research that provides a comprehensive understanding of people's experiences over their life course.

CONCLUSION 3-1: The ability to adopt a longitudinal, comprehensive perspective of an individual's journey could open new opportunities for patient-centered outcomes research. The shift could be facilitated by focusing on efforts to

- simplify integration of data across the research data ecosystem;
- address challenges posed by the limitations associated with health identifiers;
- incorporate person-generated data into health data systems; and
- leverage real-world data to expand the timeline view of a person's health-related experiences.

There is also a need for transparency and the continued refinement of best practices related to how data and methods are used. This is especially important for emerging data sources and methods that capture more lifestyle and behavioral information than traditional clinical measurements, as well as the application of artificial intelligence methods, which could have biases confounded by patterns associated with new technologies. These considerations are also important for the use of observational data.

> **CONCLUSION 3-2:** Observing scientific best practices, including those of transparency and ethical use of data, is essential to generate trust in patient-centered outcomes research among all stakeholders, including the public and researchers. This is important both for observational data and for emerging data sources and methods.

The workshop highlighted the importance of interpreting best practices in the dissemination of research broadly, to include not only sharing results but also making available other resources and components associated with the research process, such as the software developed for the analyses.

> **CONCLUSION 3-3:** The results of patient-centered outcomes research (and research in general) are only replicable and are most useful when the underlying data and comprehensive research documentation (such as analytic code) are made available for use by others.

DATA POLICY AND OTHER DATA INFRASTRUCTURE CONSIDERATIONS

A theme that emerged from the workshop was the need to involve the people and communities whose data are being used in decisions about the data collection and data use throughout the entire research lifecycle. This is essential for building trust, which increases willingness to participate and, in turn, the likelihood that the data that are obtained will be complete, reliable, representative, and relevant to diverse stakeholders. This is particularly important for data on social determinants of health.

> **CONCLUSION 4-1:** Building and maintaining trust among the people and communities whose data are being sought for research is essential for high-quality data. Including representatives of consumers and patients in the research process to understand how to measure health impacts that matter to individuals is an important component in building trust.

The existing laws and regulations that govern the use of data for research, including the Health Insurance Portability and Accountability Act of

1996, are outdated and would benefit from a critical review and updating to facilitate PCOR while preventing misuses of the data.

CONCLUSION 4-2: This is an opportune time to revisit and update the legislation and rules governing data privacy and the sharing of data for research.

1

Introduction

The Office of the Assistant Secretary for Planning and Evaluation (ASPE), in partnership with other agencies and divisions of the U.S. Department of Health and Human Services (HHS), coordinates a portfolio of projects that build data capacity for conducting patient-centered outcomes research (PCOR). The PCOR data infrastructure provides decision makers with objective, scientific evidence on the effectiveness of treatments, services, and other interventions used in health care. This research is frequently focused on analyzing existing data to address questions and provide objective information for the purpose of informing real-world health care decisions.

BACKGROUND

The legal framework that established funding for research on the outcomes and effectiveness of treatments and health care interventions dates back to the 2003 Medicare Prescription Drug, Improvement, and Modernization Act. This act provided authorization for the Agency for Healthcare Research and Quality (AHRQ) to support research comparing the outcomes and effectiveness of treatments and clinical approaches and to disseminate the findings from this research. In 2009, the American Recovery and Reinvestment Act provided additional funding to AHRQ, the National Institutes of Health, and HHS for research that compares the effectiveness of medical options. In 2010, the Patient Protection and Affordable Care Act provided further authorization for research that assists patients, clinicians, purchasers, and policy makers in making informed health decisions.

To facilitate PCOR, in 2010 Congress established the Patient-Centered Outcomes Research Trust Fund (PCOR Trust Fund) with the U.S. Department of the Treasury. The goals of the PCOR Trust Fund are to fund PCOR research, disseminate research findings, and develop a data infrastructure for PCOR. The PCOR Trust Fund has been reauthorized through 2029, through H.R.1865 of the Further Consolidated Appropriations Act of 2020. The most recent statute specified intellectual and developmental disabilities, as well as maternal mortality, as research priorities. The statute also called for PCOR studies to include consideration of the full range of outcomes data. Specifically, the law states that:

> Research shall be designed, as appropriate, to take into account and capture the full range of clinical and patient-centered outcomes relevant to, and that meet the needs of, patients, clinicians, purchasers, and policymakers in making informed health decisions. In addition to the relative health outcomes and clinical effectiveness, clinical and patient-centered outcomes shall include the potential burdens and economic impacts of the utilization of medical treatments, items, and services on different stakeholders and decision-makers respectively. These potential burdens and economic impacts include medical out-of-pocket costs, including health plan benefit and formulary design, non-medical costs to the patient and family, including caregiving, effects on future costs of care, workplace productivity and absenteeism, and healthcare utilization.[1]

The bulk of the PCOR Trust Fund funding (80%) is allocated for research and is made available through the Patient-Centered Outcomes Research Institute (PCORI), a nongovernmental organization established by Congress for this purpose. Approximately 16 percent of the PCOR Trust Fund funding is set aside for disseminating research findings, incorporating findings into clinical practice, and training researchers in PCOR. The agency overseeing this work is AHRQ.

The remaining funding, which constitutes 4 percent of the PCOR Trust Fund, is allocated for building data capacity for PCOR and is overseen by ASPE. Specifically, Section 937(f) of the Public Health Service Act instructed the Secretary of HHS to:

> … provide for the coordination of relevant Federal health programs to build data capacity for comparative clinical effectiveness research, including the development and use of clinical registries and health outcomes research networks, in order to develop and maintain a comprehensive, interoperable data network to collect, link, and analyze data on outcomes and effectiveness from multiple sources including electronic health records.[2]

---

[1] https://www.ssa.gov/OP_Home/ssact/title11/1181.htm.
[2] https://aspe.hhs.gov/collaborations-committees-advisory-groups/os-pcortf/about-os-pcortf.

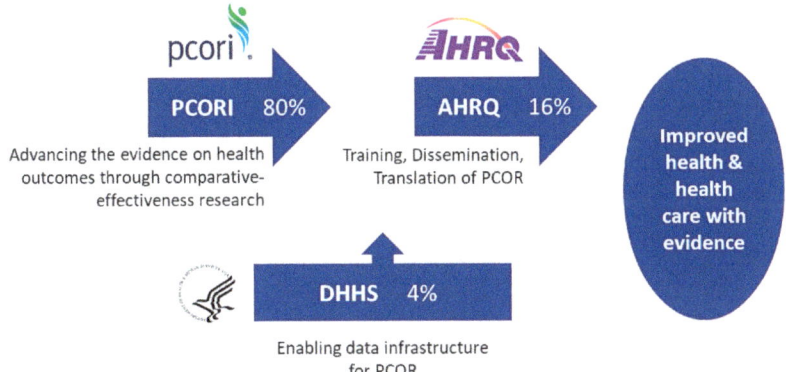

FIGURE 1-1 Patient-Centered Outcomes Research Trust Fund: Three streams of work and funding.
NOTE: AHRQ = Agency for Healthcare Research and Quality; DHHS = U.S. Department of Health and Human Services; PCOR = patient-centered outcomes research; PCORI = Patient-Centered Outcomes Research Institute.
SOURCE: Workshop presentation by ASPE, May 3, 2021.

Figure 1-1 shows how the PCOR funding and work is allocated across the three entities. This National Academies of Sciences, Engineering, and Medicine study is focused on issues relevant to ASPE's continued work on the PCOR data infrastructure, in other words, on the priorities for the use of the 4 percent of the funding that is allocated to HHS for work related to the data infrastructure for PCOR.

As the coordinating agency for the data infrastructure investment portfolio across HHS agencies, ASPE guides the PCOR data infrastructure's strategic framework and vision, sets funding priorities, and coordinates interagency workgroups. ASPE's work is assisted by a Leadership Council for the PCOR Trust Fund, which includes representatives from other HHS agencies, including the Administration for Children and Families, the Administration for Community Living, the Assistant Secretary for Preparedness and Response, AHRQ, the Centers for Disease Control and Prevention (CDC), the Centers for Medicare & Medicaid Services, the U.S. Food and Drug Administration (FDA), the Health Resources and Services Administration, the Indian Health Service, the National Institutes of Health, the Office of the Chief Technology Officer, the Office of the National Coordinator for Health Information Technology, and the Substance Abuse and Mental Health Services Administration. The Leadership Council provides input on priorities for the portfolio, including projects to fund. During the period

2010 to 2019, the PCOR Trust Fund funded 53 projects, which translated to 76 agency awards, totaling approximately $131 million.

Figure 1-2 is a visual representation of ASPE's current framework for the PCOR data infrastructure. The bottom row shows the main data sources feeding into the PCOR infrastructure. Data collected as part of clinical care include data collected for health care delivery and for billing purposes. Examples of primary data collected as part of research studies include data from clinical trials and national health surveys. Other examples of data sources include Medicare or Medicaid claims data; quality or outcomes data collected by health care providers for the purposes of improving health care value; FDA data on the safety of medications and medical devices; and CDC data on births and deaths provided by state public health authorities.

The framework describes the relationship between the data sources and the current key functionalities and focus areas (middle row) that support the research. The key functionalities are described in further detail in Box 1-1. Major building blocks are the services, standards, policies, and governance that enable the use of the data for research, described in further detail in Box 1-2. The top row shows the key data users and contributors of data. A more detailed overview of ASPE's work and the projects funded to date will be included in the final report, at the conclusion of the committee's review.

APPENDIX C

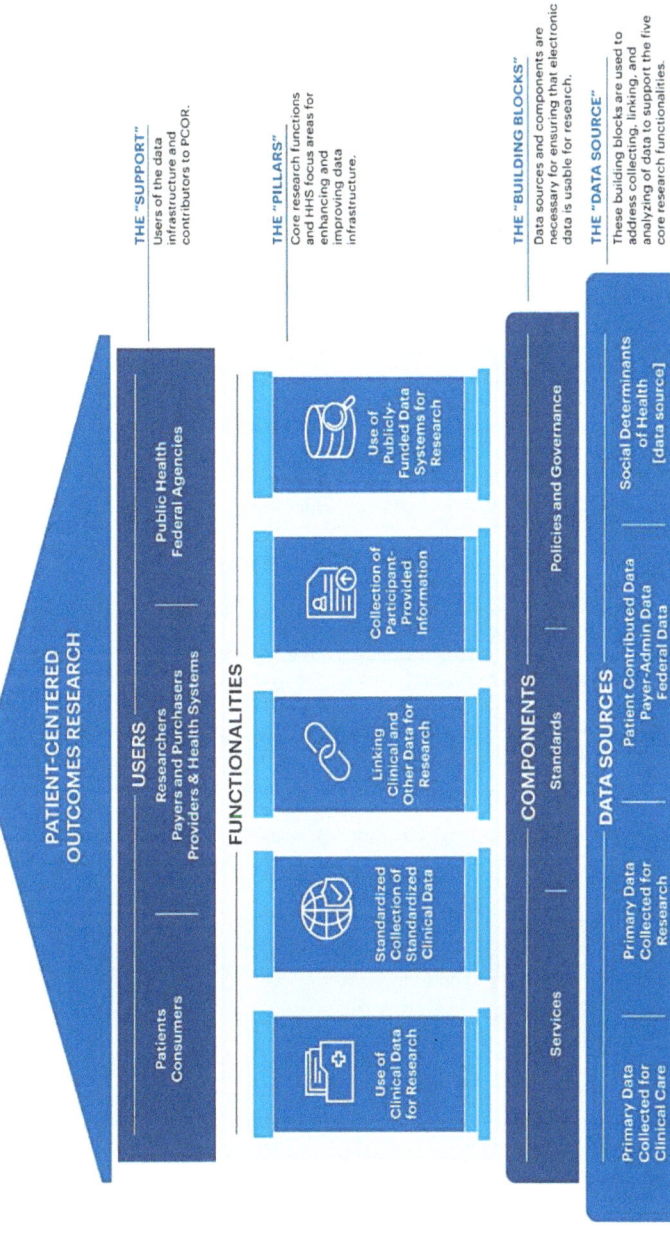

FIGURE 1-2 ASPE's strategic framework for the patient-centered outcomes research data infrastructure.
SOURCE: Workshop presentation by ASPE, May 3, 2021.

> **BOX 1-1**
> **Key Data Infrastructure Functionalities in the Existing Strategic Framework for Patient-Centered Outcomes Research**
>
> *Standardized Collection of Standardized Clinical Data*
> Researchers will be able to use standardized clinical data based on common data element standards across research projects and networks, thereby facilitating linkage and aggregation of data across data sources.
>
> *Collection of Participant-Provided Information*
> Participants, including those in safety net organizations, will be able to participate more fully in clinical research by directly providing information (i.e., data points provided by the participant such as Patient-Reported Outcomes).
>
> *Linking of Clinical and Other Data for Research*
> Researchers will be able to follow patients across the care continuum over time, including those enrolled in clinical trials. Researchers will be able to capture the range of variables influencing health outcomes and link clinical and other types of data (e.g., other clinical data, claims data, participant-provided information, and environmental data) required for research regardless of where the participant goes.
>
> *Use of Clinical Data for Research*
> Researchers will be able to utilize and analyze routinely collected clinical data for implementation of clinical studies (observational and interventional), including data relevant to assessing safety, efficacy, and adherence, as well as genetic data and Patient-Reported Outcomes.
>
> *Use of Enhanced Publicly Funded Data Systems for Research*
> Researchers will be able to readily use, retrieve, link, and aggregate publicly funded data for research due to enhancements in publicly funded data systems.
>
> SOURCE: https://aspe.hhs.gov/collaborations-committees-advisory-groups/os-pcortf/about-os-pcortf/building-data-capacity-patient-centered-outcomes-research.

> **BOX 1-2**
> **Building Blocks of the Patient-Centered**
> **Outcomes Research Data Infrastructure**
>
> *Standards* represent information and meaning to patient-centered data to ensure that health-specific information can be accurately (and securely) exchanged and used. In most cases standards should be nationally accepted, widely approved, or broadly adopted either through market forces, community approval, or regulatory requirements. These include such items as data standards for capturing, storing, representing, and exchanging data in a secure manner such that accurate information is conveyed to the recipient of the data.
>
> *Policies* are standards of behavior that participants can rely on consistently to build patient-centered data for research. Policies may include federal policies, as well as models for standardized state and local policies, that will lead to a trusted framework within the patient-centered outcomes research (PCOR) data infrastructure that ensures productivity, protects the patient and the patient's data, ensures that evidence generation remains in the center of PCOR, and ensures the use of agreed-upon standards and services.
>
> *Services* refer to resources that entities can employ on demand to capture, store, or exchange either PCOR data or evidence through a centrally hosted model provided remotely (such as through the internet) rather than provided locally or on site. Services make it easy for the research data to interoperate among different systems without having to start from scratch for every connection.
>
> *Governance* structures refer to entities that are needed to develop and apply the rules and policies needed for building an interoperable and sustainable research network. Governance structures support the efficient use of the data infrastructure for research across individuals' and organizations' boundaries of control and ownership. Governance structures are distinguished from "governance," which is what a governing body or governance structure does.
>
> SOURCE: https://aspe.hhs.gov/collaborations-committees-advisory-groups/os-pcortf/about-os-pcortf/building-data-capacity-patient-centered-outcomes-research.

ISSUES FOR THE COMMITTEE

ASPE asked the National Academies of Sciences, Engineering, and Medicine to appoint a consensus study committee and identify issues critical to building data capacity for PCOR and for generating new evidence to inform health care decisions. The input provided by the committee will contribute to ASPE's strategic planning for their work related to the data infrastructure over the next decade. The study is part of a broader initiative by ASPE intended to update the strategic plan in light of the reauthorization of the PCOR Trust Fund and advances in health information technology and interoperability tools in recent years.

The study is a collaboration of three units of the National Academies: the Committee on National Statistics, the Board on Health Care Services, and the Computer Science and Telecommunications Board. The consensus study committee has a diverse membership; its 15 members include experts with decades of experience, as well as emerging leaders, in the broad fields of (1) PCOR; (2) research methods, statistics, and demography; (3) computer science and data infrastructure; and (4) patient engagement and patient perspectives. Appendix A contains the biographical sketches of the committee members.

As part of its information-gathering activities, the committee was asked to organize three workshops to collect input from stakeholders on aspects of the charge developed in consultation with ASPE. The workshops focused on key topics that the committee believed would particularly benefit from broad input from a variety of data users and other stakeholders. The committee's conclusions from each workshop are summarized in a series of interim reports, of which the first centered on emerging data needs. This first interim report summarizes the discussion and committee conclusions from the first workshop, which focused on looking ahead at data user needs over the next decade. The second workshop in the series centered on data standards, methods, and policies that could make the PCOR data infrastructure more useful. The third workshop discussed research and data collaborations. This report summarizes the discussion and committee conclusions from the second workshop, which focused on data standards, methods, and policies that could make the PCOR data infrastructure more useful. The third report will discuss research and data collaborations.

As an interim report focused on one in a series of information-gathering activities, the scope of this report is limited to a subset of the topics relevant to the committee's charge and the conclusions reached by the committee are, at this stage, fairly high level. Some aspects of the topics discussed are examined in further detail in other workshops. After completing all of its information-gathering activities, the committee will issue a final report, which will integrate and examine these topics in further detail.

Box 1-3 shows the committee's Statement of Task for the overall study. The committee will address this charge in its final report, integrating what was learned from the workshops and from all other forms of input, including public meetings with HHS staff and background documentation available on the history and operations of the PCOR Trust Fund. The final report will contain overall findings and conclusions from the study, on the basis of the committee's further deliberations and integrated judgment on the input received and materials reviewed.

> **BOX 1-3**
> **Statement of Task for the Overall Study**
>
> The National Academies will appoint an ad hoc committee to conduct a series of three one-day public workshops and develop conclusions to help guide the data capacity development for patient-centered research from 2021 through 2030. Each workshop will seek input from key stakeholders on topics relevant to the committee charge, and the specific focus of each workshop will be determined by the committee in consultation with ASPE.
> As part of its activities, the committee will also
>
> - Consider the published review of the history and trajectory of the Office of the Secretary Patient-Centered Outcomes Research Trust Fund (OS-PCORTF) portfolio of investments and the OS-PCORTF roadmap.
> - Assess anticipated changes to health care priorities and priorities for health data and their impact on building data capacity into the foreseeable future, as identified by ASPE.
> - Evaluate the feasibility and utility of developing a phased-in approach to building the interoperable data capacity for patient-centered outcomes research with existing databases in HHS, other Federal Departments and the private sector in a phased approach, such as projects identified in the Cures Act Title III Section 4003 (Interoperability).
> - Consider other existing legislation, regulations, and the like, as deemed relevant; and
> - Receive input from individuals or groups that represent stakeholders, including patients and their caregivers or families and their health care providers.
>
> The committee will issue interim reports after each public workshop with conclusions, and will produce a final written report with findings and conclusions to help guide a future course to continue building the data capacity for patient-centered research. All reports will follow institutional guidelines and be subject to the National Academies review procedures prior to release.

Appendix B shows the agenda for the workshop, which was held on May 24, 2021. The committee's goal for this event was to bring together researchers and policy experts to

- Identify data standards and methods that can make the PCOR data infrastructure more useful for research and other data needs.
- Identify data policies that are needed to facilitate the continued development and operation of the PCOR data infrastructure.
- Discuss what HHS is best positioned to address and support, and how the agency could maximize resources available for the PCOR

data infrastructure (representing 4% of the PCOR Trust Fund), in the context of the HHS public mission, authorities, programs, and data resources.

Invited speakers in each of the sessions were asked to reflect on the general topics above. The specific questions for each session are described in Chapters 2 through 4. An obvious limitation of an activity of this type is that only a small number of stakeholders can be invited to speak. To compensate for this limitation, the invited participants included diverse experts working in a variety of areas and on a range of types of projects, including both early career researchers and experts with decades of experience. A recording of the workshop as well as the presentation slides used by the speakers are available on the National Academies website at www.nationalacademies.org/PCORData.

Prior to the workshop, information about the event was disseminated through National Academies mailing lists and on the project website. To collect additional stakeholder input, members of the public were invited to provide comments on topics related to the workshop (or any other topic related to the committee's charge), using a public input form available on the National Academies website.

OVERVIEW OF THE REPORT

This report is organized around the three main sessions of the workshop: Chapter 2 discuses data standards, Chapter 3 is centered on research methods, and Chapter 4 describes discussions focused on data policies and related infrastructure considerations. The points conveyed by the workshop participants do not necessarily reflect the views of the committee. In each chapter, a summary of the input received is followed by the committee's conclusions. The conclusions are based primarily on the input collected as part of the workshop, background documentation received from ASPE and other public sources, and the committee members' synthesis and expert judgment. Because this is an interim report, the committee's conclusions at this stage are big-picture conclusions, which will be integrated with additional input over the course of the study.

2

Patient-Centered Outcomes Research Data Standards

This chapter summarizes presentations and discussion focused on data standards. As discussed in Chapter 1, the Office of the Assistant Secretary for Planning and Evaluation (ASPE) considers standards to be one of the building blocks of the patient-centered outcomes research (PCOR) infrastructure. Specifically

> Standards represent information and meaning to patient-centered data to ensure that health-specific information can be accurately (and securely) exchanged and used. In most cases standards should be nationally accepted, widely approved, or broadly adopted either through market forces, community approval, or regulatory requirements. These include such items as data standards for capturing, storing, representing, and exchanging data in a secure manner such that accurate information is conveyed to the recipient of the data.[1]

Speakers participating in this session were asked to focus on the questions below. The brief overview of the input received from the presenters is followed by the committee's conclusions.

- What data standards could make the PCOR data infrastructure more useful for research and other data needs? What data standards are likely to become more relevant looking forward? What needs to be prioritized?

---

[1] https://aspe.hhs.gov/patient-centered-outcomes-research-trust-fund-faqs.

- What role can ASPE play in supporting effective standards to build data capacity that supports PCOR studies? What characteristics of the U.S. Department of Health and Human Services' (HHS') public mission, programs, or authorities could be leveraged?

John Halamka, Mayo Clinic, provided some context for the session by describing three ways of thinking of data standards. First, there is a need for standards for presenting content from data sources such as electronic health records or other administrative records. Second, there is a need for vocabulary standards that would provide semantic interoperability for the content (e.g., SNOMED CT, RxNorm, and LOINC). Third, standards are needed for transporting the data from one place to another in a secure way (such as HL7 Version 2, EDIFACT, X12, and XML standards of various kinds). Ultimately, this led to the development of the Fast Healthcare Interoperability Resources (FHIR), which enable provider-to-provider, provider-to-patient, and provider-to-payer workflows to be supported by FHIR/JavaScript object notation and rest parameters. Halamka said that this is a good development, though it is not enough.

Looking ahead at the next 10 years, the Mayo Clinic has an initiative to move to a digital-first approach in its operations, undertake clinical research and clinical trials with less friction, and enable global access to new kinds of ideas. To accomplish this, the Mayo Clinic needs access to more types of data, and expanding the FHIR standard is one way to enable that. Two interesting examples are the Minimal Common Oncology Data Elements (mCODE) and the Mobile Health Augmented Cardiac Rehabilitation (MCard) data sets. Taking the basic FHIR construct and adding domain-specific data elements will be useful for research, but thousands of data elements may be needed to deal with various use cases.

Halamka also discussed an example of data standards applicable to research on COVID-19 treatment. There is a need to define "ventilator days" for research on when medications versus other interventions would make a difference to COVID-19 patients, he noted; at present, ventilator days are not defined in electronic health records in a standard way. Ultimately, a working group of about 100 experts might be involved in deciding on the definitions of data elements that are needed to answer process questions.

The challenges associated with data standards are heightened, Halamka added, when the research goes beyond structured and unstructured clinical data to incorporate other forms of data, such as research data emerging from various "omics" fields (e.g., genomics). Data from wearable devices, or what he called "high-velocity continuous data," comprise another area where standards are lacking.

Halamka also discussed the topic of data de-identification. He said that the Mayo Clinic has de-identified its data for use in clinical research and scientific discovery, but de-identification is itself a science that is evolving. For example, when using information from computed tomography (CT) on a patient's head, the patient's name and medical number would be removed, but it remains possible to reconstruct the person's face from the CT with 3D reconstruction software. Halamka said that he and his colleagues found that they have been able to re-identify a person this way 27 percent of the time using publicly available images and photo matching. Because of this, they have been working to develop technologies that would prevent head CT data from being used to reconstruct a face. This area needs attention, because de-identified information that cannot lead to unique identification today could nevertheless potentially become identifiable in the future as technologies evolve. Halamka also highlighted the related consideration of ways of obtaining consent for the future use of data, and specifically the reuse of de-identified, aggregate data.

Shaun Grannis, Regenstrief Institute and Indiana University, focused on standards for data linkage, particularly for participant-provided information. Within this area, he discussed the topics of (1) patient identity strategy, (2) digital identity and federation, (3) privacy-preserving record linkage, and (4) linking of social determinants of health (SDOH) data.

Grannis noted that the patient identity strategy in the United States is evolving based on a recognition that matching patient records from different sources is one of the few remaining large holes in the electronic health data infrastructure. For this reason, Congress charged the Office of the National Coordinator for Health Information Technology with writing a report focused on effective matching methods. While the report had not been released at the time of this workshop, Grannis underscored the importance of monitoring developments in this area to understand how PCOR can benefit from any changes.

Within the digital identity framework, Grannis noted, not everyone is willing to wait for the U.S. government to develop a national strategy. He pointed out that "matching on devices" is an area where a lot of work is taking place. Organizations such as the CARIN Alliance are working to develop a digital identity and a federated trust agreement to increase and federate trust in digital identity credentials. They are also considering digital identity frameworks that work well within FHIR. Grannis noted that there are also new developments in the more technical areas of identity certification or proofing. Examples of this include the work of FIDO and DirectTrust, as well as identity assigners such as ID.me, AllClearID, and Okta. These organizations are beginning to work on identity approaches at scale in health care, so it is important to observe these developments and learn from these experiences.

Concerning privacy issues, Grannis mentioned that he is working on two projects to advance privacy-preserving record linkage. This is a maturing field, with some maturing technologies that already work well. There is a need to establish best practices, use cases, and evidence-based guidance on how to conduct this work to ensure that this field does not become too fragmented and those participating in it do not find themselves doing everything differently. Specifically, it would be helpful to have widely shared technical descriptions of what types of data, what types of tokens, and what types of information combinations work well.

Grannis also discussed his work on linking nontraditional, nonclinical SDOH data in Indiana. He noted that there are various methods for linking these types of data, including linking by person, place, or time—or some combination of those—but work remains to identify the best approaches. Grannis argued that for the SDOH data, the main considerations are granularity, standardization, and linkage. For example, in some cases using zip code-level data is valuable, but in other cases more granular information is needed. A variety of data are available on SDOH, and Grannis said that coordinating work on PCOR with the work carried out by the Office of the National Coordinator for Health Information Technology in this area would be important.

Concerning the challenge of matching data, Grannis noted that there have been sustained efforts over the years to find new approaches to matching, and many researchers have been advocating for similar things. What is needed is alignment in this area. As an example of building on evidence-based research to develop standards, Grannis mentioned a 2019 paper that showed that standardizing address and last name significantly improves matching accuracy.[2] This research led to a bipartisan Senate bill calling to address standardization, and work is now in progress on developing a universal standard.

Evelyn Gallego, EMI Advisors, discussed her work on the Gravity Project, which focuses on developing consensus-driven data standards to support use and exchange of SDOH within the health care sectors and between the health care sector and other sectors, including research. She said that even before the onset of COVID-19, there was growing awareness that SDOH information improves whole-person care and lowers health care costs, and that unmet social needs negatively impact health outcomes.

Gallego discussed several uses of social risk data, identified by the Social Interventions Research and Evaluation Network (SIREN). These areas include medical care, population health management, community health improvement, social risk interventions, risk adjustment, and

---

[2] S.J. Grannis, H. Xu, J.R. Vest, S. Kasthurirathne, N. Bo, B. Moscovitch, R. Torkzadeh, and J. Rising. (2019). Evaluating the effect of data standardization and validation on patient matching accuracy. *Journal of the American Medical Informatics Association*, 26(5), 447–456. https://doi.org/10.1093/jamia/ocy191.

research. Despite a clear business case, clinical systems face challenges in capturing and exchanging this type of data. Gallego cited a 2020 paper from the National Association of Social Determinants of Health that identified the key challenges as follows:

- Consent management.
- Standardization of SDOH data collection and storage.
- Data sharing between ecosystem parties.
- Access and comfort with digital solutions.
- Concerns about information collection and sharing.
- Social-care sector capacity and capability.
- Unnecessary medicalization of SDOH.[3]

Gallego discussed two of these areas in detail: standardization and data sharing.

The Gravity Project was launched in 2019 with the goal of developing data standards for domains that Gallego described as grounded in a 2014 National Academies report.[4] The domains include items such as education, elder abuse, environment, financial insecurity, food deserts, food insecurity, homelessness, housing instability, inadequate housing, interpersonal violence, material hardship, neighborhood safety, racism, social isolation, stress, transportation insecurity, unemployment, and veteran status.

The Gravity Project develops data standards to represent patient-level SDOH data documented across four clinical activities: screening, assessment/diagnosis, goal setting, and treatment/interventions. Described as a "public collaborative," the project convenes participants from across the health and human services ecosystem, including clinical provider groups, community-based organizations, standards development organizations, federal and state government, payers, technology vendors, and others.

Gallego described the Gravity Project as having two workstreams: work on terminology, focused on SDOH domains; and technical work, focused on specifications for Health Level Seven International (HL7) FHIRs. The terminology workstream focuses on defining data elements for each SDOH domain by asking What concepts need to be documented across the four activities of screening, diagnosis, goal setting, and interventions? What codes reflecting these concepts are currently available? and, What codes are missing? On the technical side, the HL7 SDOH clinical care FHIR implementation guide provides guidance on how to do assessment screening,

---

[3] https://www.nasdoh.org/wp-content/uploads/2020/08/NASDOH-Data-Interoperability_FINAL.pdf.
[4] https://www.nap.edu/catalog/18709/capturing-social-and-behavioral-domains-in-electronic-health-records-phase.

how to capture health concerns or problems that inform the diagnosis, goal setting, interventions, capturing consent, and aggregation for data exchange and reporting.

When the Gravity Project was launched, according to Gallego, its leaders developed a conceptual framework that accounts for various entry points for the data (e.g., a digital application used by a patient or the health care providers' electronic health records). They defined SDOH data concepts that can be documented and shared across the four activities discussed above, regardless of the initial input system. This framework emphasizes the value of these data for secondary use by public and private payers, social service providers, public health entities, and researchers.

Rachel Richesson, University of Michigan, discussed the concept of a *learning health care system*, where research influences practice and practice influences research. Standards could provide the infrastructure for turning real-world data into real-world evidence, and thereby be the foundation for enabling real-world evidence to influence practice.

Richesson shared her perspective on the key data needed for PCOR and the associated standards to consider. Box 2-1 summarizes these data types and relevant standards. She argued that there is a need for robust data that describe patients and patient populations, including patient problems, in a standard way, with up-to-date problem lists. There is also a need to capture treatments and interventions, broadly defined. Richesson said that patient goals and preferences are increasingly important. Standards exist for some clinical domains, but they are not widely used. Richesson argued that the outcomes and endpoints most useful for PCOR are those that are condition-specific.

In terms of standards (the right-hand column in Box 2-1), Richesson said that it is important to have terminology that can represent related concepts at different levels of granularity while at the same time being suitable for being combined analytically. She highlighted the Gravity Project and the Gender Harmony Project as approaches that start with the high-level question of what concepts need to be measured and then look at what data are available and how those data can be pulled together in a useful way. The information is then shared with those who need to implement the standards. She cited SNOMED CT as the recognized standard for nursing data, such as nursing goals, nursing diagnosis, and nursing-related outcomes, and also noted that a set of standards is quickly emerging from the work of BPM+ Health group, an organization that is modeling clinical pathways and clinical workflows.

Richesson summarized her perspective on the key steps for developing standards as the following:

1. Leverage processes of existing standards organizations;
2. Encourage patient engagement in standards developing organizations;

BOX 2-1
A Perspective on Data Required for Patient-Centered Outcomes Research and Standards to Consider

Data Required

Patients/Persons
- Condition/phenotype
- Status
- Problem lists
- Risk or protective factors

Treatments and Interventions
- Medical or behavioral (targeted at the level of provider, patient, or organization)
- Nursing, physical therapy, occupational therapy, dietary, education
- Coordinated care
- Person-controlled
- Fidelity

Patient Goals and Preferences, Outcomes, and Endpoints
- General and condition specific
- Calculated or summary data
- Clinical/treatment response
- Patient-reported
- Patient-delivered

Standards to Consider

SNOMED CT
- Problems
- "Normal" observations
- Medical
- Nursing
- Other clinical
- Goals, preferences
- Outcomes

LOINC (Logical Observation Identifiers Names and Codes)
- Questions/answers
- Document names

Open mHealth mobile health data interoperability standard
- Questions/answers

HL7 – Learning Health Systems care team; Gender Harmony group
HL7 FHIR
- Profiles, FHIR Accelerator projects

BPM+ Health (Business Process Management for Healthcare)
- Clinical pathways, interventions, use cases

Agency for Healthcare Research and Quality
- Outcome Measures Framework

SOURCE: Workshop presentation by Rachel Richesson, May 24, 2021.

3. Support tools for use of standards in real-world settings;
4. Promote semantic interoperability and intrinsic value sets or "groupers";
5. Use concept maps/information models (e.g., recent nursing work[5]);
6. Show value of standards for application development and dissemination;
7. Create tools to make it easy for application developers of all types;
8. Develop standards roadmaps;
9. Make use of feedback loops on standards (e.g., to understand whether they are useful or whether they are granular enough); and
10. Repeat the steps above, as needed.

Patrick Ryan, of both Janssen Research and Development and Columbia University, discussed data standards based on his experiences with the Observational Health Data Sciences and Informatics (OHDSI) collaborative. OHDSI is an open, multistakeholder, interdisciplinary collaborative whose mission is to improve health by empowering communities to collaboratively generate the evidence that promotes better health decisions and better care. OHDSI is driving development and adoption of open community data standards, open-source analysis software, and open-science best practices among regulators, academia, industry, payors, and health systems. While OHDSI is not a data standards organization, it is a heavy user of those standards and a steward of them simply because they advance the collaborative's goal of generating reliable evidence to improve health.

OHDSI has a data network that includes organizations with patient-level data in more than 150 databases. Standardization, Ryan said, is about structure, content, and learning from the differences among data sources, rather than trying to create something that is homogeneous. The data in this network are not centralized, and organizations can decide whether and how to participate in the network. Researchers can conduct "network studies" by identifying a research question and then reaching out to the data network to generate standardized aggregate results.

Ryan argued that data standards are a means to an end, not an end in itself. In this context, the key questions to ask would be (1) What evidence would be useful to improve health policy and health care, which could be reliably generated by the PCOR data infrastructure? (2) How can data standards enable real-world analytics to meet the relevant evidence needs moving forward? and (3) What needs to be prioritized?

---

[5]B.L. Westra et al. (2020). A refined methodology for validation of information models derived from flowsheet data and applied to a genitourinary case. *Journal of American Medical Informatics Association*, 27(11), 1732–1740. doi: 10.1093/jamia/ocaa166. PMID: 32940673.

Ryan said that the OHDSI community has given a lot of thought to the topic of reliable evidence. Data standards are necessary, he pointed out, to enable replicability, generalizability, and robustness, because answering questions requires that disparate data be brought together, and there is a need for a mechanism that enables examining the same question in different data sets in some reliable way. It is also clear that data standards without standardized analytics are not sufficient to ensure reliable evidence. Ryan also argued that public health questions require global data to generate global evidence, and standards that are not limited to data in the United States are more useful, even for research specific to the population in the United States.

Thinking about the specific role of standards in generating evidence, and working backward from the question of what evidence would be helpful to improve health policy and health care, Ryan discussed three analytical use cases on which the OHDSI community focuses: (1) characterization, or producing descriptive statistics to understand what is happening in the world; (2) estimation, or causal inference, to understand the effects of medical interventions and the comparative effectiveness of interventions; and (3) prediction of risks. Data standards need to be based on the evidence needed and the type of use case it needs to support.

The ecosystem of complementary standards discussed by Ryan includes data standards to enable data exchange (e.g., the FHIR from HL7), data standards to harmonize data structure and enable analytics (e.g., the Observational Medical Outcomes Partnership Common Data Model or OMOP CDM[6]), and analytics standards to generate and disseminate evidence (e.g., the Health Analytics Data-to-Evidence Suite or HADES). Underlying all of this, there are vocabulary standards that harmonize data content and also enable analytics (e.g., ATHENA). The OHDSI community works on bringing these standards together. For example, they developed a suite of open-source analytic tools that sit on top of the OMOP CDM as their open community data standard, but they are also collaborating with HL7 on the interoperability of FHIR standards and the OMOP CDM standards for enabling analytics.

Ryan said that the initial focus of the OMOP CDM was on health systems data, clinical data, and health economics data, because those are the analytical use cases and the evidence needs that OHDSI is trying to fill within their community. Underlying the data model are the infrastructure of vocabulary standards and the mappings from source codes onto standards, which enable the adoption of standards. He added that the use of vocabularies is not just an obligation, but an opportunity to expand the

---

[6] For an overview of the CDM, see https://ohdsi.github.io/TheBookOfOhdsi/CommonDataModel.html#fn20.

value of the data. The OMOP data partners have different data structures and different data contents. Each partner goes through its own journey to standardize its data under a common data model, and OMOP enables those data to be analyzed through standardized analytic routines.

Ryan said that the OHDSI community has done a lot of work to try to help policy makers, regulators, and clinicians with questions related to COVID-19. One of the first efforts was related to examining the safety of hydroxychloroquine. Starting with the need, they reached out to their data network across the world to find out who had standardized data that could meaningfully contribute to this question. They then worked on developing the right analytic approach to apply to the question. While this work ultimately resulted in academic publications,[7] the primary goal was to generate evidence that could inform policy decisions and the work of the European Medicines Agency and the U.S. Food and Drug Administration (FDA).

VG Vinod Vydiswaran, University of Michigan, focused on the role of natural language processing (NLP) in the use of PCOR data. He argued that three of the areas deserving attention to make the PCOR data infrastructure more useful are (1) the informatics infrastructure that includes clinical notes, (2) computable phenotypes as knowledge objects, and (3) looking beyond electronic health records for health data.

To illustrate the use of clinical notes, Vydiswaran discussed his work with the Patient-Centered Network of Learning Health Systems (LHSNet), a Clinical Data Research Network funded by the Patient-Centered Outcomes Research Institute. The common data model for LHSNet focuses on structured data typically available in clinical settings, such as demographic information, laboratory values, and ICD-9 and -10 codes. Vydiswaran worked on extending the common data model to include textual components and extract clinically relevant information from free text. This work built on a prior study, the Clinical Language Engineering Workbench (CLEW), developed as part of the National Program of Cancer Registries of the Centers for Disease Control and Prevention.

Figure 2-1 shows the CLEW NLP machine learning process functionalities. Vydiswaran noted that it is important to expand the component that creates a pipeline for extracting features, not only to look at individual attributes but also to look at concepts and relationships between concepts.

Vydiswaran said that the second area of work where advances could make the PCOR data infrastructure more useful is the use of computable phenotypes as *knowledge objects*, specifically standardized definitions for analysis across multiple sites. By knowledge objects, he meant the

---

[7] https://www.medrxiv.org/content/10.1101/2020.04.08.20054551v2; https://www.thelancet.com/journals/lanrhe/article/PIIS2665-9913(20)30276-9/fulltext; https://academic.oup.com/rheumatology/article/60/7/3222/6048420.

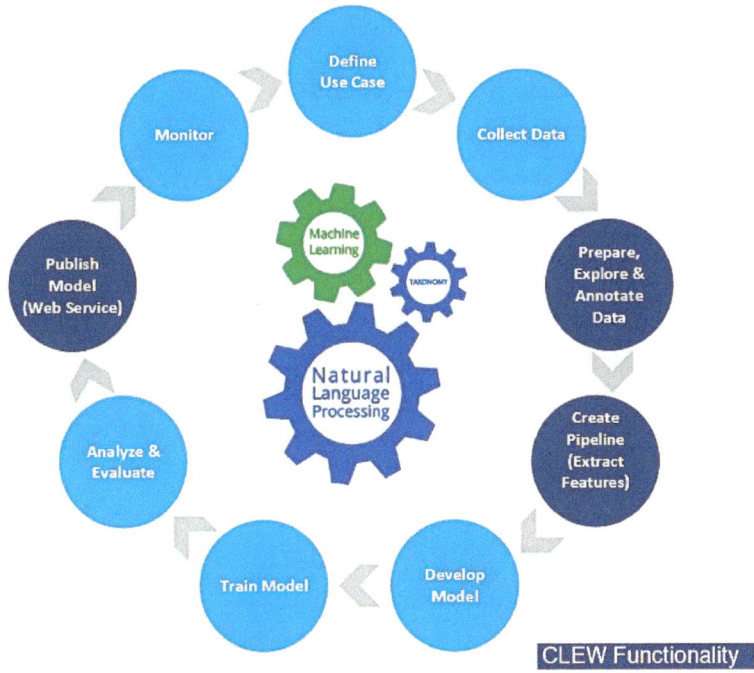

FIGURE 2-1 Clinical language engineering workbench: Key functionalities in the natural language processing machine learning process.
SOURCE: Workshop presentation by VG Vinod Vydiswaran, May 24, 2021; ASPE, 2019.[8]

computational components of research that can be used and expanded on by others. This includes standardized clinical natural language tools for processing text so that it is interpreted the same way across multiple sites.

The typical data elements in computable phenotypes, Vydiswaran said, are structured components such as ICD-9 and -10 codes, Current Procedural Terminology (CPT) codes, information about medications, and sometimes key terms and phrases, along with the frequency of their mentions. Novel areas for consideration include patient-reported outcomes such as symptoms, medication response, and adverse events in telephone notes, medication refill requests through web portal requests, and care provider information, especially for patients unable to independently manage their

---

[8]https://aspe.hhs.gov/system/files/pdf/259016/NLP-CLEW-UserGuidanceDocument-508.pdf.

health care needs. A lot of information about patient-reported outcomes is available in electronic health records in text form.

Vydiswaran mentioned his prior work on self-reporting behavior concerning the toxicity of oral anticancer agents in clinical notes.[9] In that work, he found that 23.5 percent of the clinical oral anticancer agent toxicity notes were based on telephone encounters. In another study, Vydiswaran and his colleagues are working on extracting patient-provided information on Crohn's disease symptoms, medication response, and adverse events using email and telephone notes stored in electronic medical records.

Vydiswaran also encouraged looking beyond electronic health records for health data. For example, information on the adverse effects of drugs can increasingly be found on social media. However, Vydiswaran noted that processing consumer-generated text is even more challenging than processing clinical text, due to the prevalence of grammatical errors, typos, new acronyms, and abbreviations.

Text found on social media can be useful for a variety of purposes, beyond collecting data on drugs' adverse effects. For example, geo-located social media can be useful for exploring community health information. Social media can be analyzed through the lens of communities (e.g., affluent versus disadvantaged neighborhoods), demographics (e.g., "BlackTwitter"), or patient cohorts (e.g., smoking cessation patient groups). Spatio-temporal factors that can be linked to patients include air pollution, neighborhood walkability, rurality, and "food deserts."

Vydiswaran mentioned that his current work includes the use of social media to augment information in the FDA Adverse Event Reporting System and the Vaccine Adverse Event Reporting System. NLP can be helpful for parsing text from both social media and the federal adverse event reporting databases.

As a summary of his key points, Vydiswaran emphasized (1) the need for an enhanced informatics infrastructure for processing textual clinical notes; (2) treating computable phenotypes as knowledge objects, and incorporating patient-reported outcomes derived using NLP; and (3) taking advantage of health-related social media to augment existing data.

After the presentations, participants in this session were asked to comment on what the federal government could do to accelerate work on standards for patient-centered outcomes data and research. Halamka said that one of the strengths of the federal government is that of a convener of meetings. As an example, he mentioned the role of the Office of the

---

[9] Y. Jiang, V.G.V. Vydiswaran, Y.L. Eun, H. Joo, A. Zheng, and M.R. Harris. (2018). *Feasibility of Identifying Oral Anticancer Agent Toxicity Self-Reporting and Management Advice from Clinical Notes.* AMIA Annual Symposium, November 3–7, San Francisco, CA.

National Coordinator for Health Information Technology in convening meetings to attempt to harmonize U.S. and international standards on vaccine credentials. He added that he does not believe that attempting to regulate standards would be advisable. If the federal government facilitates the harmonization of standards, those standards will be adopted because they will bring value. Grannis agreed that convening and building consensus is what the government does well. He argued that this would be especially useful for accelerating work in areas that are "hotspots" of nonstandardized data, such as SDOH.

Gallego highlighted creating incentives for testing the standards as a need that could be filled by federal or state governments, through mechanisms such as grants. Richesson argued for a library of computable phenotypes. She noted that there is a need for better organizing information on existing standards. ASPE could facilitate the sharing of tools and metadata standards and incentivize the reporting of results. She said that currently it is almost easier to develop new standards than to find something that has already been done and that would work in a particular situation. Ryan agreed with the idea of a phenotype library, and argued that the scope could be broadened to other types of information about what was learned from a study. He also agreed with Gallego on the need for testing, and with Halamka and Grannis on ASPE's potential role in community building. Vydiswaran highlighted the need for maintaining analytic tools over the years, by updating documentation to facilitate their use and progress toward eventual standardization.

DISCUSSION

During the workshop, the formal presentations were followed by additional discussion among the workshop participants, including the speakers, committee, and audience members. Among the topics that were explored in further detail were arguments for and against additional standards. One of the themes that emerged is the inherent difficulty associated with the process of agreeing on standards. It could be argued that an adequate variety of standards already exists for most situations, and the challenge is to converge around a single standard. Despite the challenges, past experience in a variety of domains indicates that convergence can be accomplished by bringing together communities and increasing communication around these topics. Participants also acknowledged that the context around standards is continuously evolving because the use cases, workflows, and information flows are always changing. This means that standards will also have to evolve over time.

Another topic that was discussed by workshop participants was the role of the federal government, and particularly HHS, in the context of standards for PCOR. Convening stakeholders emerged as a role that is especially well suited for HHS to handle. Participants cautioned against the blunt instrument of regulation, arguing that standards are most likely to be adopted when they bring value, because without a clear purpose and value for the standards, clinician frustration with electronic health records could increase. HHS could play a role in facilitating discussions to prioritize areas where standardization could be most useful and convening activities around topics such as SDOH, where there is a notable lack of standards and a common language.

Speakers also highlighted the need for a support infrastructure that would facilitate activities such as testing and enable the adoption of standards. Examples of the support infrastructure focused on building community and collaboration around standards. At the same time, views differed on a potential role for HHS in incentivizing the use of standards, and what those incentives could look like.

Workshop participants noted that there was a need for cataloging existing standards, because currently it is almost easier to develop a new approach than to figure out what already exists and whether and how it applies to a particular situation. This need extends to the cataloging of analytic tools, which are easier to use when documentation from earlier studies is maintained and updated.

Another theme addressed by the speakers and revisited as part of the discussion was that of the relationship between U.S. and international data standards. Participants noted that there are a variety of differences among countries, ranging from population differences to differences in health care systems. The use of standards also differs, but common international standards would facilitate a better understanding of the heterogeneity and could inform policy decisions everywhere, including in the United States.

CONCLUSIONS

The workshop session demonstrated that, within the context of PCOR, standardization is increasingly and ever more widely applied to the processes of collecting, storing, analyzing, and exchanging data. These standards are most useful when they are focused on addressing a specific problem or are driven by a specific use case. The needs and norms evolve over time, and because of this, standards need to evolve too. Lessons might be learned from best practices that emerge for the development of standards.

The workshop made it clear that in some areas there is a fair amount of agreement around what standards are needed and what useful standards look like. In other areas, for example, for data on SDOH, the work is just beginning, so these areas might not be ready for wide agreement on standards. In all cases, extensive testing of the potential standards is necessary.

CONCLUSION 2-1: Standards are most useful when their development is driven by their potential uses and a clear concept of the value they can contribute.

Participants in this session did not see a large role for ASPE in developing standards or deciding what the standards should be. ASPE's most valuable contributions could be in developing an architecture and an implementation strategy that facilitate common language and interoperability across data sets, as well as accessibility of the data. Other areas where ASPE could play an important role include convening stakeholder meetings to discuss and develop standards, as well as taking the lead in cataloguing existing standards.

CONCLUSION 2-2: The Office of the Assistant Secretary for Planning and Evaluation could add significant value in the area of standards for patient-centered outcomes research by

- continuing to promote the development of a data infrastructure and an implementation strategy that facilitates the use of standards and access to the data;
- convening stakeholder meetings to enhance communication and work toward developing a common language for standards;
- facilitating accessibility to the data and collaborations with existing organizations working in this area; and
- leading efforts to catalogue and exemplify data standards and analytic standards.

The speakers touched on the need for a broad interpretation of standards, to include not only the data but also the methods used to analyze PCOR data.

CONCLUSION 2-3: While data standards are important to conducting patient-centered outcomes research, applying standards to the analytic methods as well is important to facilitate the reliability and reproducibility of study results.

Speakers also highlighted the potential benefits of staying abreast of the standards development that happens not only in the United States but also internationally. Learning from experiences across the globe would further advance PCOR and benefit patients in the United States.

CONCLUSION 2-4: An international perspective is an important consideration for the patient-centered outcomes research data infrastructure, and the infrastructure focused on standards specifically would benefit from building on work that happens internationally.

3

Methods for Patient-Centered Outcomes Research

The workshop discussions summarized in this chapter cover methods that could advance patient-centered outcomes research (PCOR) and make PCOR data more useful going forward. The brief overview of the input received from the presenters is followed by the committee's conclusions. Speakers in this session were asked to focus on the following questions:

- What emerging methods are likely to be most relevant for the PCOR data infrastructure looking forward? What are the most important research and data challenges?
- What computing advances, innovative health information technologies, and methodologies might present opportunities going forward?
- What role can the Office of the Assistant Secretary for Planning and Evaluation (ASPE) play in supporting effective methods for PCOR studies? What characteristics of HHS's public mission, programs, or authorities could be leveraged?

Nigam H. Shah, Stanford University, argued that to make better use of patient-centered outcomes data, it would be useful to adopt a *patient timeline view* of the data. Typically, data are thought of as residing in tables, text files, images, and so on, but health care happens over time, and it is useful to think of the data in those terms, as events occurring over time.

Figure 3-1 illustrates Shah's patient timeline perspective. The figure shows a patient's journey, with the red dots denoting events with some health care relevance. Depending on which access point into medical data

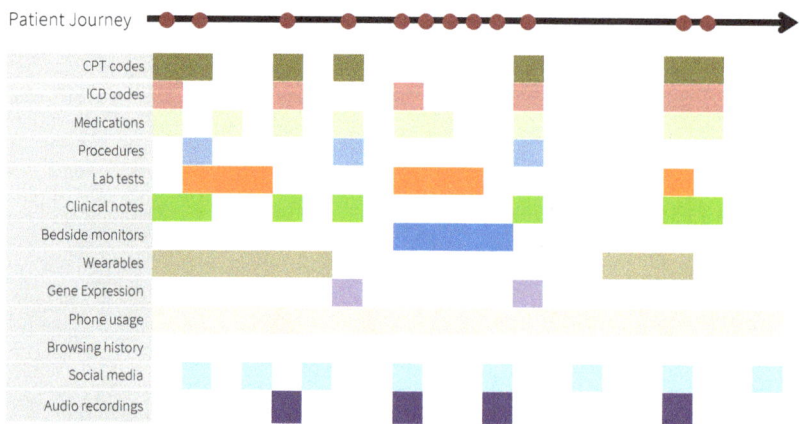

FIGURE 3-1 A patient timeline view of data.
SOURCE: Workshop presentation by Nigam Shah, May 24, 2021.

they use, researchers only get a partial view of the event that really occurred. For example, they might have access to claims filing information corresponding to a medical visit, which might have International Classification of Disease (ICD) codes, medication codes, Common Procedural Terminology (CPT) codes, and laboratory test orders. From the electronic health records, researchers might be able to access test results, the clinician's notes, and perhaps the signal streams from bedside monitors. Outside of the health system, we might get data from wearables, such as a Fitbit or an Apple watch. In a research setting, we might find gene expression data, genomic data, and perhaps more kinds of molecular measurements. Outside of the context of medical care, researchers might have access to information about online activities, such as phone usage, browsing, social media postings, audio clips, and so on.

Shah said that artificial intelligence (AI) or machine learning may make it easier to automate the processing of the types of data included in the timeline view. A more innovative use of AI is to combine multiple data modalities to trigger some proactive action.

Shah pointed out that few data source systems in routine use have native constructs for handling a task such as, for example, finding patients with a history of myocardial infarction who have pneumonia. This query has to be programmed in SQL (Structured Query Language) programming language, which is currently the dominant mechanism for interacting with this type of data. To be able to make full use of timeline data, it is also necessary to have tools that can perform interval algebra. The next step after performing interval algebra would be navigating knowledge graphs.

For example, one might want to find patients with disorders of glucose metabolism or patients with disorders of glucose metabolism treated with certain types of medications. The challenge is that current data systems do not handle medical knowledge graphs, and manual coding is necessary.

Shah also discussed the need to be able to state phenotype definitions, in other words, the necessary and sufficient conditions for believing that a particular event of interest occurred. As an example, hypertension as a phenotype might imply a different blood pressure cutoff, depending on the decade. "Ventilator days" was another example, mentioned in the workshop in connection with the COVID-19 pandemic. Shah noted that the complexity of phenotype definitions ranges from the collection of codes to elaborate Word documents that need to be translated into SQL.

Shah summarized his points as the need for technology that allows researchers to go from timelines to data frames in real time, taking timeline objects (with their as-yet unsolved storage challenges) and performing advanced analytics, satisfying the necessary and sufficient statements to conclude that a particular exposure outcome happened, and producing an analysis data frame in real time. He argued that solving these challenges would greatly accelerate PCOR.

Shah also discussed the Advanced Cohort Engine (ACE), a search engine he and his colleagues developed for patient data.[1] The search engine consists of a persistent in-memory database of patient objects and a temporal query language, both optimized for fast search, and a flexible application programming interface to access and retrieve data. Researchers can quickly find patients by searching across diagnosis and procedure codes, concepts extracted from clinical notes, laboratory test results, or vital signs, as well as by visit types and duration of inpatient stays. They can then compare the outcomes of these patients. Shah mentioned that the search engine is available with the Observational Medical Outcomes Partnership Common Data Model (OMOP CDM) version 5.3 and higher, emphasizing the importance of adhering to at least one community standard so that going from data to analyses is reproducible, reliable, and scalable.

Shah underscored the need to upgrade the collective computational infrastructure in the United States to be able to conduct the types of analyses he described in real time. There is also a need for a stronger focus on systems and software, beyond methods development.

Sharon-Lise Normand, Harvard University, highlighted data silos as one of the main challenges for PCOR data and PCOR in general. There are a large number of data sources, the usability and availability of unique IDs

---

[1] A. Callahan, V. Polony, J.D. Posada, J.M. Banda, S. Gombar, and N.H. Shah. (2021). ACE: The Advanced Cohort Engine for searching longitudinal patient records. *Journal of the American Medical Informatics Association.* https://doi.org/10.1093/jamia/ocab027.

are questionable, and linkages across databases are difficult to accomplish. She agreed with Shah that understanding what works requires longitudinal observation of patients over time.

Normand pointed at missing data as another challenge for PCOR. While missing data has always posed difficulties for statisticians, it is important to understand what this means specifically for electronic health records and to consider solutions for irregularly spaced data. She also noted the added challenges of missing data when more than one source is linked, when dealing with large volumes of data, and when using machine learning approaches.

The large number of data sets and new tools for processing the data also bring new challenges in terms of uncertainty over the precision of the estimates. One issue is selective inference, and the numerous decisions required as part of the analysis, because this ends up making the findings difficult to reproduce. Normand noted that currently no good methods exist for dealing with the propagation of differing errors associated with the use of multiple, complicated data sets. She argued that it is necessary to have an honest reflection concerning uncertainty and that there is a need for transparency regarding the assumptions and decisions that are made as part of the analyses.

Normand also discussed several areas where methodological opportunities exist for PCOR. The first such area is clinical trials. The availability of large volumes of electronic data will make it possible to streamline approaches for adaptive trials, which are difficult to conduct. Developing parallel randomized and prospective observational studies, using the same database and the same cohort receiving treatment at the same time, can also increase ability to learn about how effective certain treatments are. Finally, the usefulness of the data could be improved if adjustments were developed for reporting non-blinded outcomes, such as when participants are asked to complete a questionnaire.

The second area where opportunities exist for advancing PCOR is causal inference and the adoption of experimental thinking. Normand encouraged more emphasis on designing studies, as opposed to simply focusing on the analysis. Integrating causal inference approaches would be particularly useful in pragmatic trials. Opportunities exist to better understand the implications of missing data in sparse data settings and to better understand uncertainty and error propagation for the estimates.

Finally, Normand argued that exploiting the connectedness of information that is available from observational settings represents another methodological opportunity. She described this as a longitudinal multitask approach, sharing information across devices and across patients.

Addressing what ASPE could focus on, Normand said that the new Bridge2AI funding opportunity announcement from the National Institutes of Health (NIH) made her think that it would be useful to have "on demand" data, for example data that are already linked. Building a trial infrastructure for randomized and observational studies would be helpful. She also argued that to be able to make valid inferences about patient-centered outcomes data, it is necessary to invest in statistical methodology.

Sherri Rose, Stanford University, began by talking about data transformations in cases where it might be necessary to intervene if the information available represents structural biases in the collection of those data. Rose mentioned a recent paper she coauthored with colleagues on the ethical use of machine learning in health care.[2] The paper discusses the potential for data tools to exacerbate existing health disparities, along the different steps in the process from problem selection, through data collection and outcome definitions, and finally to algorithm development and potential postdeployment activities. She said that the preprocessing steps are where data transformations would typically be considered, but a lot of the work can also happen in the algorithm-building stage, or in the post-processing stage, where one might decide, for example, to adjust thresholds to handle concerns about the data. Rose said that questions to ask include Who decides the research questions? Who is the target population? and, What do the data reflect?

Rose discussed her prior work on using data transformation to bring causal conceptual thinking to the matter of fairness in data infrastructure.[3] The work focused on payment systems, aiming to reduce disparities in low-income neighborhoods and underprovision of services for chronic conditions, and the idea was to develop a methodology to set policies at desired levels. Rose added that thinking about how to do these types of data transformations is challenging, but this methodology is underleveraged and could benefit data infrastructure.

In the context of data linking and causality, Rose discussed a collaboration she had undertaken with Normand, in which they linked claims, registry, and vital statistics data to study the comparative effectiveness of cardiac stents.[4] Using machine learning made it possible to identify heterogeneous effects for the safety outcome in a cohort of patients receiving percutaneous coronary interventions. One piece of information they did not have was a

---

[2] I.Y. Chen, E. Pierson, S. Rose, S. Joshi, K. Ferryman, and M. Ghassemi. (2021). Ethical machine learning in healthcare. *Annual Review of Biomedical Data Science*, 4(1), 123–144. https://www.annualreviews.org/doi/abs/10.1146/annurev-biodatasci-092820-114757.

[3] S.L. Bergquist, T.J. Layton, T.G. McGuire, and S. Rose. (2019). Data transformations to improve the performance of health plan payment methods. *Journal of Health Economics*, 66, 195–207. https://doi.org/10.1016/j.jhealeco.2019.05.005.

[4] R.S. and S.-L. Normand. (2018). Double robust estimation for multiple unordered treatments and clustered observations: Evaluating drug-eluting coronary artery stents. *Biometrics*, 75, 289–296. https://doi.org/10.1111/biom.12927.

reliable estimate of the operator's skill, so they controlled for the operator in that study. She said that technology now exists to film operators doing surgery and produce an estimate of operator skill based on the footage to augment existing data. This technology might not scale well to large data sets, but it is an area with a lot of potential.

Generalizability was another topic touched on by Rose. While generalizability is typically considered in the context of inference, she argued that it is also useful to think of generalizability in prediction and clustering. The literature on generalizability from disparate data sources is spread across a variety of fields, including computer science, statistics, and health sciences. She mentioned a review she completed with one of her students and noted that there is substantial work yet to be done in this area.[5]

In some of their current work, Rose and her colleagues are focusing on integrating randomized and observational data, where each data source contains individuals who were missed by the other source with respect to the covariate distribution. In this work, they are focused on the area of overlap between randomized and observational data to develop new estimators and leverage the probability of selection into the randomized trial and the probability of receiving the treatment or receiving the intervention.

Rose echoed some of the conclusions highlighted by other speakers regarding opportunities to enhance PCOR. This includes the need to support work on developing new databases and software as well as maintaining existing software. She emphasized as well the importance of supporting the development of creative new methods for building data infrastructure. In closing, she urged researchers to consider whether their algorithms have a social impact statement. In connection with building tools for a data infrastructure, she named several social impact principles, including responsibility, explainability, accuracy, auditability, and fairness.

Nirosha Mahendraratnam Lederer, of Aetion, said that the company's Aetion Evidence Platform puts real-world data on a patient timeline, and uses transparent and scientifically validated workflows to analyze the data to generate real-world evidence. All the company's designs and analysis considerations are maintained in an audit trail.

Concerning real-world data, Lederer said that many variables of interest are available from traditional sources, such as medical and pharmacy claims, hospital chargemasters, electronic medical records, and clinical laboratory results. Additionally, newer digital tools, such as mobile health apps, sensors, and wearables enable the collection of additional patient-generated data. Linking traditional and newer digital sources makes it possible to generate a fuller picture of a patient, including the different factors

---

[5] I. Degtiar and S. Rose. (2021). *A Review of Generalizability and Transportability*. https://arxiv.org/pdf/2102.11904.pdf.

that ultimately impact the person's well-being, beyond physical health and traditional clinical outcomes. This enables researchers to study questions that patients really care about and provide information that can address issues with health care delivery, as well as structural and societal challenges.

Lederer suggested that the key for successfully using real-world data for research is to start with a well-defined research question that can be studied in the real world, and to ensure that a data source suitable for answering the question is available. However, the right data are not always available. For example, data that would allow researchers to study health disparities are rarely usable. Lederer said that there are two main reasons for challenges of this type.

The first reason why the available real-world data do not always include all the necessary data elements is that they are typically collected for purposes such as claims for billing, and not targeted for research purposes. As a result, these data sets are often missing key variables necessary to generate high-quality evidence. Lederer suggested that identifying a minimum set of core data elements to collect in routine clinical care can enable more meaningful research and facilitate data linkages. She added that building on existing tools and initiatives instead of creating new programs might be most practical. For example, instead of creating bespoke sets of required minimum data elements, perhaps the Office of the National Coordinator for Health Information Technology could collaborate with the research community to augment the United States Core Data for Interoperability (USCDI) to include essential data elements for research. Lederer acknowledged that USCDI applies only to electronic health records, and suggested that perhaps voluntary community standards could work for other types of data. To encourage adoption, it would be important to engage with digital health companies and organizations such as the Digital Medicine Society, because high-quality standardized data entry can make a big difference in the suitability of data for research.

The second reason why real-world data sometimes do not include data elements necessary for research is that privacy laws or commercial interests may be restricting the accessibility of these data, even when the data elements are captured. Lederer said that in an effort to protect privacy, frequently the tradeoffs are between information on race, geographical granularity, and place of service. All three of these data elements are essential for addressing issues with health care quality and disparities. Given technological advances, and the way data are collected, used, and linked today, Lederer said that it is important to revisit these policies in the context of research.

Another challenge highlighted by Lederer is that often only researchers within a health care system have access to certain data, and external researchers do not. This brings up the issue of parity, and the benefits that would result from more researchers with different perspectives and ideas having the opportunity to test their hypotheses using these restricted data sets.

Lederer also highlighted challenges associated with carrying out analysis using real-world data, even when the data are available. She pointed out that not all real-world data translate to high-quality evidence. However, there are some clear principles for generating high-quality evidence that is patient-centered and suitable for decision making. This includes starting with the concept of designing the target randomized controlled trial that one would conduct to answer the research question, and then emulating that trial through an observational study.

Over the longer term, Lederer said that she supports making research an infrastructure investment for state-of-the-art data curation and analytics such as AI or advanced methods to aim to quantify and adjust time-varying unobservables. However, in the more immediate term, it would be useful to think about how to refine the operationalization of valid research. Lederer suggested organizing, evaluating, and incentivizing the use of PCOR and real-world evidence tools to promote the generation of decision-grade real-world evidence. She added that this could essentially be a real-world PCOR toolbox. While many of the tools that would need to be included in such a toolbox are available today, many researchers do not know that they exist or how to find them. Making a toolbox readily available could also result in the development of a framework for conducting real-world PCOR.

Lederer noted that the development of new tools is also necessary. For example, raw data need to be transformed into variables that can be analyzed. For federal data sets that are available for public use, this could involve creating standardized, validated measures and measure sets to help operationalize and augment the use of the data. It would also be useful to create disease-specific tools, which could include master protocols for real-world evidence that centralize the relevant expertise needed for high-priority research questions. One potential model that could be leveraged is the Reagan-Udall Foundation for the U.S. Food and Drug Administration (FDA) in collaboration with Friends of Cancer Research's COVID-19 Evidence Accelerator, which convenes health care stakeholders to use a common data shell and protocol to run analyses for high-priority research questions for COVID-19.

The creation of a toolbox would not be easy, Lederer acknowledged. Part of the process would be reviewing all of the available resources, triaging them, harmonizing them, and identifying how they can be used for regulatory decision making, clinical decision making, policy decision making, or personal decision making.

Lederer also emphasized the importance of transparency for building credibility to advance the science of real-world PCOR. This includes data transparency, protocol transparency (e.g., preregistering studies to address potential concerns over hacking and data dredging), and publishing the results regardless of the outcome.

Lederer argued that science should not be proprietary. She highlighted the benefits of a culture where inferential protocols are made publicly available, not only in the interest of reproducibility and replicability, but also because otherwise one might not have access to the full scope of expertise necessary to conduct a high-quality study. She said that transparency could be accelerated through incentives, such as tying access to federal data sets or federal funding to the registration of the studies and the publication of the research protocols and results.

Lara Mangravite, Sage Bionetworks, focused on the governance component of the data infrastructure, discussing issues related to the governance structures used to enable research that typically involves data from multiple sources. She briefly described the governance structure of the National Center for Advancing Translational Sciences (NCATS) National COVID Cohort Collaborative (N3C), which assembled medical records from approximately 65 medical centers from across the country into one central repository with the purpose of using it for research.

Mangravite noted that, typically, one of the important roles within governance structures is that of a data steward. The data steward is responsible for the technology that allows the data to be managed and used and for the legal agreements between the data donors and the data users. The N3C effort, Mangravite said, illustrated the challenge of integrating data across systems. She argued that data interoperability between health systems and data linkage across sources requires increased investment in data quality standards.

Mangravite also discussed the evaluation of care, which in her view often requires integrating data on lived experience beyond the data captured in the medical system. Person-centered research necessitates data that comes directly from the patient, in part because clinical care is impacted by a variety of factors not captured in the medical record. She noted, however, that obtaining data on individuals' lived experiences increasingly involves private and sensitive information, and that it is important to consider the value proposition from the perspective of the individual providing the data. Sage Bionetworks works with a lot of sensor data, and Mangravite pointed out that a person's characteristics impact what researchers see, for example, in the accelerometry data from someone walking down the street. This has implications for how the data are analyzed, but also how the data are managed and what the privacy considerations and value proposition are.

Mangravite said that most discussions of data sharing involve researchers acting as data stewards and exchanging data. These discussions typically do not involve the individuals whose data are shared. The expectation is that these individuals would simply need to trust the data governance to happen in their interests. This might not be an acceptable situation, given that for many types of data the risks and benefits are not well understood. Mangravite argued that approaches to data governance need to change; they need to go beyond simply making the informed consent processes more dynamic and involving the people being represented in the data in the practice of the research itself, throughout the lifecycle of the studies. This is especially important because the implications of the use of the data are not always clear at the stage when the data are collected. Involving the individuals providing the data in the study would at a minimum ensure transparency about how the data are being used, and ideally would also allow room to impact decisions related to the data use.

One of Sage Bionetwork's current projects, called the MindKind Study, aims to identify self-management strategies that might work for youth with anxiety or depression. Mangravite said that to observe youths' mental health states in combination with self-management strategies or other activities they may be engaging in, and to do that dynamically over time, requires a lot of data that are not found in medical records. She and her colleagues are examining whether integrating youth into the data governance and stewardship model impacts their willingness to participate. They asked youth and researchers in several countries a series of questions related to data governance (e.g., their preferences related to who can access the data, who controls the data, what kind of research can be conducted with the data, and so on). They found agreement between the youth and researchers on responses to many of the questions, including, for example, on who can access the data. However, perspectives differed on some questions, such as, for example, on who control the data. Mangravite said that they are now conducting a study that aims to better understand differences between what is preferred and what is acceptable, and looks at how potential changes based on what they learned would impact willingness to participate.

In summary, Mangravite highlighted the need for integration of data across systems, and the integration of participants into the research lifecycle, as two of the areas that need the most attention in terms of the data infrastructure. To integrate participants, her specific suggestions were to focus on enabling richer understanding of lived experiences outside of the medical system, support the alignment of research questions with community needs, and support capacity building for translating research outcomes into action.

DISCUSSION

As with the previous session, the formal presentations on PCOR methods were followed by additional discussion among the participants.

One topic that was explored in further detail and emerged as a key theme was the need for a more holistic "timeline" view of people's experiences. The main challenges associated with developing longitudinal data sets are the costs and barriers associated with following and identifying people over time and with linking information from different sources. The fragmentation of the health care system and the lack of unique identifiers were reoccurring themes in the discussion of barriers. The limited availability of timestamps associated with the data that are available was also highlighted.

A theme that had been explored in detail in the committee's first workshop and was revisited by the participants in this one was the need to broaden research perspectives from the patient to the person in a broader sense, bringing in additional data on factors that are outside of the health care provider system. Integrating relevant data that go beyond provider databases represents its own challenges, but a timeline view that expands beyond a person's experiences within the health care system would greatly increase our ability to understand, for example, chronic diseases.

The topic of data privacy was also discussed, including concerns about the unknowns in the area of potential re-identification. The discussion echoed points made by the speakers in the previous two sessions, highlighting tensions related to different perspectives on whether fully de-identified data is a realistic goal, and whether access to identified data with strong security and penalties for misuse would be an option. This topic, and the committee's conclusions, are addressed further in Chapter 4.

Another theme that emerged during the discussion was the importance of engaging patients in the research process and being transparent about the methods used to generate findings. Participants also discussed the need to balance the goals of transparency with the interests of stakeholders who would like to keep some of the information proprietary, and there are efforts under way to develop approaches that achieve this balance. However, widespread adoption would be more likely if there were incentives and a central repository in place.

CONCLUSIONS

One theme that emerged from the session on methods for PCOR was the potential usefulness of adopting a timeline or longitudinal perspective on understanding a person's journey through the health care system, and through life events that have a relevance to health more broadly. Several changes could facilitate this shift, as summarized in Conclusion 3-1.

CONCLUSION 3-1: The ability to adopt a longitudinal, comprehensive perspective on an individual's journey could open new opportunities for

patient-centered outcomes research. The shift could be facilitated by focusing on efforts to
- simplify the integration of data across the research data ecosystem;
- address challenges posed by the limitations associated with health identifiers;
- incorporate person-generated data into health data systems; and
- leverage real-world data to expand the timeline view of a person's health-related experiences.

Speakers emphasized the need for transparency and for consideration of related scientific principles, such as reproducibility of the data and methods used for PCOR. These considerations are important for all types of data and analysis, but the increasing use of tools such as machine learning and natural language processing raises the question of whether best practices can ensure that these tools do not have negative social impacts.

CONCLUSION 3-2: Observing scientific best practices, including those of transparency and ethical use of data, is essential to generate trust in patient-centered outcomes research among all stakeholders, including the public and researchers. This is important both for observational data and for emerging data sources and methods.

The session on methods highlighted the importance of interpreting best practices around the dissemination of the research broadly. That is, best practices apply not only to the sharing of results but also to other resources and components associated with the research process, such as the software developed for analyses. Sharing all these resources ensures that the data can be widely used and that the research can be replicated. Ultimately the goal of patient-centered outcomes research is to benefit people, so the question of what happens to the research after it is done, and the sharing of the information with those whose data are being used, also deserves further attention.

CONCLUSION 3-3: The results of patient-centered outcomes research (and research in general) are only replicable and are most useful when the underlying data and comprehensive research documentation (such as analytic code) are made available for use by others.

4

Data Policies and Other Data Infrastructure Considerations

This chapter summarizes the workshop discussions centered on data policies and other data infrastructure considerations. Speakers in this session were asked to focus on the questions below. The chapter concludes with the committee's conclusions.

- What data policies are likely to be most relevant for the patient-centered outcomes research (PCOR) data infrastructure looking forward?
- What role can the Office of the Assistant Secretary for Planning and Evaluation (ASPE) play in supporting these policies for PCOR studies?
- What characteristics of HHS' public mission, programs, or authorities could be leveraged?

Pamela Riley, District of Columbia Department of Healthcare Finance, discussed policy considerations to support PCOR on the social determinants of health (SDOH). She focused on ways to address unmet social needs in health care systems and health care settings in order to improve health care delivery. This includes addressing basic resource needs both in the clinical setting and at an individual patient level, as well as using data to address population health issues. Riley noted that the District of Columbia Medicaid agency is currently working to help develop a community-level social needs screening referral and resource inventory and is also working on ways to support data collection, sharing, and use to improve clinical care delivery and population health.

Riley emphasized the importance of being aware of considerations specific to data on SDOH, including sensitivities around data collection, such as the issue of what the data are going to be used for. She noted that collecting data on social needs, such as whether a person has enough food to eat or has unmet financial needs, can be particularly sensitive from the perspective of those who are being asked to provide the data. Because of this, it is important to think about best practices for collecting these types of data to assure that the information is complete and can be reliably used to inform practice. Riley highlighted the related need to involve stakeholders at both the community and patient levels, as well as the need for transparency, noting that lack of trust often hinders efforts of this type and that involving stakeholders could potentially help address this. It is necessary, she said, to engage people, patients, communities, and other stakeholders every step of the way in designing and implementing data collection approaches and research strategies that people are actually onboard with and that will be reliable and useful.

Riley also noted the importance of considering ahead of time how the data will be used. Is it to inform clinical care delivery? Is it to inform population health at the health-system, national, state, or local level? Is it for academic research? The uses of the data need to be considered when thinking about policies around data infrastructures. A related consideration is what specific data are needed depending on the intended purpose. For example, what data does a hospital need in order to evaluate community-level interventions? What does a state need for planning purposes?

Data sharing was another topic discussed by Riley. Approaches to data sharing need to consider the sensitivities, and balance the need to reduce how many times people are being asked to provide the same information with the need to ensure that those who provide the data have confidence in giving permission for the intended uses, which could range from improving their own care to fulfilling a broader purpose.

In terms of interoperability and combining data from multiple data sources, Riley argued that clinical claims data that are being collected from nonclinical entities is one area that represents a challenge.

Concerning consent management, Riley considered this to be an area whose challenges need to be addressed in a systematic way that is broadly applicable. This is particularly important if the goal is to support whole-person studies that include data on physical health, SDOH, and behavioral health. She argued that an infrastructure needs to be put in place for consent management, to facilitate best practices in data sharing for research, and to improve patient care.

Riley pointed to a particular need to identify best practices that work at the local level, because data collection, data sharing, and interventions often have a local focus. She also emphasized the need to develop an infrastructure for data collection by nonhealth care entities. Community-based behavioral health providers and mental health and substance abuse disorder providers, she said, are especially likely to be lagging behind in their capacity to implement electronic health records. Community-based organizations, in general, would benefit both from being able to participate in health information exchanges and from being able to share data in a standardized way.

Touching on the role of the federal government, Riley said there is a need to build an evidence base for what works. There is room for a federal voice in this, she argued, specifically concerning interventions that work to address SDOH related to health care delivery, what works to address needs and in what settings, and what works among which populations. There is also a need to better understand what data collection approaches are most effective in obtaining complete, reliable data. Related to that, there is a need to understand what gives people confidence and comfort in how the data will be used so that they are willing to share the information. More broadly, there is a need for an infrastructure that facilitates the involvement, at every step of the way, of those who are providing the data.

Abel Kho, Northwestern University, argued for a need to improve the quality of the identifying information being collected, something particularly important because the need for record linkages is becoming increasingly common. As an example, Kho mentioned the use of speeding cameras by the police and how that information is linked to other databases before a speeding ticket is mailed. He also discussed the City of Chicago's use of Clearview AI for facial recognition, which has then been linked to additional data sets to identify potential criminal activity. Kho said that the use of these technologies raises questions that also have implications for health research. For example, in Chicago, areas with high crime rates also have high rates of chronic disease. Kho echoed Riley's points related to being thoughtful about why the data are collected, who they are collected from, and what the needs of the communities are. He also emphasized the need for community input on data collection, for example in the case of whether and where to use street cameras.

Kho noted that the way people identify themselves impacts researchers' ability to perform record linkages. He said that it is important to consider not only the implications of research bias, but also social bias. For example, gender information has historically not been considered useful for record linkages, because this information typically has binary values in electronic health records. However, the concept of gender identity has changed dramatically over the years, and it is now considered to be a much more complex construct. Data systems are not set up for capturing a lot of this information yet, but Kho said that collecting detailed data that reflects how people self-identify is important for a variety of reasons, including understanding their sense of self-identity and to avoid discriminatory practices.

Those who are interested in data need to be thoughtful about identity concepts, which are evolving and are shaped by the social context, Kho argued. The information available in health records to identify a person for the purposes of record linkages is also constantly changing. While binary gender is captured in virtually all electronic health records, Kho and his colleagues have been noticing an increase in the availability of data on sex assigned at birth and sexual orientation. They also found that social security numbers are less and less likely to be available in electronic health records, while email addresses are increasingly available, and are becoming more useful for record linkage. Other types of information that might be captured and useful for record linkages include driver's license images and information about the person's occupation. Kho said that the latter is largely driven by COVID-19. He argued that it is important to think about how to balance considerations such as privacy versus a "big brother" approach, or category labels versus self-identity, in a dynamic, constantly shifting environment.

In Kho's view, the data available today are subject to historical and social biases, even as the data and identities themselves are constantly changing. Therefore, it is necessary to understand when and how the data were collected. Kho said that policies can help with data hygiene, that is, with standardizing data collections, which is easier to do than addressing data bias. He underscored that data bias is not solely a technical issue. To address it requires engaging stakeholders early and often, particularly among at-risk or hidden populations.

Julia Adler-Milstein, University of California, San Francisco, focused her remarks on the need to use policy levers to advance interoperability, which she described as applicable to many of the topics discussed throughout the day, including data standards, consent management, approaches to identification and patient matching, governance, and incentives to share data. She said that the main lesson from her work in this area is that meaningful progress cannot be made on interoperability if policy efforts, and in particular federal policy efforts, are limited to convening activities. She argued that there is a need for policy actions to address some of the market failures, in particular the lack of incentives to invest in the types of infrastructure discussed throughout the workshop. While recognizing that policy is a blunt instrument, Adler-Milstein said that the types of policies the federal government and states need to focus on are those that create strong incentives to engage in interoperable data sharing.

Although many capabilities have been developed for interoperability supporting PCOR, Adler-Milstein argued, the challenge remains getting those capabilities adopted at scale. She said that to facilitate such adoption,

DATA POLICIES AND OTHER DATA INFRASTRUCTURE CONSIDERATIONS

there is a need to measure and incentivize conformance to existing standards. An example, she mentioned the patient-reported outcomes Fast Healthcare Interoperability Resources implementation guides. These standards are available, but they are not federally required, and there are no test tools that would make it possible to determine whether someone is actually conforming to the standards.

Adler-Milstein also discussed the United States Core Data for Interoperability (USCDI) as a policy vehicle to promote scale. USCDI is a set of data elements that health systems must make available through an application programming interface (via their electronic health records), and that set of data elements will, by definition, expand over time. Thus, Adler-Milstein said that data that are included in USCDI are expected to become available at scale. She added that the data also need to conform to specified standards, but that it is not clear to what extent this will be measured and enforced. Without such measurement and enforcement, there is a risk that a lot of manual work will be required to make use of the data, despite widespread availability.

Adler-Milstein provided several examples of how the framework she suggested could work in several domains. In the case of patients, robust identity data are needed, because when these data exist and they are conformant, it is possible to perform data matching across sources. Demographic data exist within USCDI, and they have been part of the first wave of required data elements. What is needed now is ongoing conformance assessment and incentives to address poor conformance.

On the patient-centered side, there is a need to support efforts that advance robust identity matching across data sources, in part to overcome the challenges posed by data fragmentation, but also to address the need for longitudinal data. Some examples of projects that are targeting identity matching to support more comprehensive and longitudinal data are Gravity and the Da Vinci Payer Coverage Decision Exchange. Adler-Milstein argued that the first step toward developing policies that support scaling PCOR activities would be to identify which use cases are important to prioritize. In turn, this would facilitate adding patient-centered outcomes data that support those use cases into USCDI.

Deven McGraw, Ciitizen, provided an overview of the existing privacy laws that govern how data are accessed, used, and shared for research. The four laws that are most relevant are

1. The Health Insurance Portability and Accountability Act of 1996 (HIPAA).
2. "Part 2", which relates to regulations on substance abuse data confidentiality.

3. The Family Educational Rights and Privacy Act (FERPA), which covers educational institutions.
4. The Privacy Act, which covers federal government data resources.

In the case of some entities, more than one of these laws might apply.

McGraw said that HIPAA has the most impact on PCOR data. She noted that HIPAA does not cover all health data, only the data of covered entities and their business associates. This coverage, however, is broad, and it includes most doctors and hospitals, health plans, and contractors. Exceptions might be some doctors practicing concierge medicine and some mental health professionals.

McGraw noted that HIPAA only governs identifiable data, which is known as protected health information (PHI). The disclosure of PHI is permitted for uses that fall in the category that combines treatment, payment, and operations. Public health disclosures are included among the permitted uses. McGraw said that in general, HIPAA was designed to enable data flows within a health care system, and data flows that are usual, expected, and customary, but it might be important to disclose only the minimum information necessary, particularly when the data are not used for treatment.

PHI can also be disclosed for research. This use of identifiable data was not considered to be standard and usual, but rather something that would require the consent of the person whose data would be used. However, regulators have recognized that requiring authorization for all research might not be feasible, so provisions exist that allow for a privacy board or an institutional review board to waive the consent requirement. Recent guidance from HHS enables an entity that is covered by HIPAA to obtain broad consent for research, instead of study-specific consent, for future uses of data. There are also provisions for the use of limited data sets, which involves removing some identifying information but allowing some identifying data elements to be left in.

McGraw said that the Common Rule is not included among the laws that govern data disclosure, because the Common Rule is a research ethics rule, not a privacy rule. However, there are many similarities between how HIPAA and the Common Rule govern research uses of data.

Data that are de-identified are not covered by HIPAA, and McGraw noted that it is also typical for privacy laws globally to only apply to identifiable data. One approach to de-identification is the Safe Harbor method, which involves the removal of identifiers that fall into 18 categories. It is also possible to rely on expert opinion (such as that of a statistician) to determine whether there is a risk of re-identification for a particular data set.

McGraw said that the use of data that are not identifiable falls outside of the realm of privacy regulations and that is why this type of data is

DATA POLICIES AND OTHER DATA INFRASTRUCTURE CONSIDERATIONS

widely used in research, but it is also why there is a robust commercial trade of unidentified data. She noted that data that are not identifiable are not aggregated data, but individual-level data that have been stripped of identifiers or manipulated in some other way (e.g., by noise being introduced) to reduce the risk of re-identification. She emphasized that the standard is very low risk, rather than zero risk, and that there are no penalties to protect those data against re-identification.

Some state laws provide stronger data protections than HIPAA, and McGraw said that HIPAA does not preempt such laws. State laws typically govern access to data on minors, with minors in some states holding the right to consent to the disclosure of certain types of data for research, to third parties, or to their parents. Other states have robust consent laws that are not limited to minors, but as with HIPAA, they typically cover only identifiable data.

McGraw also noted that while HIPAA addresses permitted disclosures of data, it does not *require* the sharing of data for research purposes. However, the new information blocking rules[1] that went into effect in April 2021 create a presumption for sharing electronic health information for any lawful purpose, including research. These rules apply to health care providers, certified electronic health records vendors, and health information exchanges. Initially they will cover the USCDI data elements, but eventually they will cover all electronic health information. The penalties for "blocking" the sharing are up to $1 million per incident for electronic health records vendors and health information exchanges. The providers are referred to the Centers for Medicare & Medicaid Services (CMS) for "appropriate disincentives." There are eight Safe Harbor provisions that allow an entity covered by these rules to decline a request for data sharing. These provisions are related to concerns such as privacy, security, harm, and infeasibility.

McGraw said that there has not yet been any enforcement since the rules went into effect (approximately 2 months prior to the workshop), and the rules around enforcement are still under consideration. McGraw noted that providers who want to decline a request for data have to attest to CMS that they are not information blocking, and if that claim does not hold up it could result in a False Claims Act penalty.

Another area where there are new developments concerns patients' rights to their own data. Patients already have the right to their data under HIPAA, but this is now being more robustly enforced. Information blocking rules prioritize access by patients or apps acting on their behalf. There are also provisions to allow people to send data from their electronic health

---

[1] For more on information blocking, see https://www.healthit.gov/topic/information-blocking.

records directly to third parties, such as researchers, but these are still pending implementation.

Don Detmer, University of Virginia, shared his views on policy reforms necessary for robust data sharing for PCOR. He noted that HIPAA was passed into law in 1996, before use of the Internet became widespread. Today the use of data for health research is still defined by the rules that were developed based on "pre-Internet thinking," with some minor regulatory tweaks taking place over the years. Detmer said that while there are some promising developments, it is time to ask whether this system is working.

The societal context today differs from what it was before the Internet. A large volume of new forms of data is available, and there is growing interest in goals such as equity, engaging patients and citizen-scientists, supporting precision medicine, and supporting precision health. Detmer said that continuing to do things within the current framework is going to be less than optimal. He argued that the basic structure for conducting research needs a reset to allow for informed public policy development that addresses new societal desires, with citizen-scientists, patients, and health providers as primary players in the data system, along with covered entities and business associates.

Detmer argued for reviving and enacting the HIPAA changes included in section 1124 in H.R.6, the initial 21st Century Cures Act. The revisions proposed at the time were to expand the access, use, and sharing of PHI from treatment, payment, and health care operations to also include "data research." In 2015, H.R.6 passed the House by a vote of 344 to 77, but it did not pass the Senate.

Detmer described several current prevailing options for data sharing, clinical registries, and de-identified data sets, each of which he considers flawed. Registries with individuals donating their data are time-consuming to build and maintain and typically do not contain enough information. The aggregating of data sets that are limited to begin with has limited use when diverse data are sought. Using de-identified data poses additional challenges because authentication is difficult or impossible with diverse data sets.

Looking at potential solutions, Detmer wondered whether regulations could allow the use of text or e-mail for the sharing of PHI for research, and in particular the use of text or e-mail for obtaining approval from individuals. This would address the burden and challenges associated with obtaining written consent. He also wondered whether authorization could be created that would allow specified entities, such as the Patient-Centered Outcomes Research Institute, to securely access PHI in relevant databases, without individual consent. Detmer observed that while this is probably not realistic within the current system, it is allowed in some countries. He also suggested developing a system for unique patient identifiers, which becomes especially important for the use of longitudinal data. Secure options for handling this type of information exist today.

Detmer argued for the need for a National Academies study that would develop a vision and a plan for a sound functional replacement for HIPAA. He mentioned a prior study that could serve as a model.[2] His desired goals and capabilities for the new framework would include robust system security for all data and "no-questions-asked opt-in" privacy for sharing personal data. He added that the data sharing would assure (1) system trust, (2) compassionate care, (3) scientific health care practice and evaluation for individuals and populations, (4) support for citizen-science and special populations, (5) secure unique personal identifiers, (6) pandemic data fitness and management, and (7) automation of all business operations and other administrative functions to reduce the time investment required.

DISCUSSION

One topic that was discussed by workshop participants in additional detail related to the role of the federal government in incentivizing the adoption of standards and assuring conformance. Participants cautioned about the burden associated with requirements of this type, and the potentially disproportionate burden on smaller health care providers.

A theme that emerged from the discussion was the need to better understand what type of information is truly important to people. Participants discussed projects such as *Pastors 4 PCOR* that involved community-based organizations to facilitate community engagement in research, identify specific disease priorities, and build trust.

Another topic that was revisited was the desire to link data from different sources and the consent and privacy challenges associated with this. In many cases complications related to consent prevent data sharing and linking, even when people are interested in making their data available for research. There was debate about the extent of public support for the concept of a unique identifier and whether the potential benefits are becoming more widely recognized. Technical solutions, such as tokenization, are creating new options that did not exist before, and this presents an opportunity to reassess these questions in new light.

Participants discussed the need to revisit HIPAA, which was passed in 1996, before the spread of social media, apps that require broad consent for data sharing, and expansive databases that are publicly available or can be purchased. HIPAA, in its current form, is not focused on privacy, and it

---

[2] Institute of Medicine. (1997). *The Computer-Based Patient Record: An Essential Technology for Health Care* (revised edition). Washington, DC: National Academy Press. https://doi.org/10.17226/5306.

only covers a small slice of health data. Many aspects of the regulation are outdated. Solutions could range from updating HIPAA "at the margins" to comprehensive privacy legislation. Participants commented that ASPE could have an enormously influential role in bringing stakeholders together on this issue.

CONCLUSIONS

This session echoed discussions from previous sessions about the importance of transparency in how the data will be used. Speakers also echoed the need to involve the people whose data are being used, as well as their communities, in decisions at each stage of the process, from data collection through research and dissemination. Building and maintaining trust with those whose data are being sought is essential to ensure that the data obtained are representative, complete, and reliable. This is especially important when the data could be perceived as sensitive, as is the case with some SDOH information.

> **CONCLUSION 4-1: Building and maintaining trust among the people and communities whose data are being sought for research is essential for high-quality data. Including representatives of consumers and patients in the research process to understand how to measure health impacts that matter to individuals is an important component in building trust.**

The workshop made it clear that there are concerns about the laws and rules governing data access and data sharing. HIPAA, in particular, was developed several decades ago, and its approach to setting thresholds for data disclosures makes it outdated. There is a need for a new framework with guardrails that balance the risk of disclosure with the need for research that improves peoples' health. This includes a need for a critical review of current privacy legislation, an understanding of public perspectives, and the development of recommendations for revisions or reform that would be applicable to the protection of health data in the post-Internet world, with a focus on preventing misuses of the data.

> **CONCLUSION 4-2: This is an opportune time to revisit and update the legislation and rules governing data privacy and the sharing of data for research.**

Appendix A

Biographical Sketches of Committee Members

GEORGE ISHAM (NAM) (*Chair*) is a senior fellow at the HealthPartners Institute and a senior advisor for the Alliance of Community Health Plans. Previously, he served as a senior advisor to the board of directors and the senior management team of HealthPartners, and prior to that, he was HealthPartners' medical director and chief health officer, responsible for quality of care and health and health care improvement. He has been active in health policy, serving as a member of the Centers for Disease Control and Prevention's Task Force on Community Preventive Services, a member of the Agency for Healthcare Research and Quality's United States Preventive Services Task Force, as a founding co-chair of the National Committee for Quality Assurance's committee on performance measurement as well as founding co-chair of the National Quality Forum's Measurement Application Partnership. He has an M.D. from the University of Illinois at Chicago and an M.S. in preventive medicine and administrative medicine from the University of Wisconsin–Madison.

JOHN F.P. BRIDGES is professor and vice chair of academic affairs in the Department of Biomedical Informatics at The Ohio State University (OSU) College of Medicine. He is also a professor in the Department of Surgery and an adjunct professor in both the Division of Epidemiology at the OSU College of Public Health and Department of Health Behavior and Society at the Johns Hopkins Bloomberg School of Public Health. Prior to joining OSU he was on the faculty of the Johns Hopkins Bloomberg School of Public Health, the Department of Tropical Hygiene and Public Health within University of Heidelberg School of Medicine, and the Department of

Epidemiology and Biostatistics within the Case Western Reserve University School of Medicine. He has previously held positions in the Department of Economics at the Weatherhead School of Management at Case Western Reserve University, the National Bureau of Economic Research, Center for Medicine in the Public Interest, and the Center for Health Economics, Research and Evaluation in Australia. He has a Ph.D. in economics from the City University of New York.

JULIE BYNUM is the Margaret Terpenning Professor of Medicine in the Division of Geriatric Medicine and vice chair for Faculty Affairs in the Department of Internal Medicine at the University of Michigan. She is also a research professor in the Institute of Gerontology, Geriatric Center Associate Director for Health Policy and Research, and a member of the Institute for Healthcare Policy and Innovation. She currently leads a portfolio of National Institutes of Health–funded research that examines the quality of care, diagnosis, and treatment of people with Alzheimer's disease and related dementia in the community, nursing homes, and assisted living and is the director of the Center to Accelerate Population Research in Alzheimer's. She is currently a member of the National Academies of Sciences, Engineering, and Medicine's Forum on Aging, Disability, and Independence and was a member of a National Academies committee that authored *Vital Signs: Core Metrics for Health and Health Care Progress*. She has an M.P.H. from the Johns Hopkins University School of Hygiene & Public Health and an M.D. from the Johns Hopkins University School of Medicine.

ANGELA DOBES is vice president of the Crohn's & Colitis Foundation's IBD Plexus Program, a research-information exchange platform designed to centralize data and biosamples from diverse research initiatives to advance science, accelerate precision medicine, and transform the care of Inflammatory Bowel Disease (IBD) patients. She has previously worked for clinical technology and pharmaceutical organizations, where she has led implementation of various technology solutions focused on business optimization and accelerating the delivery of new therapies to patients safely. She is currently serving as principal investigator on a study to enhance engagement, research participation, and collaboration through the IBD Partners Patient Powered Research Network. She has an M.A. in public health from the Icahn School of Medicine at Mount Sinai.

OLUWADAMILOLA FAYANJU is the Helen O. Dickens Presidential Associate Professor of Surgery at the Perelman School of Medicine at the University of Pennsylvania. She is also chief of breast surgery at Penn Medicine. Previously, she was associate professor of surgery and population health sciences in the Duke University School of Medicine and director of the

Durham VA Breast Clinic. She was also associate director for Disparities & Value in Healthcare with Duke Forge, Duke University's center for actionable data science. In 2019, she was recognized by the National Academy of Medicine as an Emerging Leader in Health and Medicine Scholar. She received an M.A. in comparative literature from Harvard University and her M.D. and M.P.H.S. from the Washington University in St. Louis.

DEBORAH ESTRIN (NAE/NAM) is a professor of computer science at Cornell Tech where she holds the Robert V. Tishman founder's chair, serves as the associate dean for impact, and is an affiliate faculty at Weill Cornell Medicine. Her research activities include technologies for caregiving, immersive health, small data, participatory sensing, and public interest technology. Estrin was an Amazon Scholar, and before joining Cornell University she was founding director of the National Science Foundation's Center for Embedded Networked Sensing at the University of California, Los Angeles, pioneering the development of mobile and wireless systems to collect and analyze real-time data about the physical world. Estrin cofounded the nonprofit startup, Open mHealth, and has served on several scientific advisory boards for early-stage mobile health startups. She has a Ph.D. in electrical engineering and computer science from the Massachusetts Institute of Technology.

CONSTANTINE GATSONIS is the Henry Ledyard Goddard University Professor of Statistical Sciences, director of statistical sciences, and professor of biostatistics at Brown University. He was founding director of the Center for Statistical Sciences and founding chair of the Department of Biostatistics at Brown University. He is a leading authority on the evaluation of diagnostic and screening tests and has made major contributions to the development of methods for medical technology assessment and health services and outcomes research. He is a world leader in methods for applying and synthesizing evidence on diagnostic tests in medicine and is currently developing methods for comparative effectiveness research in diagnosis and prediction and radiomics. Since 2016 he has served as a statistical consultant for the *New England Journal of Medicine* and was the founding editor-in-chief of *Health Services and Outcomes Research Methods*. He has a Ph.D. in mathematical statistics from Cornell University.

ROBERT GOERGE is a senior research fellow at Chapin Hall at the University of Chicago. He is also a senior fellow and founder of the Master's Degree in Computational Analysis in Public Policy at the University of Chicago Harris School of Public Policy. His research is focused on improving the available data and information on children and families, particularly those who require specialized services related to maltreatment, disability,

poverty, or violence. At Chapin Hall, he is principal investigator for the Family Self-Sufficiency Data Center, the Linking Federal Data to Local Data project, and the National Survey for Early Care and Education. He currently serves on the National Academies of Sciences, Engineering, and Medicine's Committee on National Statistics. He has a Ph.D. in social policy from the University of Chicago.

GEORGE HRIPCSAK (NAM) is the Vivian Beaumont Allen Professor and chair of the Department of Biomedical Informatics at Columbia University. He is also the director of medical informatics services for New York Presbyterian Hospital. He is also a board-certified internist. He led the effort to create the Arden Syntax, a language for representing health knowledge that has become a national standard. As chair of the American Medical Informatics Association Standards Committee, he coordinated the medical informatics community response to the Department of Health and Human Services for the health informatics standards rules under the Health Insurance Portability and Accountability Act of 1996. His current research is on the clinical information stored in electronic health records. Using data mining techniques, he is developing the methods necessary to support clinical research and patient safety initiatives. He has an M.D. and an M.S. in biostatistics from Columbia University.

LISA IEZZONI (NAM) is professor of medicine at Harvard Medical School and the Health Policy Research Center at Massachusetts General Hospital, where she served as director in the past. She was previously co-director of research in the Division of General Medicine and Primary Care at Beth Israel Deaconess Medical Center in Boston. Her research focuses on risk adjustment methods for predicting cost and clinical outcomes of care, and on health care experiences and outcomes of persons with disabilities. She has served on the editorial boards of the *Annals of Internal Medicine*, the *Journal of General Internal Medicine*, *Health Affairs*, *Medical Care*, *Health Services Research*, and the *Disability and Health Journal*, among others. She has an M.D. from Harvard Medical School and an M.Sc. from the Harvard T.H. Chan School of Public Health.

S. CLAIBORNE JOHNSTON (NAM) is the inaugural dean of Dell Medical School, vice president for medical affairs, and the Frank and Charmaine Denius Distinguished Dean's Chair in medical leadership at The University of Texas at Austin. Previously, Johnston was associate vice chancellor for research at the University of California, San Francisco (UCSF). He also directed the Clinical and Translational Science Institute and founded the UCSF Center for Healthcare Value. His research is focused on clinical trials and health services research in stroke. He is also an expert in medical education, research administration, health care value, and population health. He has led several large-cohort studies of cerebrovascular disease and three international multicenter randomized trials. He has an M.D. from Harvard Medical School and a Ph.D. in epidemiology from the University of California, Berkeley.

MIGUEL MARINO is an associate professor with joint appointments in the School of Public Health Division of Biostatistics and the Department of Family Medicine at Oregon Health & Science University. His research focuses on the development and implementation of novel statistical methodology to address complexities associated with the use of electronic health records (EHRs) to study changes in policy, using EHRs to study health disparities, validation of EHRs as a reliable source for observational studies, pragmatic randomized trials, and preventive health maintenance. He was selected by the National Academy of Medicine as an Emerging Leader in Health and Medicine Scholar. He has a Ph.D. in biostatistics from Harvard University.

ELIZABETH McGLYNN (NAM) is vice president for Kaiser Permanente Research and executive director for the Center for Effectiveness & Safety Research at Kaiser Permanente. She is also interim senior associate dean for research and scholarships at the Kaiser Permanente Bernard J. Tyson School of Medicine. She is an internationally known expert on methods for evaluating the appropriateness and quality of health care delivery. She has led major initiatives to evaluate health reform options under consideration at the federal and state levels. She is the lead of Kaiser Permanente & Strategic Partners Patient Outcomes Research To Advance Learning (PORTAL) Network. She was a member of the Strategic Framework Board, which provided a blueprint for the National Quality Forum on the development of a national quality measurement and reporting system. She chaired the board of AcademyHealth, served on the board of the American Board of Internal Medicine Foundation, and served on the Board of Providence-Little Company of Mary Hospital Service Area in Southern California. She has a Ph.D. in public policy from RAND Graduate School.

DAVID MELTZER (NAM) is the Fanny L. Pritzker Professor in the Department of Medicine, chief of the section of Hospital Medicine and faculty in the Department of Economics and Harris School of Public Policy at the University of Chicago. He is also director of the Center for Health and the Social Sciences and of the Urban Health Lab at the University of Chicago. His research explores problems in health economics and public policy with a focus on the theoretical foundations of medical cost-effectiveness analysis and the cost and quality of hospital care. Since 1997, he has developed the inpatient general medicine services at the University of Chicago as a Learning Health Care System to produce knowledge on how to improve the care of hospitalized patients, mobilizing the clinical care process to generate and learn from diverse data from electronic health records, claims data, patient interviews, and biospecimens on more than 100,000 patients. He is the lead of the University of Chicago network site as part of the Chicago Area Patient-Centered Outcomes Research Network. He has an M.D. and a Ph.D. in economics from the University of Chicago.

PAUL C. TANG (NAM) is an adjunct professor in the Clinical Excellence Research Center at Stanford University and an internist at the Palo Alto Medical Foundation. He was formerly chief innovation and technology officer at the Palo Alto Medical Foundation and vice president, chief health transformation officer at IBM Watson Health. He has more than 25 years of executive leadership experience in health information technology within medical groups, health systems, and corporate settings. He has directed innovation and technology teams in provider organizations, academic institutions, corporate research organizations, and product development organizations. Most recently, he led the creation, development, deployment, and evaluation of the application of artificial intelligence to physician point-of-care solutions integrated within an electronic health record system. He also led a corporate enterprise-wide design team. He has chaired numerous federal and private-sector advisory and professional association groups related to health information technology and policy. He received an M.S. in electrical engineering from Stanford University and his M.D. from the University of California, San Francisco.

Appendix B

Workshop Agenda

Building Data Capacity for Patient-Centered Outcomes Research:
An Agenda for 2021 to 2030

Virtual Workshop 2: Data Standards, Methods, and Policy

May 24, 2021, 11 am–5 pm EDT

OBJECTIVES FOR THE WORKSHOP
- Identify data standards and methods that can make the PCOR data infrastructure more useful for research and other data needs.
- Identify data policies that are needed to facilitate the continued development and operation of the PCOR data infrastructure.
- Discuss what HHS is best positioned to address and support, and how the agency could maximize resources available for the PCOR data infrastructure (representing 4% of the PCOR trust fund), in the context of the HHS public mission, authorities, programs, and data resources.

11:00–11:05 am EDT   **Goals for the Workshop**

GEORGE ISHAM (Committee Chair), HealthPartners Institute

11:05 am–1:05 pm EDT	**PCOR Data Standards** Discussion questions: • What data standards could make the PCOR data infrastructure more useful for research and other data needs? What data standards are likely to become more relevant looking forward? What needs to be prioritized? • What role can ASPE play in supporting effective standards to build data capacity that supports PCOR studies? What characteristics of HHS's public mission, programs, or authorities could be leveraged? **Moderators:** GEORGE HRIPCSAK, Columbia University, and DAVID MELTZER, University of Chicago **Speakers:** JOHN HALAMKA, Mayo Clinic SHAUN GRANNIS, Regenstrief Institute EVELYN GALLEGO, EMI Advisors RACHEL RICHESSON, University of Michigan PATRICK RYAN, Janssen Research and Development VG VINOD VYDISWARAN, University of Michigan
1:05–1:20 pm EDT	**Break**
1:20–3:00 pm EDT	**PCOR Methods** Discussion questions: • What emerging methods are likely to be most relevant for the PCOR data infrastructure looking forward? What are the most important research and data challenges? • What computing advances, innovative health information technologies, and methodologies might present opportunities going forward? • What role can ASPE play in supporting effective methods for PCOR studies? What characteristics of HHS's public mission, programs, or authorities could be leveraged?

Moderators:
MIGUEL MARINO, Oregon Health & Science University, and CONSTANTINE GATSONIS, Brown University

Speakers:
NIGAM SHAH, Stanford University
SHARON-LISE NORMAND, Harvard University
SHERRI ROSE, Stanford University
LARA MANGRAVITE, Sage Bionetworks
NIROSHA MAHENDRARATNAM LEDERER, Aetion

3:00–3:15 pm EDT	**Break**
3:15–4:55 pm EDT	**Data Policies and Other Data Infrastructure Considerations**

Discussion questions:
- What data policies are likely to be most relevant for the PCOR data infrastructure looking forward?
- What role can ASPE play in supporting these policies for PCOR studies? What characteristics of HHS's public mission, programs, or authorities could be leveraged?

Moderators:
DEBORAH ESTRIN, Cornell Tech and
PAUL TANG, Palo Alto Medical Foundation and Stanford Clinical Excellence Research Center

Speakers:
PAMELA RILEY, Government of the District of Columbia
ABEL KHO, Northwestern University
JULIA ADLER-MILSTEIN, University of California, San Francisco
DEVEN MCGRAW, Ciitizen
DON DETMER, University of Virginia

4:55-5:00 pm EDT	**Wrap-up**

GEORGE ISHAM (Committee Chair), HealthPartners Institute

Appendix C

Biographical Sketches of Workshop Speakers

JULIA ADLER-MILSTEIN (NAM) is a professor of medicine and director of the Center for Clinical Informatics and Improvement Research at the University of California, San Francisco (UCSF). She spent 6 years on the faculty at the University of Michigan prior to joining UCSF. She is a leading researcher in health information technology policy, with a specific focus on electronic health records (EHRs) and interoperability. She has examined policies and organizational strategies that enable effective use of EHRs and promote interoperability. She is also an expert in EHR audit log data and their application to studying clinician behavior. Her research—used by researchers, health systems, and policy makers—identifies obstacles to progress and ways to overcome them. She has served on an array of influential committees and boards, including the NHS National Advisory Group on Health Information Technology, the Health Care Advisory Board for Politico, and the Interoperability Committee of the National Quality Forum. Adler-Milstein holds a Ph.D. in health policy from Harvard University.

DON EUGENE DETMER (NAM) is professor of medical education at the University of Virginia. He has served as vice president for health sciences at the University of Virginia and the University of Utah, as the Dennis Gillings professor for health management at Cambridge University, as president/chief executive officer of the American Medical Informatics Association, and as medical director of policy for the American College of Surgeons. Professorial appointments have included university professor of health policy, professor of surgery, business administration, public health sciences, preventive medicine, as well as visiting professor at University College London. He is past chair of the Board of Regents of the National Library of Medicine; the National Committee on Vital and Health Statistics; the National Academies of Sciences, Engineering, and Medicine's Board of Health Care Services; and Blue Ridge Academic Health Group, which he founded. Current boards include the Corporation for National Research Initiatives, the American College of Medical Informatics, and the International Academy of Health Sciences Informatics. He helped envision the national health information infrastructures of the United States and Hong Kong, as well as shaped policy for direct electronic communications of health records with patients in the United States and Europe. He earned an M.A. from Cambridge University and an M.D. from the University of Kansas. He completed postgraduate training at Johns Hopkins University, the National Institutes of Health, Duke Medical Center, and Harvard Business School.

EVELYN GALLEGO is the chief executive officer and founder of EMI Advisors LLC, an 8(a) certified Small Minority-Owned Business, founded to deliver value-driven health data management advisory services to government and commercial clients. She helps clients to bridge the gap between health information technology policy and standards and business requirements. She has a strong ability to work across and build consensus with diverse stakeholder groups to include multidisciplinary providers, policy makers, health care payers, researchers, system vendors and implementers, and standard development organizations. Gallego provides specialized expertise in digital health interoperability and health policy with a focus on alignment of regulatory, technical, and process improvement requirements to enable the effective adoption and use of technology. She is a thought leader in the areas of care coordination, social determinants of health, health information technology (IT) policy analysis and development, health information exchange and interoperability, and health IT standards development. She currently serves as the program manager and subject matter expert for three leading interoperability projects including the HL7 Gravity Project, the ONC STARS HIE Technical Assistance Program, and the NIH/AHRQ Multiple Chronic Care Electronic Care Plan Project. Gallego earned her international M.B.A. from the Schulich School of Business in Toronto, Canada, and her M.P.H. in health policy from George Washington University.

SHAUN GRANNIS is the vice president of data analytics and a medical informatics research scientist at the Regenstrief Institute. He is also the Sam Regenstrief professor of medical informatics and professor of family medicine at the Indiana University School of Medicine. In these roles, he collaborates with national and international health stakeholders seeking to advance health data technical infrastructure and data-sharing capabilities. He has provided identity management consultancy to organizations, including the World Health Organization and the Office of the National Coordinator for Health Information Technology. Grannis also supports health information exchange (HIE) activity among more than 120 hospitals in Indiana for use in clinical research and disease surveillance. His recent research focuses on developing and testing large-scale HIE-based solutions in support of population health and public health informatics; integrating clinical and social determinants of health (SDH) to identify at-risk patients in need of SDH services, which include nutrition counseling, financial planning, and medical-legal partnership assistance; developing and testing novel patient matching methods; and leveraging machine learning–based models to improve discovery and decision support in a variety of contexts. Grannis holds an M.D. from Michigan State University and bachelor's degree in aerospace engineering from the Massachusetts Institute of Technology.

JOHN HALAMKA (NAM) is the president of Mayo Clinic Platform. Prior to the Mayo Clinic, he served as the executive director of the Health Technology Exploration Center for Beth Israel Lahey Health in Massachusetts. During his tenure at Beth Israel Lahey Health, he oversaw digital health relationships with industry, academia, and government worldwide. Previously, he was chief information officer at Beth Israel Deaconess Medical Center for more than 20 years. In his role at Beth Israel Deaconess Medical Center, Halamka was responsible for all clinical, financial, administrative and academic information technology (IT). As a Harvard Medical School professor, he served the George W. Bush administration, the Obama administration, and governments around the world planning their health care IT strategies. In addition, he was the international healthcare innovation professor at Harvard Medical School. He remains chairman of New England Healthcare Exchange Network Inc. and is a practicing emergency medicine physician. Halamka received his B.S. in medical microbiology and his B.A. in public policy from Stanford University, his M.D. from the University of California, San Francisco, and his M.S. from Harvard University.

ABEL KHO is professor of medicine and preventive medicine in the Feinberg School of Medicine at Northwestern University and founding director of the Center for Health Information Partnerships and the Institute for Augmented Intelligence in Medicine. He has served as principal investigator for several regional or national projects including the Office of the National Coordinator for Health Information Technology–funded Chicago Health IT Regional Extension Center, the Patient-Centered Outcomes Research Institute–funded Chicago Area Patient Centered Outcomes Research Network, and the Agency for Healthcare Research and Quality–funded Health Hearts in the Heartland consortium within the EvidenceNOW initiative. His research focuses on developing regional electronic health record–enabled data sharing platforms for a range of health applications including high throughput phenotyping, cohort discovery, estimation of population level disease burden, and quality improvement. Kho received his M.D. from the Medical College of Wisconsin and completed a residency and chief residency in internal medicine at the University of Wisconsin–Madison.

NIROSHA MAHENDRARATNAM LEDERER is director of real-world evidence strategy at Aetion, where she leads the engagement of federal accounts and advises clients on generating decision-grade evidence. Previously, she was a managing associate at the Duke-Margolis Center for Health Policy, where she led the Center's real-world evidence portfolio. Prior to this position, she was a subject matter expert in the Oncology Center of Excellence at the U.S. Food and Drug Administration. While there, Lederer helped to implement patient-focused drug development in cancer products including clinical trial study design and product review, as well as foster consensus across U.S. and ex-U.S. health care stakeholders on best practices for patient-reported outcome capture, analysis, and communication. She has more than 15 years of pharmaceutical policy and health economics and outcomes research experiences, including providing evidence-generation advisory services at Avalere Health, working in commercial and medical roles at Genentech and Bristol-Myers Squibb, respectively, and serving on Capitol Hill during the passage of the Affordable Care Act. Lederer received her Ph.D. in health outcomes and policy from the University of North Carolina at Chapel Hill with a focus on large database analyses and decision-sciences. She received an M.S.P.H. in health policy and management from the Johns Hopkins Bloomberg School of Public Health and a B.A. in public health from the Johns Hopkins University.

LARA MANGRAVITE is president of Sage Bionetworks, an organization focused on the development and implementation of practices for large-scale collaborative biomedical research. Sage Bionetworks' work is centered on new approaches to scientific process that use open systems to enable community-based research regarding complex biomedical problems. Previously, she served as director of the systems biology research group at Sage Bionetworks where she focused on the application of collaborative approaches to advance understanding of disease biology and treatment outcomes at a systems level with the overriding goal of improving clinical care. Mangravite has a B.S. in physics from the Pennsylvania State University and a Ph.D. in pharmaceutical chemistry from the University of California, San Francisco. She completed a postdoctoral fellowship in cardiovascular pharmacogenomics at the Children's Hospital Oakland Research Institute.

DEVEN McGRAW is general counsel and chief regulatory officer for Ciitizen, a consumer health technology start-up. Previously, she directed U.S. health privacy and security as deputy director, Health Information Privacy at the U.S. Department of Health and Human Services' Office for Civil Rights and chief privacy officer (acting) of the Office of the National Coordinator for Health Information Technology. Widely recognized for her expertise in health privacy, she directed the Health Privacy Project at the Center for Democracy & Technology for 6 years and led the privacy and security policy work for the HITECH Health IT Policy Committee. She also served as the chief operating officer of the National Partnership for Women and Families. She advised health industry clients on Health Insurance Portability and Accountability Act of 1996 (HIPAA) compliance and data governance while a partner at Manatt, Phelps & Phillips, LLP. McGraw graduated magna cum laude from Georgetown University Law Center and has an M.P.H. from Johns Hopkins University.

SHARON-LISE NORMAND is S. James Adelstein professor of health care policy (biostatistics) in the Department of Health Care Policy at Harvard Medical School and professor in the Department of Biostatistics at Harvard School of Public Health. Her research focuses on the development of statistical methods for health services and outcomes research, including the evaluation of medical devices, causal inference, provider profiling, evidence synthesis, item response theory, and latent variables analyses. Her application areas include cardiovascular disease, severe mental illness, medical device safety and effectiveness, and medical technology diffusion. Normand was the 2010 president of the Eastern North American Region of the International Biometrics Society and inaugural vice chair of the Patient-Centered Outcomes Research Institute's Methodology Committee (2010–2012). She was awarded the ASA 2011 Health Policy Statistics Section's Long Term Excellence Award, the 2012 American Heart Association's Distinguished Scientist Award, the 2017 American Heart Association Council on Quality of Care and Outcomes Research Outstanding Lifetime Achievement Award, and the 2018 Mosteller Statistician of the Year. She is a fellow of the American Statistical Association, the American Heart Association, the American College of Cardiology, and the American Association for the Advancement of Science. Normand earned her Ph.D. in biostatistics, and M.Sc. and B.Sc. in statistics, and completed a postdoctoral fellowship in health care policy.

RACHEL RICHESSON is a professor in the Department of Learning Health Sciences, School of Medicine at the University of Michigan. She conducts original research on the quality and usability of data from electronic health records (EHRs) for research and has fostered numerous interdisciplinary research collaborations. She has directed implementation of data standards for a number of multinational multisite clinical research and epidemiological studies, including the National Institutes of Health (NIH) Rare Diseases Clinical Research Network, Type 1 Diabetes TrialNet, and The Environmental Determinants of Diabetes in the Young study, and the national distributed Patient-Centered Outcomes Research Network. Richesson currently leads the EHR Core for the NIH Health Systems Research Collaboratory, which is developing standards and quality metrics for clinical phenotyping using EHR data in pragmatic clinical trials. In addition, she and Department of Learning Health Science chair Charles Friedman colead the multi-stakeholder "Mobilizing Computable Biomedical Knowledge" community charged with establishing the standards, policies, and governance needed for biomedical knowledge to be widely disseminated and applied. Richesson holds a Ph.D. and an M.S. in health informatics and an M.P.H. from the University of Texas.

PAMELA RILEY is medical director of the District of Columbia Department of Health Care Finance, overseeing medical administration and quality of care in the District of Columbia's Title XIX (Medicaid), CHIP, and Alliance Programs. She previously served as vice president for delivery system reform at The Commonwealth Fund, developing and managing grants focused on transforming health care delivery systems for vulnerable populations, including low-income groups, racial/ethnic minorities, and uninsured populations. She also served as program officer at the New York State Health Foundation, where she developed and managed grant-making programs in the areas of integrating mental health and substance use services, addressing the needs of returning veterans and their families, and diabetes prevention and management. Earlier in her career, Riley served as clinical instructor in the Division of General Pediatrics at the Stanford University School of Medicine. She served as a Duke University Sanford School of Public Policy Global Health Policy fellow at the World Health Organization in Geneva, Switzerland, and has served as a volunteer physician in Peru and Guatemala. Riley has an M.D. from the University of California, Los Angeles (UCLA) David Geffen School of Medicine, and completed her internship and residency in pediatrics at Harbor-UCLA Medical Center in Torrance, California. She received an M.P.H. from the Harvard School of Public Health as a Commonwealth Fund fellow in minority health policy.

SHERRI ROSE is an associate professor at Stanford University in the Center for Health Policy and Center for Primary Care and Outcomes Research. She is also codirector of the Health Policy Data Science Lab.

Her research is centered on developing and integrating innovative statistical machine-learning approaches to improve human health. Within health policy, she works on risk adjustment, comparative effectiveness research, and health program evaluation. She has published interdisciplinary projects across varied outlets, including *Biometrics*, the *Journal of the American Statistical Association*, the *Journal of Health Economics*, *Health Affairs*, and the *New England Journal of Medicine*. Rose is the coeditor of *Biostatistics* and chair of the American Statistical Association's Biometrics Section. Her honors include a National Institutes of Health Director's New Innovator Award, the ISPOR Bernie J. O'Brien New Investigator Award, and Mid-Career Awards from the American Statistical Association's Health Policy Statistics Section and Penn-Rutgers Center for Causal Inference. She was also named a fellow of the American Statistical Association in 2020. In 2011, she coauthored the first book on machine learning for causal inference, with a sequel text released in 2018. Rose has a B.S. in statistics from George Washington University, and a Ph.D. in biostatistics from the University of California, Berkeley.

PATRICK RYAN is vice president of observational health data analytics at Janssen Research and Development, where he is leading efforts to develop and apply analysis methods to better understand the real-world effects of medical products. He is an original collaborator in Observational Health Data Sciences and Informatics, a multistakeholder, interdisciplinary collaborative to create open-source solutions that bring out the value of observational health data through large-scale analytics. Ryan served as a principal investigator of the Observational Medical Outcomes Partnership, a public-private partnership chaired by the U.S. Food and Drug Administration, where he led methodological research to assess the appropriate use of observational health care data to identify and evaluate drug safety issues. He has worked in various positions within the pharmaceutical industry at Pfizer and GlaxoSmithKline and also in academia at the University of Arizona Arthritis Center. Ryan received his undergraduate degrees in computer science and operations research at Cornell University, his M.Eng. in operations research and industrial engineering at Cornell, and his Ph.D. in pharmaceutical outcomes and policy from University of North Carolina at Chapel Hill.

NIGAM H. SHAH is a professor of medicine (biomedical informatics) at Stanford University, associate chief information officer for data science at Stanford Healthcare, and a member of the Biomedical Informatics Graduate Program as well as the Clinical Informatics Fellowship. His research focuses on combining machine learning and prior knowledge in medical ontologies to enable use cases of the learning health system. He received the AMIA New Investigator Award for 2013 and the Stanford Biosciences Faculty Teaching Award for outstanding teaching in his graduate class on data-driven medicine. He was elected into the American College of Medical Informatics in 2015 and was inducted into the American Society for Clinical Investigation in 2016. Shaw holds an M.B.B.S. from Baroda Medical College, India, and a Ph.D. from Penn State University, and completed his postdoctoral training at Stanford University.

VG VINOD VYDISWARAN is an assistant professor in the Department of Learning Health Sciences with a secondary appointment in the School of Information at the University of Michigan, Ann Arbor. His research focuses on developing and applying text mining, natural language processing, and machine-learning methodologies for extracting relevant information from health-related text corpora. This includes medically relevant information from clinical notes and biomedical literature, and studying the information quality and credibility of online health communication (via health forums and tweets). His previous work includes developing novel information retrieval models to assist clinical decision making, modeling information trustworthiness, and addressing the vocabulary gap between health professionals and laypersons. Vydiswaran received his Ph.D. from the University of Illinois at Urbana-Champaign and his M.Tech from the Indian Institute of Technology Bombay.

Appendix D

Building Data Capacity for Patient-Centered Outcomes Research: Interim Report 3– A Comprehensive Ecosystem for PCOR

(Full text of the committee's third interim report released on January 11, 2022.)[1]

---

[1] https://www.nap.edu/catalog/26396/building-data-capacity-for-patient-centered-outcomes-research-interim-report.

APPENDIX D

Building Data Capacity for Patient-Centered Outcomes Research

INTERIM REPORT 3 – A Comprehensive Ecosystem for PCOR

Committee on Building Data Capacity for
Patient-Centered Outcomes Research:
An Agenda for 2021 to 2030

Committee on National Statistics
Division of Behavioral and Social Sciences and Education

Board on Health Care Services
Health and Medicine Division

Computer Science and Telecommunications Board
Division on Engineering and Physical Sciences

A Consensus Study Report of

The National Academies of
SCIENCES · ENGINEERING · MEDICINE

THE NATIONAL ACADEMIES PRESS
Washington, DC
www.nap.edu

THE NATIONAL ACADEMIES PRESS   500 Fifth Street, NW   Washington, DC 20001

This activity was supported by a contract between the National Academy of Sciences and the U.S. Department of Health and Human Services (award # HHSP233201400020B/75P00120F37102). Any opinions, findings, conclusions, or recommendations expressed in this publication do not necessarily reflect the views of any organization or agency that provided support for the project.

International Standard Book Number-13: 978-0-309-27366-4
International Standard Book Number-10: 0-309-27366-8
Digital Object Identifier: https://doi.org/10.17226/26396

Additional copies of this publication are available from the National Academies Press, 500 Fifth Street, NW, Keck 360, Washington, DC 20001; (800) 624-6242 or (202) 334-3313; http://www.nap.edu.

Copyright 2022 by the National Academy of Sciences. All rights reserved.

Printed in the United States of America

Suggested citation: National Academies of Sciences, Engineering, and Medicine. (2022). *Building Data Capacity for Patient-Centered Outcomes Research: Interim Report 3– A Comprehensive Ecosystem for PCOR*. Washington, DC: The National Academies Press. https://doi.org/10.17226/26396.

The National Academies of
SCIENCES • ENGINEERING • MEDICINE

The **National Academy of Sciences** was established in 1863 by an Act of Congress, signed by President Lincoln, as a private, nongovernmental institution to advise the nation on issues related to science and technology. Members are elected by their peers for outstanding contributions to research. Dr. Marcia McNutt is president.

The **National Academy of Engineering** was established in 1964 under the charter of the National Academy of Sciences to bring the practices of engineering to advising the nation. Members are elected by their peers for extraordinary contributions to engineering. Dr. John L. Anderson is president.

The **National Academy of Medicine** (formerly the Institute of Medicine) was established in 1970 under the charter of the National Academy of Sciences to advise the nation on medical and health issues. Members are elected by their peers for distinguished contributions to medicine and health. Dr. Victor J. Dzau is president.

The three Academies work together as the **National Academies of Sciences, Engineering, and Medicine** to provide independent, objective analysis and advice to the nation and conduct other activities to solve complex problems and inform public policy decisions. The National Academies also encourage education and research, recognize outstanding contributions to knowledge, and increase public understanding in matters of science, engineering, and medicine.

Learn more about the National Academies of Sciences, Engineering, and Medicine at **www.nationalacademies.org**.

The National Academies of
SCIENCES · ENGINEERING · MEDICINE

Consensus Study Reports published by the National Academies of Sciences, Engineering, and Medicine document the evidence-based consensus on the study's statement of task by an authoring committee of experts. Reports typically include findings, conclusions, and recommendations based on information gathered by the committee and the committee's deliberations. Each report has been subjected to a rigorous and independent peer-review process and it represents the position of the National Academies on the statement of task.

Proceedings published by the National Academies of Sciences, Engineering, and Medicine chronicle the presentations and discussions at a workshop, symposium, or other event convened by the National Academies. The statements and opinions contained in proceedings are those of the participants and are not endorsed by other participants, the planning committee, or the National Academies.

For information about other products and activities of the National Academies, please visit www.nationalacademies.org/about/whatwedo.

COMMITTEE ON BUILDING DATA CAPACITY FOR PATIENT-CENTERED OUTCOMES RESEARCH: AN AGENDA FOR 2021 TO 2030

GEORGE ISHAM (*Chair*), HealthPartners Institute
JOHN F.P. BRIDGES, The Ohio State University
JULIE BYNUM, University of Michigan
ANGELA DOBES, IBD Plexus, Crohn's & Colitis Foundation
DEBORAH ESTRIN, Cornell Tech
OLUWADAMILOLA FAYANJU, The University of Pennsylvania
CONSTANTINE GATSONIS, Brown University
ROBERT GOERGE, Chapin Hall, University of Chicago
GEORGE HRIPCSAK, Columbia University
LISA IEZZONI, Massachusetts General Hospital
S. CLAIBORNE JOHNSTON, The University of Texas at Austin
MIGUEL MARINO, Oregon Health & Science University
ELIZABETH McGLYNN, Kaiser Permanente
DAVID MELTZER, University of Chicago
PAUL TANG, Stanford University and Palo Alto Medical Foundation

KRISZTINA MARTON, *Study Director*
CRYSTAL BELL, *Associate Program Officer*
RUTH COOPER, *Associate Program Officer*
MARY GHITELMAN, *Senior Program Assistant*
BRIAN HARRIS-KOJETIN, *Director, Committee on National Statistics*
SHARYL NASS, *Director, Board on Health Care Services*
JON EISENBERG, *Director, Computer Science and Telecommunications Board*

SAUL RIVAS (*National Academy of Medicine Fellow*), University of Texas Rio Grande Valley

COMMITTEE ON NATIONAL STATISTICS

ROBERT M. GROVES, (*Chair*), Georgetown University
LAWRENCE D. BOBO, Harvard University
ANNE C. CASE, Princeton University, *Emeritus*
MICK P. COUPER, University of Michigan
JANET M. CURRIE, Princeton University
DIANA FARRELL, JPMorgan Chase Institute, Washington, DC
ROBERT GOERGE, Chapin Hall, University of Chicago
ERICA L. GROSHEN, Cornell University
HILARY HOYNES, University of California-Berkeley
DANIEL KIFER, The Pennsylvania State University
SHARON LOHR, Arizona State University, *Emeritus*
JEROME P. REITER, Duke University
JUDITH A. SELTZER, University of California-Los Angeles, *Emeritus*
C. MATTHEW SNIPP, Stanford University
ELIZABETH A. STUART, Johns Hopkins University
JEANNETTE WING, Columbia University

BRIAN HARRIS-KOJETIN, *Director*
MELISSA CHIU, *Deputy Director*
CONSTANCE F. CITRO, *Senior Scholar*

APPENDIX D

BOARD ON HEALTH CARE SERVICES

DAVID BLUMENTHAL (*Chair*), The Commonwealth Fund
ANDREW BINDMAN, Kaiser Foundation Health Plan, Inc.
NIRANJAN BOSE, Gates Ventures
MELINDA J. BEEUWKES BUNTIN, Vanderbilt University School of Medicine
NEIL S. CALMAN, The Institute for Family Health
PAUL CHUNG, Kaiser Permanente School of Medicine
PATRICIA M. DAVIDSON, Johns Hopkins University School of Nursing
MARTHA DAVIGLUS, University of Illinois at Chicago
JENNIFER E. DeVOE, Oregon Health & Science University
R. ADAMS DUDLEY, University of Minnesota
RICHARD G. FRANK, Harvard Medical School
TERRY FULMER, John A. Hartford Foundation
CINDY GILLESPIE, Arkansas Department of Human Services
ELMER HUERTA, The George Washington University Cancer Center
SHARON INOUYE, Harvard Medical School
JOHN LUMPKIN, Blue Cross Blue Shield of North Carolina Foundation
FAITH MITCHELL, The Urban Institute
DAVID B. PRYOR, Ascension Health
TRISH RILEY, National Academy for State Health Policy
WILLIAM SAGE, The University of Texas at Austin
HARDEEP SINGH, Baylor College of Medicine

SHARYL NASS, *Director*

COMPUTER SCIENCE AND TELECOMMUNICATIONS BOARD

LAURA HAAS (*Chair*), University of Massachusetts, Amherst
DAVID CULLER, University of California, Berkeley
ERIC HORVITZ, Microsoft Corporation
CHARLES ISBELL, Georgia Institute of Technology
BETH MYNATT, Georgia Institute of Technology
CRAIG PARTRIDGE, Colorado State University
DANIELA RUS, Massachusetts Institute of Technology
FRED B. SCHNEIDER, Cornell University
MARGO SELTZER, University of British Columbia
NAMBIRAJAN SESHADRI, University of California, San Diego
MOSHE VARDI, Rice University

JON EISENBERG, *Senior Board Director*

Acknowledgments

This Consensus Study Report was reviewed in draft form by individuals chosen for their diverse perspectives and technical expertise. The purpose of this independent review is to provide candid and critical comments that will assist the National Academies of Sciences, Engineering, and Medicine in making each published report as sound as possible and to ensure that it meets the institutional standards for quality, objectivity, evidence, and responsiveness to the study charge. The review comments and draft manuscript remain confidential to protect the integrity of the deliberative process.

We thank the following individuals for their review of this report: Robert M. Califf, Verily Life Sciences, Google Health, and Duke University; Steven B. Cohen, Statistical and Data Sciences, RTI International; Heidi M. Crane, Clinical Cohort and Comorbidity Research Core and Center for AIDS Research, University of Washington; Beth Jarosz, U.S. Programs and KidsData, Population Reference Bureau; and Russell L. Rothman, Institute for Medicine and Public Health, Vanderbilt University.

Although the reviewers listed above provided many constructive comments and suggestions, they were not asked to endorse the conclusions of this report, nor did they see the final draft before its release. The review of this report was overseen by Andrew B. Bindman, chief medical officer, Kaiser Foundation Health Plan and Hospitals, and Alicia L. Carriquiry, Department of Statistics, Iowa State University. They were responsible for making certain that an independent examination of this report was carried out in accordance with the standards of the National Academies and that all review comments were carefully considered. Responsibility for the final content rests entirely with the authoring committee and the National Academies.

Contents

Summary	1
1 Introduction	5
2 Federal Partnerships	17
3 State-Level Data and Collaborations	33
4 Clinical Trial Networks and Collaborations	43
5 Public-Private Partnerships	51
6 Collaborations with Patient Groups	57

Appendixes

A	Biographical Sketches of Committee Members	63
B	Workshop Agenda	69
C	Biographical Sketches of Workshop Speakers	73

Boxes and Figures

BOXES

1-1 Key Data Infrastructure Functionalities in the Existing Strategic Framework for Patient-Centered Outcomes Research, 10
1-2 Building Blocks of the Patient-Centered Outcomes Research Data Infrastructure, 11
1-3 Statement of Task for the Overall Study, 13

2-1 Collaborations Between the Centers for Medicare & Medicaid Services Office of Minority Health and Federal Partners, 23

FIGURES

1-1 Patient-Centered Outcomes Research Trust Fund: Three streams of work and funding, 7
1-2 The Office of the Assistant Secretary for Planning and Evaluation's strategic framework for the patient-centered outcomes research data infrastructure, 9

2-1 Prevalence of diabetes in 2018, 22

4-1 National Cancer Institute National Clinical Trials Network structure, 44

APPENDIX D   253

Summary

The Office of the Assistant Secretary for Planning and Evaluation (ASPE), in partnership with other agencies and divisions of the U.S. Department of Health and Human Services (HHS), coordinates a portfolio of projects that build data capacity for conducting patient-centered outcomes research (PCOR). PCOR focuses on producing scientific evidence on the effectiveness of prevention and treatment options to inform the health care decisions of patients, families, and health care providers, taking into consideration the preferences, values, and questions patients face when making health care choices. The data infrastructure includes data sources and functionalities that support the research. Major building blocks are the services, standards, policies, and governance that enable the use of the data.

ASPE asked the National Academies of Sciences, Engineering, and Medicine to appoint a consensus study committee to identify issues critical to the continued development of the data infrastructure for PCOR. The committee's work will contribute to ASPE's development of a strategic plan that will guide its work related to PCOR data capacity over the next decade.

As part of its information-gathering activities, the committee organized three workshops to collect input from stakeholders on the PCOR data infrastructure, which includes a variety of types of data, such as clinical data, research data, administrative data from payer records, and patient-provided data. This report, the third in a series of three interim reports, summarizes the discussion and committee conclusions from the third workshop, which focused on ways of enhancing collaborations, data linkages, and the interoperability of electronic databases to make the PCOR data infrastructure more useful in the years ahead. Participants in the workshop included researchers and policy experts working in these areas. The first report centered on emerging data needs[1] and the second report on data standards, methods, and policy.[2]

The conclusions included in this interim report are based primarily on the input collected as part of the workshop, background documentation received from ASPE and other public sources, and the committee members' synthesis and expert judgment regarding the input received. As an interim report based on one in a series of information-gathering activities, the scope of this report is narrowly focused on a subset of key topics relevant to the committee's charge. The conclusions reached by the committee are, at this stage, fairly high-level. After completing all of its information-gathering activities, which include but are not limited to the three workshops, the committee will also issue a final report containing the study's overall findings and conclusions.

FEDERAL PARTNERSHIPS

The workshop discussed in this report included several stakeholder groups that are involved in collaborations focused on PCOR. While it was not possible to discuss many important collaborative projects, the first session, which was held with federal agency representatives, highlighted several key areas where additional collaborative work could continue to build and strengthen the PCOR data infrastructure.

CONCLUSION 2-1: Collaboration among federal agencies and between federal agencies and other partners (such as states, patient groups, and others) is essential for continuing to build the patient-centered outcomes research data infrastructure. The areas where additional collaboration would be particularly useful include the following:

- Increasing consistency in the use of standards for data interoperability and element definitions;
- Addressing barriers that hinder data linkages, such as the limitations associated with health identifiers and mitigating potential selection biases resulting from linkage error;

---

[1] https://www.nap.edu/catalog/26297/building-data-capacity-for-patient-centered-outcomes-research-interim-report.

[2] https://www.nap.edu/catalog/26298/building-data-capacity-for-patient-centered-outcomes-research-interim-report.

- Balancing the burden of the data collections and disclosure risks with the value of the datasets;
- Communicating the usefulness of the data collections to those who are asked to provide data about themselves and those who collect the data;
- Promoting discussion and education about fitness for use of the data; and
- Working with stakeholders and patients to promote sharing of data.

While there is frequent collaboration among HHS partners on PCOR data infrastructure work, and ASPE's public website contains a comprehensive list of past and current projects funded from the Patient-Centered Outcomes Research Trust Fund, additional dissemination efforts focused on external stakeholders could further increase the usefulness of these investments.

CONCLUSION 2-2: There is a need to increase awareness among all stakeholders about new data infrastructure developments funded by the Patient-Centered Outcomes Research Trust Fund. Increased awareness will enhance the efficiency and effectiveness of research, which will increase the impact of the investments made in infrastructure development.

STATE-LEVEL DATA AND COLLABORATIONS

Many states have robust data collection systems and can produce information that is useful to state and local policy makers. State-generated data are also valuable at the national level, including for answering broader questions about issues that may be influenced by local policy, such as health care access and disparities.

CONCLUSION 3-1: There are opportunities to learn from what states have accomplished in building data capacity.

The data collected, their quality, and ease of access to the data vary by state. Challenges associated with access make it particularly difficult to use state-generated data for research at the national level.

CONCLUSION 3-2: The usefulness of data available for Patient-Centered Outcomes Research could be increased by the sharing and adoption of best practices among the states for the data collected, their quality, and ease of access.

CLINICAL TRIAL NETWORKS AND COLLABORATIONS

The session on clinical trial networks and collaborations illustrated the need for better integration between clinical care and research in ways that align differing interests and are mutually beneficial. Better integration can improve the data available for patient care as well as the data available for research.

> CONCLUSION 4-1: Infrastructure investments could enhance the utility of data routinely generated in the course of care for clinical trials.

PUBLIC-PRIVATE PARTNERSHIPS

While the benefits of data sharing are clear, the workshop also underscored the risks involved for the organizations providing the data.

> CONCLUSION 5-1: Successful partnerships across health care systems require participant trust, clear evidence of mutual benefit, and the ability to control risk.

COLLABORATIONS WITH PATIENT GROUPS

Collaborations with patient organizations can help to address patient concerns about participating in research studies and to build patient engagement, which is important for achieving a patient-centered approach. Disease registries directed by patient groups can be a particularly useful additional source of data, one that provides information that would not be available to researchers otherwise.

> CONCLUSION 6-1: Patient groups can be helpful partners in all aspects of Patient-Centered Outcomes Research, including engaging patients in order to improve research participation and the impact of results.

> CONCLUSION 6-2: Patient-directed disease registries can be a source of in-depth, longitudinal, prospective clinical and patient-reported data that are not available from other data sources.

1

Introduction

The Office of the Assistant Secretary for Planning and Evaluation (ASPE), in partnership with other agencies and divisions of the U.S. Department of Health and Human Services (HHS), coordinates a portfolio of projects that build data capacity for conducting patient-centered outcomes research (PCOR). The PCOR data infrastructure provides decision makers with objective, scientific evidence on the effectiveness of treatments, services, and other interventions used in health care. This research is frequently focused on analyzing existing data to address questions and provide objective information for the purpose of informing real-world health care decisions.

BACKGROUND

The legal framework that established funding for research on the outcomes and effectiveness of treatments and health care interventions dates back to the 2003 Medicare Prescription Drug, Improvement, and Modernization Act. This act provided authorization for the Agency for Healthcare Research and Quality (AHRQ) to support research comparing the outcomes and effectiveness of treatments and clinical approaches and to disseminate the findings from this research. In 2009, the American Recovery and Reinvestment Act provided additional funding to AHRQ, the National Institutes of Health, and HHS for research that compares the effectiveness of medical options. In 2010, the Patient Protection and Affordable Care Act provided further authorization for research that assists patients, clinicians, purchasers, and policy makers in making informed health decisions.

6   *INTERIM REPORT 3—A COMPREHENSIVE ECOSYSTEM FOR PCOR*

To facilitate PCOR, in 2010 Congress established the Patient-Centered Outcomes Research Trust Fund (PCOR Trust Fund) within the Department of the Treasury. The goals of the PCOR Trust Fund are to fund PCOR, disseminate research findings, and develop a data infrastructure for PCOR. The PCOR Trust Fund has been reauthorized through 2029, through H.R.1865 of the Further Consolidated Appropriations Act of 2020. The most recent statute specified intellectual and developmental disabilities, as well as maternal mortality, as research priorities. The statute also called for PCOR studies to include consideration of the full range of outcomes data. Specifically, the law states that

> research shall be designed, as appropriate, to take into account and capture the full range of clinical and patient-centered outcomes relevant to, and that meet the needs of, patients, clinicians, purchasers, and policy-makers in making informed health decisions. In addition to the relative health outcomes and clinical effectiveness, clinical and patient-centered outcomes shall include the potential burdens and economic impacts of the utilization of medical treatments, items, and services on different stakeholders and decision-makers respectively. These potential burdens and economic impacts include medical out-of-pocket costs, including health plan benefit and formulary design, non-medical costs to the patient and family, including caregiving, effects on future costs of care, workplace productivity and absenteeism, and healthcare utilization.[1]

The bulk of the PCOR Trust Fund funding (80 percent) is allocated for research and is made available through the Patient-Centered Outcomes Research Institute, a nongovernmental organization established by Congress for this purpose. Approximately 16 percent of the PCOR Trust Fund is set aside for disseminating research findings, incorporating findings into clinical practice, and training researchers in PCOR. The agency overseeing this work is AHRQ.

The remaining funding, which constitutes 4 percent of the PCOR Trust Fund, is allocated for building data capacity for PCOR and is overseen by ASPE. Specifically, Section 937(f) of the Public Health Service Act instructed the Secretary of HHS to

> … provide for the coordination of relevant Federal health programs to build data capacity for comparative clinical effectiveness research, including the development and use of clinical registries and health outcomes research networks, in order to develop and maintain a comprehensive, interoperable data network to collect, link, and analyze data on out-

---

[1] https://www.ssa.gov/OP_Home/ssact/title11/1181.htm.

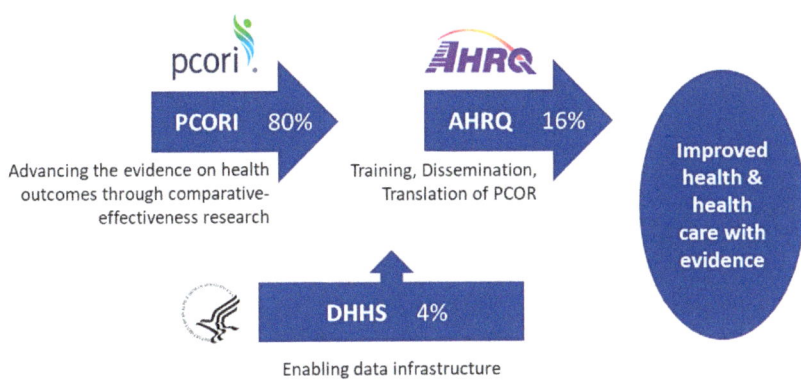

FIGURE 1-1 Patient-Centered Outcomes Research Trust Fund: Three streams of work and funding.
NOTE: AHRQ = Agency for Healthcare Research and Quality; DHHS = Department of Health and Human Services; PCOR = patient-centered outcomes research; PCORI = Patient-Centered Outcomes Research Institute.
SOURCE: Workshop presentation by ASPE, May 3, 2021.

comes and effectiveness from multiple sources including electronic health records.[2]

Figure 1-1 shows how the PCOR funding and work are allocated across the three entities. This National Academies of Sciences, Engineering, and Medicine (National Academies) study is focused on issues relevant to ASPE's continued work on the PCOR data infrastructure, in other words, on the priorities for the use of the 4 percent of the funding that is allocated to HHS for work related to the data infrastructure for PCOR.

As the coordinating agency for the data infrastructure investment portfolio across HHS agencies, ASPE guides the PCOR data infrastructure's strategic framework and vision, sets funding priorities, and coordinates interagency workgroups. ASPE's work is assisted by a Leadership Council for the PCOR Trust Fund, which includes representatives from other HHS agencies, including the Administration for Children and Families; the Administration for Community Living; AHRQ; the Assistant Secretary for Preparedness and Response; the Centers for Disease Control and Prevention (CDC); the Centers for Medicare & Medicaid Services; the Food and Drug Administration (FDA); the Health Resources and Services Administration; the Indian Health Service; the National Institutes of Health; the Office of

---

[2] https://aspe.hhs.gov/collaborations-committees-advisory-groups/os-pcortf/about-os-pcortf.

the Chief Technology Officer; the Office of the National Coordinator for Health Information Technology; and the Substance Abuse and Mental Health Services Administration.

The Leadership Council provides input on priorities for the portfolio, including projects to fund. During the period from 2010 to 2019, the PCOR Trust Fund funded 53 projects, which translated to 76 agency awards, totaling approximately $131 million.

Figure 1-2 is a visual representation of ASPE's current framework for the PCOR data infrastructure. The bottom row shows the main data sources feeding into the PCOR infrastructure. Data collected as part of clinical care include data collected for health care delivery and for billing purposes. Examples of primary data collected as part of research studies include data from clinical trials and data from national health surveys. Other examples of data sources include

- Medicare or Medicaid claims data,
- quality or outcomes data collected by health care providers for the purposes of improving health care value,
- FDA data on the safety of medications and medical devices, and
- CDC data on births and deaths provided by state public health authorities.

The framework describes the relationship between the data sources and the current key functionalities and focus areas (middle row) that support the research. The key functionalities are described in further detail in Box 1-1. Major building blocks are the services, standards, policies, and governance that enable the use of the data for research, described in further detail in Box 1-2. The top row shows the key data users and contributors of data. A more detailed overview of ASPE's work and the projects funded to date will be included in the final report, at the conclusion of the committee's review.

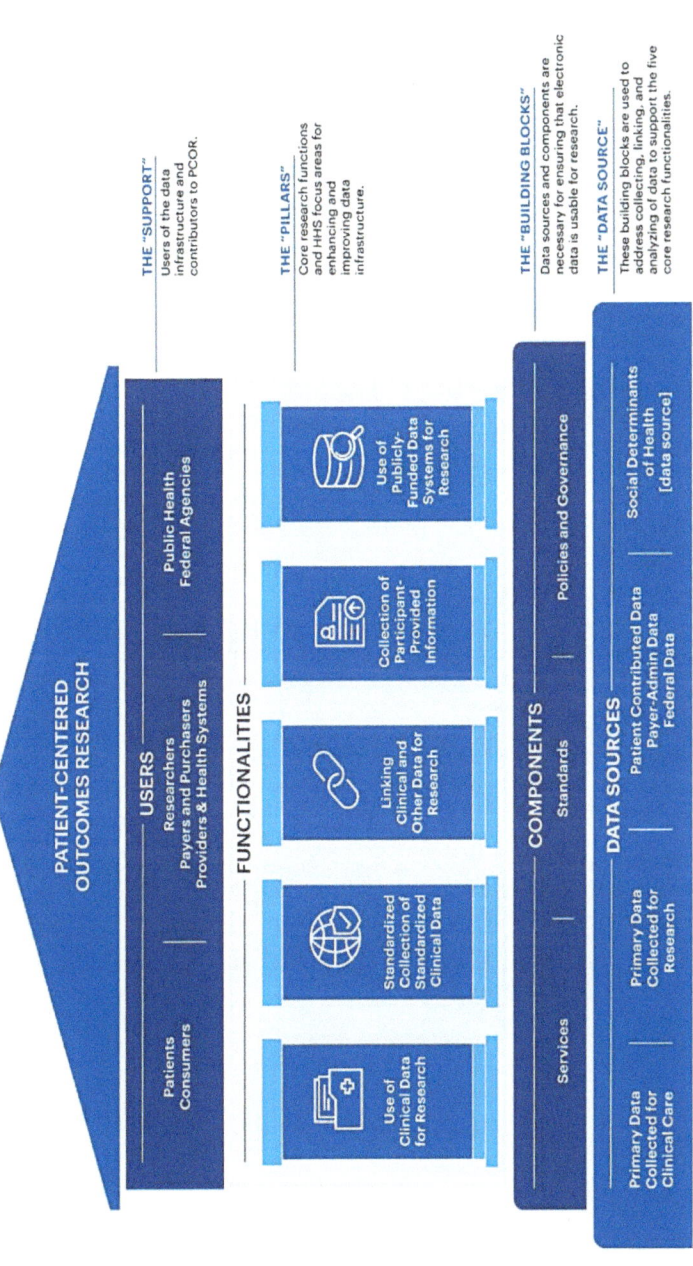

FIGURE 1-2 The Office of the Assistant Secretary for Planning and Evaluation's strategic framework for the patient-centered outcomes research data infrastructure.
SOURCE: Workshop presentation by ASPE, May 3, 2021.

> **BOX 1-1**
> **Key Data Infrastructure Functionalities in the Existing Strategic Framework for Patient-Centered Outcomes Research**
>
> *Standardized Collection of Standardized Clinical Data*
> Researchers will be able to use standardized clinical data based on common data element standards across research projects and networks, thereby facilitating linkage and aggregation of data across data sources.
>
> *Collection of Participant-provided Information*
> Participants, including those in safety net organizations, will be able to participate more fully in clinical research by directly providing information (i.e., data points provided by the participant, such as patient-reported outcomes).
>
> *Linking of Clinical and Other Data for Research*
> Researchers will be able to follow patients across the care continuum over time, including those enrolled in clinical trials. Researchers will be able to capture the range of variables influencing health outcomes and link clinical and other types of data (e.g., other clinical data, claims data, participant-provided information, and environmental data) required for research regardless of where the participant goes.
>
> *Use of Clinical Data for Research*
> Researchers will be able to utilize and analyze routinely collected clinical data for implementation of clinical studies (observational and interventional), including data relevant to assessing safety, efficacy, and adherence, as well as genetic data and patient-reported outcomes.
>
> *Use of Enhanced Publicly Funded Data Systems for Research*
> Researchers will be able to readily use, retrieve, link, and aggregate publicly funded data for research due to enhancements in publicly funded data systems.
>
> SOURCE: https://aspe.hhs.gov/collaborations-committees-advisory-groups/os-pcortf/about-os-pcortf/building-data-capacity-patient-centered-outcomes-research.

> **BOX 1-2**
> **Building Blocks of the Patient-Centered Outcomes Research Data Infrastructure**
>
> *Standards* represent information and meaning to patient-centered data to ensure that health-specific information can be accurately (and securely) exchanged and used. In most cases standards should be nationally accepted, widely approved, or broadly adopted either through market forces, community approval, or regulatory requirements. These include such items as data standards for capturing, storing, representing, and exchanging data in a secure manner such that accurate information is conveyed to the recipient of the data.
>
> *Policies* are standards of behavior that participants can rely on consistently to build patient-centered data for research. Policies may include federal policies, as well as models for standardized state and local policies, that will lead to a trusted framework within the patient-centered outcomes research (PCOR) data infrastructure that ensures productivity, protects the patient and the patient's data, ensures that evidence generation remains in the center of PCOR, and ensures the use of agreed upon standards and services.
>
> *Services* refer to resources that entities can employ on demand to capture, store, or exchange either PCOR data or evidence through a centrally hosted model provided remotely (such as through the Internet) rather than provided locally or on-site. Services make it easy for the research data to interoperate among different systems without having to start from scratch for every connection.
>
> *Governance* structures refer to entities that are needed to develop and apply the rules and policies needed for building an interoperable and sustainable research network. Governance structures support the efficient use of the data infrastructure for research across individual and organizations' boundaries of control and ownership. Governance structures are distinguished from "governance," which is what a governing body or governance structure does.
>
> SOURCE: https://aspe.hhs.gov/collaborations-committees-advisory-groups/os-pcortf/about-os-pcortf/building-data-capacity-patient-centered-outcomes-research.

12 INTERIM REPORT 3—A COMPREHENSIVE ECOSYSTEM FOR PCOR

ISSUES FOR THE COMMITTEE

ASPE asked the National Academies to appoint a consensus study committee and identify issues critical to building data capacity for PCOR and for generating new evidence to inform health care decisions. The input provided by the committee will contribute to ASPE's strategic planning for its work related to the data infrastructure over the next decade. The study is part of a broader initiative by ASPE intended to update the strategic plan in light of the reauthorization of the PCOR Trust Fund and advances in health information technology and interoperability tools in recent years.

The study is a collaboration of three units of the National Academies: the Committee on National Statistics, the Board on Health Care Services, and the Computer Science and Telecommunications Board. The 15-person consensus study committee has a diverse membership, including experts with decades of experience, as well as emerging leaders, in the broad fields of (1) PCOR; (2) research methods, statistics, and demography; (3) computer science and data infrastructure; and (4) patient engagement and patient perspectives. Appendix A contains the biographical sketches of the committee members.

As part of its information-gathering activities, the committee was asked to organize three workshops to collect input from stakeholders on aspects of the charge developed in consultation with ASPE. The workshops focused on key topics that the committee believed would particularly benefit from broad input from a variety of data users and other stakeholders. The committee's conclusions from each workshop are summarized in a series of interim reports, the first of which centered on emerging data needs. That first interim report summarized the discussion and committee conclusions from the first workshop, which focused on looking ahead at data user needs over the next decade.[3] The second interim report in the series centered on data standards, methods, and policies that could make the PCOR data infrastructure more useful.[4] This report summarizes the discussion and committee conclusions from the third workshop, which focused on ways of enhancing collaborations, data linkages, and the interoperability of electronic databases to make the PCOR data infrastructure more useful in the years ahead.

As an interim report focused on one in a series of information-gathering activities, the scope of this report is limited to a subset of the topics relevant to the committee's charge, and the conclusions reached by the committee are, at this stage, fairly high-level. Some aspects of the topics discussed are

---

[3] https://www.nap.edu/catalog/26297/building-data-capacity-for-patient-centered-outcomes-research-interim-report.

[4] https://www.nap.edu/catalog/26298/building-data-capacity-for-patient-centered-outcomes-research-interim-report.

examined in further detail in other workshops. After completing all of its information-gathering activities, the committee will issue a final report, which will integrate and examine these topics in further detail.

Box 1-3 shows the committee's Statement of Task for the overall study. The committee will address this charge in its final report, integrating what was learned from the workshops and from all other forms of input, including public meetings with HHS staff and background documentation available on the history and operations of the PCOR Trust Fund. The final report will contain overall findings and conclusions from the study, on the

---

BOX 1-3
Statement of Task for the Overall Study

The National Academies will appoint an ad hoc committee to conduct a series of three 1-day public workshops and develop conclusions to help guide the data capacity development for patient-centered research from 2021 through 2030. Each workshop will seek input from key stakeholders on topics relevant to the committee charge, and the specific focus of each workshop will be determined by the committee in consultation with Assistant Secretary for Planning and Evaluation.

As part of its activities, the committee will also

- Consider the published review of the history and trajectory of the Office of the Secretary, Patient-Centered Outcomes Research Trust Fund (OS-PCORTF) portfolio of investments and the OS-PCORTF roadmap.
- Assess anticipated changes to health care priorities and priorities for health data and their impact on building data capacity into the foreseeable future, as identified by ASPE.
- Evaluate the feasibility and utility of developing a phased-in approach to building the interoperable data capacity for patient-centered outcomes research with existing databases in Department of Health and Human Services, other federal departments, and the private sector in a phased approach, such as projects identified in the Cures Act Title III Section 4003 (Interoperability).
- Consider other existing legislation, regulations, and the like, as deemed relevant.
- Receive input from individuals or groups that represent stakeholders, including patients, their caregivers or families, and their health care providers.

The committee will issue interim reports after each public workshop with conclusions, and will produce a final written report with findings and conclusions to help guide a future course to continue building the data capacity for patient-centered research. All reports will follow institutional guidelines and be subject to the National Academies review procedures prior to release.

basis of the committee's further deliberations and integrated judgment on the input received and materials reviewed.

Appendix B shows the agenda for the workshop, which was held on June 14, 2021. The committee's goal for this event was to bring together researchers and policy experts to

- discuss how research and data collaborations can evolve to meet PCOR and data capacity challenges, and how HHS can support effective research and data collaborations;
- identify barriers and potential solutions to the access and use of linked public data, as well as to the access and use of linked public and private/proprietary data; and
- discuss the feasibility and utility of developing a phased-in approach to building the interoperable data capacity for PCOR with existing databases in HHS, other federal departments, and the private sector.

Invited speakers in each of the sessions were asked to reflect on the general topics above. An obvious limitation of an activity of this type is that only a small number of stakeholders can be invited to speak. To compensate for this limitation, the invited participants included diverse experts working in a variety of areas and on a range of types of projects, including both early career researchers and experts with decades of experience. A recording of the workshop as well as the presentation slides used by the speakers are available on the National Academies website at www.nationalacademies.org/PCORData.

Prior to the workshop, information about the event was disseminated through National Academies mailing lists and on the project website. To collect additional stakeholder input, members of the public were invited to provide comments on topics related to the workshop (or any other topic related to the committee's charge), using a public input form available on the National Academies website.

OVERVIEW OF THE REPORT

This report is organized around the main sessions of the workshop and discusses the following topics: federal partnerships and collaborations with other stakeholders (Chapter 2); state-level data and collaborations (Chapter 3); clinical trial networks and collaborations (Chapter 4); public-private partnerships (Chapter 5); and collaborations with patient groups (Chapter 6). The points conveyed by the workshop participants do not necessarily reflect the views of the committee. In each chapter, a summary of the input received is followed by the committee's conclusions.

INTRODUCTION

The conclusions are based primarily on the input collected as part of the workshop, background documentation received from ASPE and other public sources, and the committee members' synthesis and expert judgment. Because this is an interim report, the committee's conclusions at this stage are big-picture conclusions, which will be integrated with additional input over the course of the study.

APPENDIX D

2

Federal Partnerships

This chapter summarizes workshop presentations and discussion focused on federal partnerships and collaborations with other stakeholder groups. The brief overview of the input received from the presenters is followed by the committee's conclusions.

Micky Tripathi, National Coordinator for Health Information Technology, discussed the work that the Office of the National Coordinator for Health Information Technology (ONC) is doing to support activities related to patient-centered outcomes research (PCOR). He noted that more than a decade after the passage of the Health Information Technology for Economic and Clinical Health Act of 2009, the United States has several well-functioning electronic health records (EHR) systems that are widely used by health care providers and represent a common foundation for capturing and sharing clinical data, even if not all providers are satisfied with their EHRs. Tripathi argued that this is a good time to consider the opportunities offered by EHRs, beyond their core functions of supporting medical records and payment processing, stating that EHRs are still a barely tapped source of information for research.

One area of focus for ONC in recent years has been the advancement and harmonization of data standards, including supporting the use of common data models, looking at research-data models as well as clinical data-models, and thinking about data integration. ONC has supported work on patient matching, aggregating, and linking through the development of tools and advancement of data standards. Tripathi also mentioned structured data capture as another area of past work aimed at facilitating the reuse of these data for clinical research.

Another area of work at ONC focuses on real-world data. Projects included testing a standards-based approach to establishing a coordinated registry network for data regarding women's health technologies, collecting patient-reported outcomes (PROs) through health IT and leveraging Fast Healthcare Interoperability Resources (FHIR), and using privacy preserving machine learning techniques to enable health information exchanges to support COVID-19-focused PCOR.

Tripathi said that ONC has done work related to creating a privacy and security framework for PCOR by developing resources that support the protection of privacy and the security of electronic health data. The agency also worked on identifying limitations in developing machine learning training datasets when pursuing complex health related research questions. ONC also collaborated with MITRE Corporation to increase the variety of reliable and robust synthetic data, particularly for opioid, pediatric, and complex care use cases. The project focuses on enhancing an open-source synthetic data engine that uses publicly available data to generate synthetic health records. Such tools can safeguard patient privacy and support appropriate stewardship practices in which real patient data are only accessed and used when necessary. These and other mentioned projects have been funded through the Patient-Centered Outcomes Research Trust Fund (PCORTF).[1]

Looking ahead, Tripathi said that ONC has several initiatives that will directly support PCOR and patient engagement in PCOR. One initiative is focused on standards for EHR data. ONC will be releasing a new version of the U.S. Core Data for Interoperability, which is a standardized set of health data classes and constituent data elements for EHRs and for nationwide, interoperable health information exchanges. The data are supposed to be available not only for provider-to-provider and provider-to-payer exchanges but also for patients.

Allison Oelschlaeger, Office of Enterprise Data & Analytics, Centers for Medicare & Medicaid Services (CMS), discussed CMS data and data linkages. For context, Oelschlaeger noted that more than 130 million Americans receive health coverage through programs administered by CMS—including Medicare, Medicaid, and the Children's Health Insurance Program—and the health insurance marketplace. As a result, CMS collects large amounts of data, which are an invaluable resource for comparative clinical effectiveness research. The data include information on enrollment and patient characteristics; utilization and cost of health care services, such as treatments and therapies; and diagnoses.

---

[1] For more information on some of the ONC PCOR data infrastructure projects, see https://www.healthit.gov/topic/scientific-initiatives/building-data-infrastructure-support-patient-centered-outcomes-research.

Despite the wealth of data collected by CMS, Oelschlaeger said this information is often insufficient on its own for research on clinical effectiveness. Much information is missing, including

- cause of death data;
- clinical data (for example, lab results);
- certain patient demographic data (for example, income and high-quality race/ethnicity data);
- data related to social determinants of health;
- health behaviors data;
- patient-generated health information; and
- human services data.

Oelschlaeger said that options for enhancing the CMS data with the missing information could include undertaking new data collection, imputation, or linkages to other data sources.

The PCOR Trust Fund funded several CMS projects throughout the years. One of these projects was Blue Button 2.0,[2] which is an application programming interface (API) that allows beneficiaries to connect their data to applications and services they trust and enables them to contribute their data to research projects. Blue Button leverages FHIR standards, also discussed by Tripathi. CMS data linkage projects that have been funded by the PCOR Trust Fund include[3]

- Augmenting the National Hospital Care Survey Data through Linkages with Administrative Records;
- National COVID-19 Longitudinal Research Database, which is linked to CMS data; and
- National Death Index—Medicare Enrollment Data Linkage.

Oelschlaeger said that CMS also has other projects funded through other agencies to link CMS data and data from other sources, including

- Surveillance, Epidemiology, and End Results;
- U.S. Renal Data System;
- Health and Retirement Survey; and
- National Health and Aging Trends Study.

---

[2] https://bluebutton.cms.gov/.
[3] For more information on specific projects, see https://aspe.hhs.gov/collaborations-committees-advisory-groups/os-pcortf/explore-portfolio.

Oelschlaeger discussed several barriers to data linkages that involve CMS data. She said that for privacy reasons, personal information is collected less often, and datasets are increasingly lacking patient identifiers that are sufficient for linkages. Private and proprietary datasets, such as registries, have additional limitations for sharing identifiers. She also noted that the volume of patient records necessary to access in order to perform the linkages is often larger than what is needed once the linkage is complete.

According to Oelschlaeger, researchers increasingly want to use tokenization solutions. These are methods that assign unique keys to the datasets being linked, enabling the linkage to happen without the sharing of patient identifiers. The challenge CMS encountered is that there are a variety of tokenization solutions, and researchers have a variety of preferences about what to use. Oelschlaeger noted that the lack of consistency (the differences in degree of difficulty across different populations) is also a challenge in probabilistic matching, specifically the question of how good the match needs to be in order for the linkage to happen.

Oelschlaeger also discussed the CMS Virtual Research Data Center (VRDC), which is meant to provide a secure and efficient mechanism for researchers to virtually access and analyze CMS data and potentially address some of the challenges. The VRDC allows researchers to access CMS data and perform their own analyses and manipulation of those data virtually, from their independent workstations, and it allows them to download aggregate results from the analyses they perform. The VRDC enables faster access at a lower cost to the CMS data that are already linked by a unique beneficiary ID. Researchers also have the ability to upload other data to the VRDC to perform additional linkages.

Meagan Khau, CMS Office of Minority Health, described the mission of her office as serving as the principal advisor to the agency on the needs of minority populations, including racial and ethnic minorities; people with disabilities; the LGBTQ+ community; individuals with limited English proficiency; rural populations; and persons otherwise adversely affected by persistent poverty or inequality. She highlighted two sections of Executive Order 13985, which are focused on the role of data in meeting the needs of these populations. Specifically, Section 4(a) focuses on methods for assessing equity, which underscores the need to collect demographic data in order to fully assess the extent of existing health disparities and the impact of health equity responses. Section 9(a) establishes a workgroup to gather necessary data to measure and advance equity.

Khau noted that federal datasets often are not disaggregated by key demographic variables, such as race, ethnicity, gender, disability, income, and veteran status. CMS is working on gaining a better understanding of what datasets contain data elements of interest, and what standards are being used. As an example, for race, the Office of Management and Budget

1997 standards use five categories, whereas the 2011 Department of Health and Human Services (HHS) standards[4] use 14 categories. Various standards and approaches are used in various EHRs.

Detailed, disaggregated data are needed to target interventions, in Khau's view. As an example (Figure 2-1), she noted that in 2018 the prevalence of diabetes in the population as a whole was around 11 percent. Using five race categories, the prevalence was highest among Native Hawaiian and other Pacific Islanders, at 15 percent. However, when the data are further disaggregated, it becomes clear that within this group the prevalence of diabetes is particularly high among Samoans, at 22 percent.

In terms of the ability to assess equity with respect to demographic data elements identified in Executive Order 13985, such as race, ethnicity, religion, income, geography, gender identity, sexual orientation, and disability, Khau pointed out that not all these data elements are collected across the different HHS programs. This means that in some cases new data collections may be necessary, and it will be important to apply the right standards to each of the data elements, in light of how the data are anticipated to be used.

Khau highlighted several projects that the CMS Office of Minority Health is working on, using CMS data. The Mapping Medicare Disparities Tool[5] is an interactive map that allows users to identify areas of disparities between subgroups of Medicare beneficiaries (for example, by race or ethnicity), chronic disease prevalence, health outcomes, spending, and utilization. The tool uses Medicare fee-for-service data. The office has also released two reports that use stratified data to look at health disparities.[6]

Khau highlighted several collaborations between the CMS Office of Minority Health and other federal partners. These projects are summarized in Box 2-1. She also called attention to the office's Minority Research Grant Program, which provides funding for principal investigators at minority-serving institutions to conduct research focused on opportunities to embed health equity into CMS programs.

Mitra Rocca, Center for Drug Evaluation and Research of the Food and Drug Administration (FDA), said that the FDA has 13 projects that are funded by the PCOR Trust Fund.[7] The projects are as follows:

---

[4] https://aspe.hhs.gov/basic-report/hhs-implementation-guidance-data-collection-standards-race-ethnicity-sex-primary-language-and-disability-status.

[5] https://data.cms.gov/mapping-medicare-disparities.

[6] See https://www.cms.gov/files/document/racial-ethnic-gender-disparities-health-care-medicare-advantage.pdf and https://www.cms.gov/files/document/omh-rural-urban-report-2020.pdf.

[7] https://aspe.hhs.gov/collaborations-committees-advisory-groups/os-pcortf/explore-portfolio.

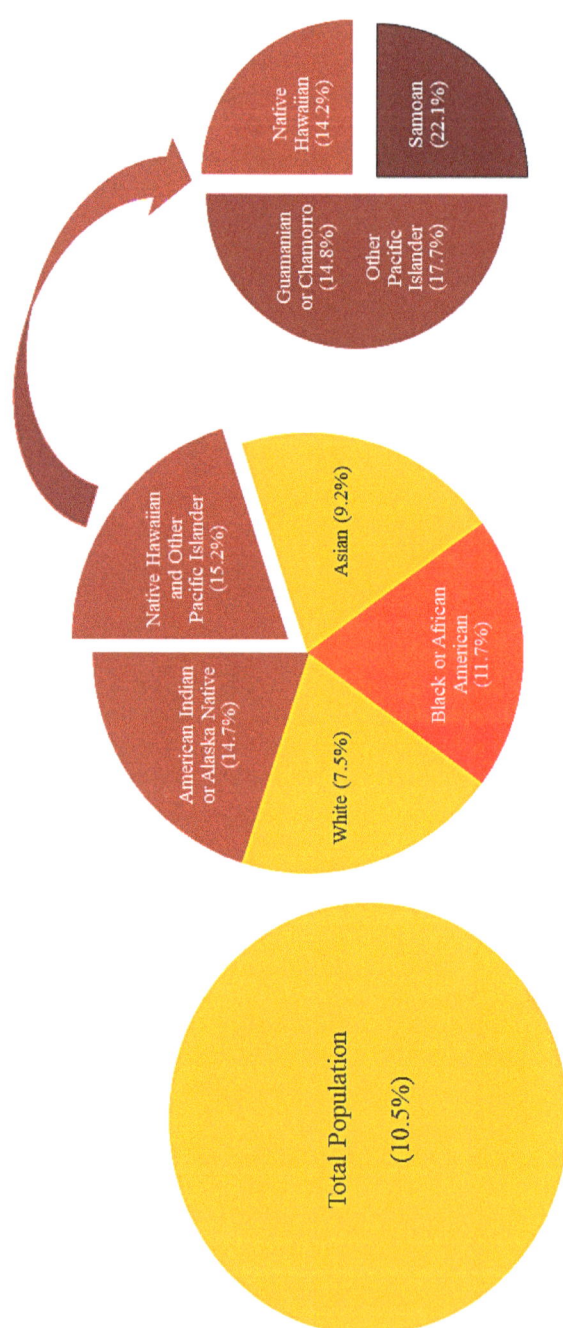

FIGURE 2-1 Prevalence of diabetes in 2018.
SOURCE: Workshop presentation by Meagan Khau, June 14, 2021.

> **BOX 2-1**
> **Collaborations Between the Centers for Medicare & Medicaid Services Office of Minority Health and Federal Partners**
>
> Trust Fund Projects
> - Building Data Capacity for Patient-Centered Outcomes Research related to Intellectual and Developmental Disabilities
> - Validate and Expand Claims-Based Algorithms, Identifying Patients with Frailty and Functional Disabilities across Payer and Patient Populations
>
> Office of Management and Budget
> - released a blog and a video showcasing how the agency uses collected data via the Mapping Medicare Disparities Tool visualization
>
> Administration on Community Living
> - worked on COVID-19 accessibility concerns and also released a paper on characteristics of Medicare beneficiaries with intellectual or developmental disabilities
>
> Department of Health and Human Services Office of Women's Health
> - promoted physical and behavioral health resources
>
> The Centers for Disease Control and Prevention (CDC), Health Resources and Services Administration, and Office of Women's Health, as well as external organizations
> - hosted the Forum on Improving Access to Maternity Health Care in Rural Communities
>
> National Institutes of Health and CDC
> - develop diabetes prevention and management resources that are culturally and linguistically tailored for the underserved populations
>
> SOURCE: Workshop presentation by Meagan Khau, June 14, 2021.

- Collection of Patient-Provided Information through a Mobile Device Application for Use in Comparative Effectiveness and Drug Safety Research;
- Common Data Model Harmonization (CDMH) and Open Standards for Evidence Generation;
- Cross-Network Directory Service;
- CURE ID: Aggregating and Analyzing COVID-19 Treatments from EHRs & Registries Globally;
- Developing a Strategically Coordinated Registry Network (CRN) for Women's Health Technologies;

- Development of a Natural Language Processing (NLP) Web Service for Public Health Use;
- Enhancing Data Resources for Studying Patterns and Correlates of Mortality in Patient-Centered Outcomes Research: Linking National Death Index (NDI) and Commercial Claims;
- Making Medicaid Data More Accessible Through Common Data Models and FHIR APIs;
- SHIELD - Standardization of Lab Data to Enhance Patient-Centered Outcomes and Value-Based Care;
- Source Data Capture from Electronic Health Records (EHRs): Using Standardized Clinical Research Data;
- Standardization and Querying of Data Quality Metrics and Characteristics for Electronic Health Data;
- Utilizing Data from Various Data Partners in a Distributed Manner; and
- WHT-CRN Project: Bridging the PCOR Infrastructure and Innovation through Coordinated Registry Network (CRN) Community of Practice.

One of the projects that Rocca leads is the Source Data Capture from EHRs. The goal of the project, which is a collaboration with the University of California, San Francisco (discussed in additional detail by Laura Esserman, Chapter 4), is to develop methods and tools to automate the flow of structured EHR data into external systems. The second project, co-led by Rocca in collaboration with the National Institutes of Health (NIH), is Common Data Model Harmonization and Open Standards for Evidence Generation. This project is a collaboration among five agencies, focusing on harmonizing across multiple common data models and generating real-world evidence from real-world data. An FDA project that is focused on data linkages in particular is the Enhancing Data Resources for Studying Patterns and Correlates of Mortality in PCOR, a project that links commercial claims data to data from the National Death Index, which is a centralized database of death records from state vital statistics offices. A collaboration among the Centers for Disease Control and Prevention (CDC), CMS, and FDA, the goal of this project is to increase the availability of information on the cause of death.

With input from the leads of the various PCOR Trust Fund projects at FDA, Rocca identified several ways collaborations could evolve to meet PCOR and data challenges going forward:

- Develop an infrastructure to support research.
- Adopt Findable, Accessible, Interoperable, and Reusable (FAIR) principles as a goal and use metrics to measure the progress.

- Use distributed data models to conduct analyses across multiple institutions, with data remaining behind data-partner firewalls.
- Build trust and validation so they are engineered into the system, which would enable collaborators to run analytic software for one another.
- Develop open-source tools to support sharing, discovering, and reusing research data.
- Convene workshops with internal and external stakeholders around particular problems.
- Improve the quality and completeness of EHR data.

In terms of the barriers and potential solutions to the access and use of linked public data, Rocca said that there is a need for a strategy and a set of standards at the HHS level that address the challenges associated with lacking a master identifier to help link several sources of data. Related to that, there is a need for standards that address the issue of re-identification. Rocca said there is also a need for a systematic review of HHS data sources with an eye toward transparency and a need to develop informed consent guidelines that enable the sharing of both public- and private-sector data.

Rocca also mentioned the need to establish a formal ontology at the HHS level to make it easier to find data, and for establishing a metadata registry and repository for data elements, controlled terminologies, and mapping for controlled terminologies. She also highlighted the need for interoperability, and challenges associated with the lack of standardization for the data that are collected. She argued that the integration of health care and clinical research will require a change in culture that begins at the point of care, where data are generated.

Regarding suggestions for building an interoperable data capacity for PCOR, Rocca highlighted the following:

- Linking existing databases within HHS and other federal government agencies and the private sector;
- Developing a universal data use agreement;
- Applying tools, standards, and services developed as part of PCOR Trust Fund projects to other types of HHS data;
- Encouraging the development of common architectures and integration frameworks to enable interoperability, rather than developing single solutions; and
- Focusing the PCOR Trust Fund investments on cutting-edge solutions that may result in technical leaps.

Adi Gundlapalli, Public Health Informatics Office, CDC, said that patient-level data with sufficient granularity are essential for improving health outcomes and that these data need to be made available in a way that preserves privacy. He argued that current laws and policies around the use of patient-level data are nuanced, and sometimes conflicting, which creates confusion for researchers, providers, and patients. This issue needs to be addressed in a way that balances individual privacy considerations, the risk of re-identification, and the utility of the datasets.

Making disease-specific datasets available for public use is an area where balancing the considerations discussed by Gundlapalli would be particularly important. He noted that recently CDC made available three COVID-19 datasets for public use, and this was accomplished by working closely with HHS to apply privacy preserving measures, including, in some cases, suppression algorithms, due to the small cell sizes. Gundlapalli said that the work done at CDC over the past year to acquire, store, provide secure access to, and analyze large datasets with high dimensionality will be an enduring resource for data capacity.

Regarding barriers and potential solutions for increased access to linked public data, Gundlapalli reiterated the risks of privacy breaches and re-identification, which, he said, have to be addressed. He noted that CDC receives only de-identified data. However, there are use cases where linking individuals within a dataset or across datasets, such as vaccination and case records for COVID-19, has tangible benefits for public health action. Because of this, CDC, in collaboration with the HHS Office of the Chief Information Officer, has been evaluating the feasibility of implementing privacy preserving record linkage (PPRL) techniques for public health data at the state, tribal, local, and territorial levels before the data are sent to CDC, with the COVID-19 vaccination data as a use case. These techniques can ensure that personally identifiable information remains within the jurisdictions' firewalls.

PPRL solutions are now available through commercial vendors, and PPRL algorithms have been applied to large, commercially available health datasets, such as laboratory data, pharmacy data, claims information, and EHRs. There are also many published examples of real-world applications of PPRL and their associated benefits, and Gundlapalli argued that these benefits have to be balanced with the risk to privacy and the efforts required to implement PPRL solutions. He added that potential linkages of publicly available data with private, proprietary data are especially interesting, and these opportunities merit detailed consideration.

As far as building interoperable data capacity, Gundlapalli said that CDC also has ongoing projects that address this issue, and it may be useful to consider what can be learned from that work. CDC has been actively working on public health data modernization, an effort that was given a boost with recent COVID-19-related funding. Through a set of targeted investments across three priority thematic areas, CDC aims to promote the reporting of clinical and laboratory data to ensure that core public health surveillance systems are interoperable, and the agency supports crosscutting upgrades such as the migration of the data to the cloud and access to new data sources. CDC is hoping that these efforts will also support the interoperable data capacity for PCOR. Gundlapalli summarized the three priority areas as (1) data sharing across the public health ecosystem, (2) using CDC systems for ongoing data modernization, and (3) adopting new standards and approaches for public health reporting.

Alison Cernich, Eunice Kennedy Shriver National Institute of Child Health and Human Development (NICHD), said that NICHD, as well as NIH more broadly, are heavily invested in ensuring that research incorporates PCOR to the greatest extent possible, and that data gathered through their research are available to other researchers for further analyses. She pointed out that NIH issued a new policy on data sharing for NIH-funded research.[8] The policy will go into effect on January 25, 2023, and it is based on an understanding that sharing scientific data accelerates biomedical research discovery by enabling validation of research results, providing accessibility to high-value datasets, and promoting data reuse for future studies. The policy is intended to ensure that there is a plan in place for the sharing of data from NIH-funded research. It also specifies allowable costs for data management and sharing, and discusses ways of selecting a repository for the data.

Cernich noted that NIH supports several domain-specific data repositories that are open for both submitting and accessing data. An example is the NICHD Data and Specimen Hub, which allows clinical research data, including PROs, to be posted and shared. NICHD also funds the Data Sharing for Demographic Research infrastructure, which provides curation and archiving services for data relevant to health policy and health systems research as well as broader demographic research.

Concerning barriers, Cernich said that data sharing might be limited by either the parameters of the initial consent provided by the participant or based on NIH policies aimed at protecting the individual. Data sharing has to be balanced with these considerations as a first step. Beyond that, she said, it is important to ensure that data that are shared comply with guiding principles, such as the FAIR data principles and the Transparency, Responsibility, User focus, Sustainability, and Technology (TRUST) data repository principles.

Cernich noted that the COVID-19 pandemic accelerated the need for data that are based on common standards and can quickly be aggregated to produce new knowledge. Tools and resources available for use in public health emergencies and disasters through the Disaster Research Response

---

[8] https://grants.nih.gov/grants/guide/notice-files/NOT-OD-21-013.html.

Resource were useful to address this need initially. The PhenX Toolkit was another resource of data standards, clinical report forms, measurement protocols, and survey instruments, some of which included patient-centered outcome variables, such as life changes, household events, and overall impact.

NICHD has also been working on pointing the community toward standard data models, such as the Observational Medical Outcomes Partnership (OMOP) or HL7 FHIR. Cernich said that adopting standard data models can be challenging, because not all of them can accommodate every type of data, but NICHD has been encouraging the use of these standards. The agency has also been developing common data elements where those are lacking. For example, early in the pandemic, NICHD convened a group of stakeholders to specify common data elements for pregnancy as part of a large-scale study to look at the effects of COVID-19 in the context of pregnancy. These data elements were intended to be generalizable to other studies of pregnancy so they could be harmonized and aggregated for more robust analyses.

Cernich also discussed the Gabriella Miller Kids First Data Resource, which is supported by NICHD in collaboration with the National Heart, Lung, and Blood Institute; the National Cancer Institute; and the Common Fund. This resource will use FHIR standards to integrate EHR data, and it is also expanding to include genomic data on conditions in children.

Another NICHD collaboration with ONC, CDC, and the National Center for Health Statistics (NCHS) is focused on developing an HL7 FHIR implementation guide for maternal health, which will specify models for using EHR data standards to identify individual women and their individual pregnancies over time and across health systems. NICHD would also like to be able to link the records of parents and their children. These linkages would make it possible to monitor the impact of emerging public health concerns, such as infectious diseases, to examine the adverse effects of commonly used medications during pregnancy and postpartum on the pregnant person and the infant, and to determine predictive models that can help address various inequities such as inequalities in maternal morbidity and mortality. Cernich noted that NICHD is leading a consortium of projects focused on maternal health to enable coordination and collaboration within this portfolio through the PCOR Trust Fund.

NIH was a pioneer in developing PCOR measures, Cernich said, through projects such as the PROMIS Initiative and the Quality-of-Life Initiative, but she argued that there is a need to continue to refine and implement standard measures of patient perception and evolve with technology. She highlighted the All of Us project, which includes participants in developing some of the project's modules and is also integrating wearables and other data sources to describe the group of people who are participating.

Cernich pointed to a need for new linkages for data within HHS. For example, NIH and NCHS reached an agreement on the use of data from the National Death Index for research, but other data on vital statistics remain difficult to integrate because of costs and challenges associated with establishing these types of agreements. She also said that access to HHS data needs to be expanded for NIH intramural investigators and that opportunities for doing this exist.

Jacob Kean, Salt Lake City Veterans Affairs Health Care System in the Department of Veterans Affairs (VA), and University of Utah, began by discussing the Department of Defense (DoD) and Department of Veterans Affairs Infrastructure for Clinical Intelligence (DaVINCI) as an example of notable progress on infrastructure for PCOR over the past 5 to 10 years. DaVINCI is a data warehouse and analytic platform that combines DoD and VA health care data, and it serves as an interface between the systems supporting the EHRs at the two agencies. The project began in 2014 and has been building on early successes to achieve scale. To date, DaVINCI has supported more than 60 operations and research projects, and transferring data between the two agencies is a key aspect of this.

Kean discussed lessons learned in several areas, including governance and compliance, data standardization, data quality, education, and partnerships. In the area of governance and regulatory compliance, DoD and VA explored several potential collaborative project governance options and resources for the navigation of regulatory policy, before they settled on an arrangement that was suitable for the DaVINCI project. Kean underscored the time and effort needed to complete this process and noted that establishing partnerships between federal agencies and other entities, such as states or private organizations, can be even more challenging.

In terms of data standardization, DaVINCI uses the OMOP Common Data Model, which Kean described as an enabler and an accelerator. For example, without the OMOP, a data user would need to look at separate data sources for inpatient, outpatient, and surgical encounters, and possibly look at seven or eight different tables for information on medications. OMOP provides researchers with an advantage because they can approach the dataset with an understanding of its structure. While a complete alignment is probably impossible, HHS efforts to harmonize standards are helping remove the barriers posed by the lack of standardization. Kean also underscored the value of HHS support for the development of open-source tools around agreed-upon standards and data models so that the consistency of the work around clinical data improves and also reduces the barrier to entry.

DaVINCI has maintained a focus on data quality throughout project development and execution. This facilitates the use of the data, for example by providing information on fitness for use. Kean said that among the most effective DaVINCI efforts so far are those related to education. Educational outreach targets current and potential data users and focuses on the structure and provenance of the data. He encouraged HHS to continue to develop and enhance existing educational efforts on the appropriate management and use of data resources.

Kean also discussed challenges and opportunities associated with linked data, including both public and private data. The past few years have witnessed great advances in PPRL technologies and in the scaling of these technologies in a variety of contexts. These advances are happening in parallel with a new set of challenges. One challenge is that there are now thousands of datasets available, and it is difficult to gain a comprehensive understanding of this ecosystem. Kean said that HHS could assist with these efforts by promoting standards, standards education, and tool development. These standards and tools can help with a comparison of similar datasets and the appreciation of strengths and limitations.

Another challenge is related to the costs of linking datasets on a large scale. Kean noted that it is difficult to assign value to the different datasets, but HHS could consider cloud-hosting solutions that enable research and make it possible to shift some of the work from a project level to an agency level. For instance, a PCOR sponsor could sponsor the cost of many data sources and allow others to access the data.

In the future, technology solutions such as blockchain technologies could greatly advance the PCOR data infrastructure. Inherent in every blockchain technology is a distributed ledger, which documents all manipulation and use of data and helps to prevent any unauthorized use. Moreover, these technologies promote federated learning models, which eliminate data transfer. Blockchain technologies could promote the assignment of value to data through combinations of data attributes and data provenance. Furthermore, these technologies could enable data self-sovereignty, which may be a pinnacle of patient centeredness, because it would allow individuals to control access to and use of their data. Kean encouraged HHS to promote regulatory and policy solutions around these transformative technologies.

HHS can play a role in helping to develop and promote use cases, according to Kean. One such use case would be a situation where decentralized models are superior to centralized models for regulatory security and other reasons. Another one could be a situation where trust between entities is a paramount concern. Kean said that the DaVINCI project shows the feasibility of building interoperable data capacity. To date, HHS has played an essential role and could in the future prioritize efforts to advance regulatory guidance, align standards, and foster knowledge of the appropriate use of the growing PCOR ecosystem.

DISCUSSION

During the workshop, the formal presentations were followed by additional discussion among the workshop participants, including the speakers, committee, and audience members. Among the topics that were explored in further detail were the need to harmonize data collections, and data elements in particular, across the federal government. The importance of increasing the adoption of standards and leveraging new opportunities for collaboration made possible by standardized health information technology was also highlighted as part of the discussion. Speakers expressed a desire for coordinating efforts to increase the interoperability of data systems, which would serve as a foundation for the scalability of common approaches in areas such as informed consent.

Speakers acknowledged that increasing the consistency and the use of standards will be a slow and gradual process. In some cases, it might be necessary to accept that heterogeneity exists and consider ways of working within those parameters. It is also important to note that the existing datasets tend to focus on specific populations that are only a subset of the population as a whole and might differ from the overall population on a variety of dimensions.

The discussion also echoed conversations about the challenges resulting from the differing data collection goals in clinical care and research contexts. A related issue is the burden placed on providers and patients who are asked to provide the data. To mitigate these challenges, more clarity is needed about the potential uses and value of the data.

Participants also discussed the usefulness of data that originate from sources other than the context of patient care (such as population surveys) and the potential conceptual limitations that result from focusing on the patient, rather than the individual, regardless of whether the person has a disease, diagnosis, or interaction with a health care provider. This discussion echoed the conversations and committee conclusions that emerged from the first workshop in this series.[9]

Another theme that emerged centered on the challenge of prioritizing projects, given the complexity and broad scope of the PCOR data infrastructure. Priorities are set by legislation or by the agencies, and there are mechanisms for input from committees and workgroups. However, the discussion also made it clear that awareness about the data infrastructure projects is limited among external stakeholders and end users.

---

[9] https://www.nap.edu/catalog/26297/building-data-capacity-for-patient-centered-outcomes-research-interim-report.

CONCLUSIONS

The session with federal agency representatives highlighted several key areas where additional work, and in particular collaborative work, is especially needed to continue to build and strengthen the PCOR data infrastructure.

CONCLUSION 2-1: Collaboration among federal agencies and between federal agencies and other partners (such as states, patient groups, and others) is essential for continuing to build the patient-centered outcomes research data infrastructure. The areas where additional collaboration would be particularly useful include the following:

- Increasing consistency in the use of standards for data interoperability and element definitions;
- Addressing barriers that hinder data linkages, such as the limitations associated with health identifiers and mitigating potential selection biases resulting from linkage error;
- Balancing the burden of the data collections and disclosure risks with the value of the datasets;
- Communicating the usefulness of the data collections to those who are asked to provide data about themselves and those who collect the data;
- Promoting discussion and education about fitness for use of the data; and
- Working with stakeholders and patients to promote sharing of data.

While there is frequent collaboration among HHS partners on PCOR data infrastructure work, and the Office of the Assistant Secretary for Planning and Evaluation's public website contains a comprehensive list of past and current projects funded from the PCOR Trust Fund, additional dissemination efforts focused on external stakeholders could further increase the usefulness of these investments.

CONCLUSION 2-2: There is a need to increase awareness among all stakeholders about new data infrastructure developments funded by the Patient-Centered Outcomes Research Trust Fund. Increased awareness will enhance the efficiency and effectiveness of research, which will increase the impact of the investments made in infrastructure development.

3

State-Level Data and Collaborations

Lynn Blewett of the State Health Access Data Assistance Center (SHADAC), which is located at the University of Minnesota, noted that SHADAC works with states to leverage state and federal data in the interest of informing policy. Blewett said that large federal data projects using electronic health records (EHRs) and linked data are critical to patient outcomes research, but the time lags in the availability of these data make the results less actionable for state health policy. State analysts are dependent on federal agencies for data access, and congressional objectives may trump state needs. For these reasons and others, local data collaboratives informed by communities of patients, providers, and payers are key to informing state health policy. These data collaboratives make timely and targeted data projects possible, resulting in information that is focused on state needs and priorities and that state policy makers can use.

Blewett discussed several examples of state initiatives. The first example she discussed was the All-Payer Claims Data (APCD) databases. These databases collect and harmonize claims data from public and private payers and include patient demographics and provider codes as well as clinical, financial, and utilization information. The purposes and mechanisms enabling these databases vary across states. The primary objectives are to better understand the financing of health care at the state level, to inform state health reform activities, and to evaluate the outcomes of state reform strategies. The APCD Council provides a forum for states implementing APCDs to share information, expertise, and insight on their development and use. Blewett said that 23 states have all-payer claims databases, and 6 more are being implemented.[1]

Advantages of APCDs include the following:

- Cover the majority of residents in each state;
- Include geographic representation;
- Capture longitudinal information on a wide range of individual patients, providers, and payers;
- Offer comprehensive utilization and spending data at the state level;
- Are mandated by state legislation; and
- Receive federal funding through various initiatives.

Challenges among APCDs include the following:

- Data access for researchers varies by state.
- They provide no data on use of services by the uninsured.
- States cannot require a self-funded insurer and its third-party administrator to share claims data with a state APCD.
- They lack standardization of encounter-level claims from capitated health plans.

Another example discussed by Blewett was a voluntary local health system collaboration, the Minnesota EHR consortium COVID-19 project. There are 11 health systems that are voluntarily participating in this consortium to provide public health surveillance data in close to real time for decision makers. While discussions have been ongoing related to a variety of diseases, the collaboration quickly materialized at the beginning of the pandemic. Blewett said that no patient-level data are shared between systems. Vaccination information is reported by the state and then linked to participating EHR systems; summary data are aggregated at a central site. The project captures about 90 percent of the initial 1.5 million first and second vaccine doses administered in the state.

The following are what has worked in the data sharing consortium:

- Skilled and innovative researchers are embedded in the health systems.
- A distributed data network model is followed (avoids concerns about data privacy and simplifies data use agreements).

---

[1] https://www.apcdcouncil.org/state/map.

Challenges in the data-sharing consortium include the following:

- There is interest in adding smaller independent clinics and Federally Qualified Health Centers, but that is more difficult and it is costly to build up infrastructure for data submissions.
- Race/ethnicity data need improvement.
- The consortium needs sustainable funding.
- There is a need for improving communications, engagement, and dissemination.

Blewett also discussed the Medicaid Outcomes Distributed Research Network (MODRN), a collaboration to analyze Medicaid data across multiple states to facilitate learning among Medicaid agencies. Participants include AcademyHealth's State-University Partnership Learning Network and the Medicaid Medical Director Network. This distributed data network allows states to retain their own data and analytic capacity while being able to compare their outcomes data to those from other states. As part of this initiative, 11 university–state partnerships now participate to provide a comprehensive assessment of Medicaid treatment quality in addressing opioid use disorders.

The following are what has worked in MODRN:

- Distributed data network model (avoids concerns about data privacy and simplifies data use agreements);
- Engagement of local universities that have analytic expertise with state Medicaid analysts; and
- Collaboration around policy priorities and closer to real-time analysis.

Challenges with MODRN include the following:

- State participation is limited.
- Data sharing agreements and data use agreements are still required for university-based research access to data files unless all of the analysis is run by the state.
- Financing is needed to support sustainability of network/models.

Blewett offered four overall conclusions based on her experiences: (1) Locally based collaborations that are close to policy makers and decision makers are more feasible and more actionable for state health policy; (2) State regulatory requirements can be leveraged to facilitate data collection and then develop infrastructure for research capacity; (3) Collaborative distributed data networks with motivated and interested researchers embedded within health systems and public agencies can lead efforts to support targeted data and analytic needs; and (4) Federal financing of local models can be used to inform other activities across the states.

She added that SHADAC collaborates with federal partners to obtain state-level data from the National Health Interview Survey, but it is a "heavy lift." Among the challenges, she listed the need to have analysts who know how to interact with the National Center for Health Statistics and have special sworn status (from the Census Bureau), and the need for a new proposal every year.

Marsha Lillie-Blanton, George Washington University, focused her remarks related to state-level data and collaborations on broadening the concept of equity to include equity across states. She noted that the policies, practices, and characteristics of geopolitical areas, such as states, matter in the efforts to improve access and quality and to achieve person-centered care.

While the federal role has increased, states continue to be the main drivers of coverage and care for low-income population groups, with Medicaid being the major player in the landscape. Lillie-Blanton pointed out that the states that decided not to expand Medicaid during the early part of the expansion were disproportionately southern states, which have large Black or African American and Hispanic or Latinx populations. This illustrates how states can become drivers of inequities in access to quality care and person-centered care.

Lillie-Blanton discussed the Nationwide Adult Medicaid Consumer Assessment of Healthcare Providers and Systems Survey (NAM CAHPS), a survey that she worked on while she was at the Centers for Medicare & Medicaid Services.[2] A nationally representative survey of adult Medicaid recipients with state-specific samples, NAM CAHPS is a collaboration among several federal partners as well as 46 states and DC. The data produced include state-specific NAM CAHPS files, which states can get access to on the basis of a data-use agreement. Lillie-Blanton echoed Blewett's comment about frequent lags in making these types of data available to the states.

Considering both challenges and opportunities associated with collaborations of this type, Lillie-Blanton highlighted the following as some of the areas that need attention:

- *Aligning priorities*: Both federal and state partners need to identify the data collection effort as a priority.
- *Cost issues*: Funding needs to be allocated for this type of data collection and analysis.

---

[2]https://www.medicaid.gov/medicaid/quality-of-care/quality-of-care-performance-measurement/nationwide-adult-medicaid-consumer-assessment-of-healthcare-providers-and-systems/index.html.

- *Longitudinal data*: While the baseline data have value, ongoing data collection (even if only every 3 to 5 years) is needed.
- *Methodological issues*: Comparative analysis across states requires adjustments for state variations in variables that may be unmeasured or not well-measured.
- *Data linking*: Future federal/state Medicaid surveys will need to include permission in the consumer consent form to link personally identifiable information.

Lillie-Blanton underscored the need for developing partnerships based on trust. Some of the potential partners for federal agencies include Medicaid Agencies, the Medicaid Medical Directors Network, and Public Health and Behavioral Health Agencies. Other stakeholders to consider are professional associations, clinicians and provider groups, advocacy groups, and consumer groups. Academic institutions, policy research organizations, and foundations could also serve as partners.

In terms of building data capacity, two areas emphasized by Lillie-Blanton are (1) supporting the development of state Medicaid infrastructure for data collection, analysis, and reporting; and (2) developing training opportunities and funding for researchers for collecting and analyzing Medicaid data. She noted that some state Medicaid agencies already have strong infrastructures for data collection (e.g., MA, MI, NY, AL) or partnerships with academic institutions (e.g., PA, AR).

Todd Gilmer, University of California, San Diego, made three key points about state-level data and collaborations. First, state-level data are useful for understanding health disparities, because lower-income individuals and families, including those with a significant disability, are underrepresented in many national and commercial datasets, while Medicaid data can provide comprehensive coverage on diverse populations. Second, state-level data can be challenging to work with and to acquire. The learning curves can be steep due to complex and bureaucratic systems, and a path for accessing protected data is not always clear. Furthermore, a high prevalence of Medicaid managed care may result in uneven data quality. Due to these challenges, long-term collaborations can facilitate the interpretation of and access to data. Third, promising opportunities also exist at the county level.

Among the types of data available at the state level, Gilmer highlighted the following:

- *Medicaid data:*
  — Provide information on health insurance coverage for low-income families and individuals (in expansion states), low-income elderly, and people with disabilities; and

- Cover a racially/ethnically diverse population with complex health conditions.
- *Inpatient and emergency department discharge data:*
  - Are available in most states;
  - In California, are provided by the Office of Statewide Health Planning and Development; and
  - Are aggregated by the Agency for Healthcare Research and Quality (AHRQ), which maintains a national database Healthcare Cost and Utilization Project (HCUP) for these data, although with less detail than is available in the state data.
- *State-level surveys and indices:*
  - Can provide local-area information;
  - Have a greater focus on health disparities compared to national surveys and are potentially more customizable; and
  - In California, are derived from the California Health Interview Survey and the Healthy Places Index.

Gilmer highlighted Medicaid datasets as especially valuable. These datasets have fairly comprehensive coverage, including on medical care and pharmaceuticals. They also have good coverage of mental health and substance use care, particularly for those who are in high need of these services. The datasets also cover home- and community-based services and custodial long-term care. Due to these characteristics, the Medicaid datasets provide a unique platform for studying special populations and topics of interest.

Medicaid programs are uniquely innovative, in Gilmer's view. Among the innovations, he highlighted the comprehensive, statewide multipayer delivery system and payment reforms that reward value as opposed to volume and support improvements in population health delivery system and payment reform. He also noted that Medicaid provides integrated services for people with complex needs, such as high-risk children and youth; adults eligible for Medicare and Medicaid, including those with long-term care needs; and people with complex physical health, behavioral health, and social service needs. Gilmer also highlighted experimentation with alternative delivery strategies, such as the use of community health workers to build health literacy and peer providers with lived experience to increase engagement in health care.

Gilmer described the Transformed Medicaid Statistical Information System (T-MSIS), which aims to provide Medicaid data on all U.S. states and territories in a more timely way than the previous information system. While there have been some delays in implementing T-MSIS, all states are now reporting data, so it is now starting to become possible to do the types of analyses discussed above. There are also efforts underway to improve data quality, targeting 21 indicators, such as reasonableness of eligible counts, beneficiary demographics, and completeness of key claims service data elements.

Gilmer also highlighted several challenges associated with using state-level data:

- *Data access:*
  — Each state will have a unique process and Institutional Review Board (IRB) requirements to access data.
  — Data are fragmented, and memoranda of agreement are required for multiple systems.
  — A significant investment is needed for a single study.

- *Data quality:*
  — Each state dataset will have some unique characteristics.
  — The high prevalence of managed care may affect data quality.
  — There are limitations associated with data on race/ethnicity, language, and sexual orientation.

State data access and quality would benefit from long-term collaborations and investment, Gilmer argued. This would mean maintenance of merged datasets, a standardized process for data access, and a shared understanding of data elements.

Gilmer also briefly discussed examples of data available at the county level. There are many large counties in California, and elsewhere, and they often manage some parts of the health care system. For example, in California mental health and substance use services are managed at the county level. Gilmer said that county-level data may have more detail than data at the state level. For example, San Diego county records include detailed data on race, ethnicity, language, and sexual orientation. When these records are combined at the state level, some of the details are lost due to missing data. It is also important to note that counties provide other social and public safety services, and linking to those datasets presents additional opportunities.

Claudia Steiner, Kaiser Permanente Colorado, discussed datasets produced by AHRQ based on inpatient, emergency department, and ambulatory surgery discharge data. Discharge data are available in all states except Alabama. AHRQ creates five nationwide databases, using a sampling technique that allows estimation to the nation. The nationwide databases are the National (Nationwide) Inpatient Sample; the Kids' Inpatient Database; the Nationwide Ambulatory Surgery Database; the Nationwide Emergency Department Database; and the Nationwide Readmissions Database. AHRQ also creates three statewide databases, available for some states that allow the distribution of the data: the State Inpatient Databases; the State Ambulatory Surgery Databases; and the State Emergency Department Databases.

The state-level databases include some identifiers that make it possible to link to other databases. Identifiers could include hospital identifiers, encrypted physician identifiers, patient state/county Federal Information Processing Standards codes, and patient zip codes. In some cases, for some states, AHRQ can link additional data at the hospital, physician, or patient level, with permission from the state data organization. State data organizations often have more restricted and fully identified data, and they can perform linkages to additional restricted data available within the state. Examples include linking to birth or death certificates, state-level surveys, patient-reported outcomes, and social determinants of health data collections. Steiner noted that AHRQ is currently actively exploring links to social determinants of health data as well as physician practice variables for Medical Expenditure Panel survey and HCUP data.

Steiner echoed a point made by other speakers, namely that access to state-level data can be challenging because each state has its own process and IRB requirements for accessing the data. She added that the AHRQ HCUP supports a consistent approach to accessing state-level data, and costs are mitigated in many cases. Unique characteristics of the data in some of the states was another challenge discussed by Steiner. AHRQ standardizes the data across all states with a consistently defined set of variables, so state data access and quality have benefited from long-term collaborations with AHRQ. Steiner argued that additional funding and collaboration across federal agencies and within the state partnerships could yield additional value and versatility.

DISCUSSION

The brief discussion that followed the presentations further highlighted the inconsistencies in the availability and quality of the data produced by the states. Comments echoed prior observations that the data collected are not necessarily collected for research purposes and research considerations might not be a priority. For example, while zip-code information is useful, the purpose of zip codes is primarily administrative, which often does not represent the "on the ground" characteristics of an area. In addition, zip codes are sometimes changed. Speakers highlighted the need to develop partnerships built on mutual trust and benefit and to support state data collection systems and analytic efforts.

Participants discussed the additional time needed to aggregate state data at the national level. The delays affect some types of data more than others, and the extent to which having up-to-date data is necessary also varies by the type of data or question, but increased consistency among the states and automation could reduce the time necessary to produce national datasets.

CONCLUSIONS

Many states have robust data collection systems and can produce information that is useful to state and local policy makers. State-generated data are also valuable at the national level, including for answering broader questions about issues that may be influenced by local policy, such as health care access and disparities.

CONCLUSION 3-1: There are opportunities to learn from what states have accomplished in building data capacity.

The data collected, their quality, and ease of access all vary by state. Challenges associated with access, ranging from how the data are stored to the processes involved in accessing them, make the use of state-generated data for research at the national level particularly difficult. The lack of standardization and lag times in data availability present additional challenges.

CONCLUSION 3-2: The usefulness of data available for patient-centered outcomes research could be increased by the sharing and adoption of best practices among the states for the data collected, their quality, and ease of access.

4

Clinical Trial Networks and Collaborations

Ruth Carlos, University of Michigan, said that two prime organizations that generate large volumes of clinical trials data are those within the National Cancer Institute (NCI), National Clinical Trials Network (NCTN), and the NCI Community Oncology Research Program (NCORP). Figure 4-1 shows the structure of the NCTN. The five core NCTN research bases conduct therapeutic and cancer control and outcomes research with imaging-based screening and diagnostic trials housed within ECOG-ACRIN (formed as a merger between the Eastern Cooperative Oncology Group [ECOG] for cancer therapy and the American College of Radiology Imaging Network [ACRIN] for cancer imaging). These research bases individually host extensive multidimensional data from their clinical trials. Academic centers and community oncology practices can participate in these clinical trials only through specific base affiliation, and each practice can belong to multiple bases. Carlos noted that no data are routinely shared across research bases.

Two additional research bases conduct only cancer control and outcomes research, such as research on symptom science, patient-reported outcomes, and cancer care delivery, through the NCORP with more than 1,000 practices throughout the United States. Carlos described the NCORP as a valuable setting for cancer clinical trials, because 80 percent of cancer patients receive their treatment in community oncology practices.

Carlos said that while the ECOG-ACRIN datasets are small compared to the national and state datasets discussed, they contain a lot more clinical information, including data on therapeutics, clinical outcomes, potential adverse events, treatment tolerability, treatment adherence, and survival.

43

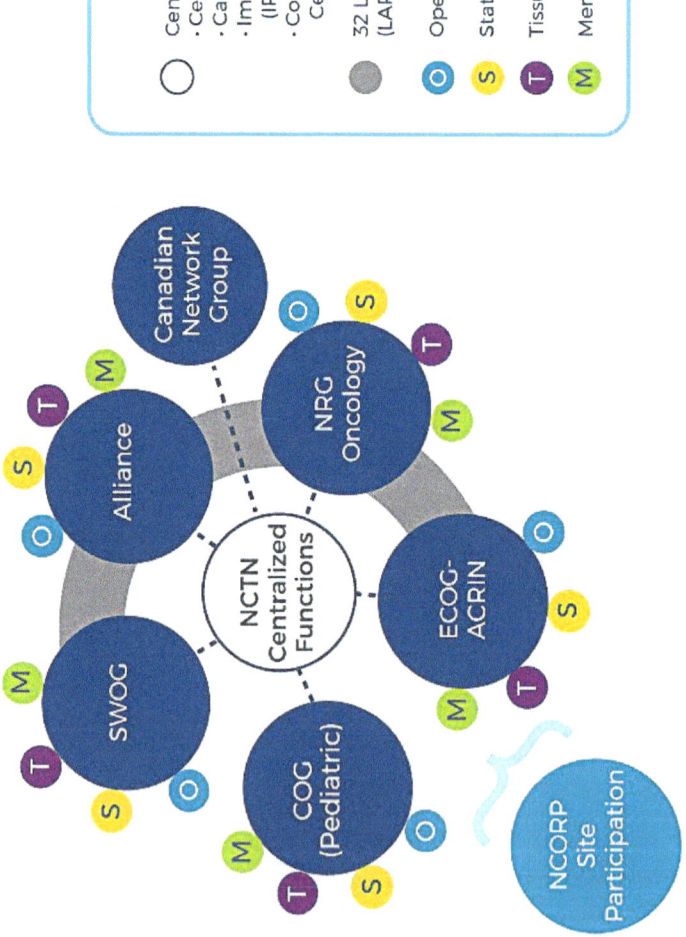

FIGURE 4-1 National Cancer Institute National Clinical Trials Network structure.
SOURCE: Workshop presentation by Ruth Carlos, June 14, 2021; CDC, 2021, https://www.cancer.gov/research/infrastructure/clinical-trials/nctn.

Some of the recent studies included the MATCH trial, the National Lung Screening Trial, and the Tomosynthesis and Mammographic Imaging Screening Trial. In addition to these large trials, they also conduct a variety of trials on cancer care delivery, such as an observational trial on financial toxicity (financial distress), an intervention trial on remote delivery of smoking cessation, and a trial on guideline-concordant optimization (de-implementation) of care. Carlos noted that the goal of many of the trials that collect patient-reported outcomes, such as those concerning treatment tolerability, adherence, or quality of life, is to produce information that is actionable and allows clinicians to make decisions on altering, modifying, or otherwise providing supportive care for their patients.

Health equity has also been a particular emphasis within ECOG-ACRIN, with data on ancestry and race, insurance and access, neighborhood deprivation, stress/physiologic dysregulation (allostatic load), and outcome disparities. Carlos and her colleagues conducted retrospective analyses of some of the data from prior trials and noted the absence of information that reflects contemporary thinking about the topics of health equity, structural racism, and discrimination. Addressing an earlier discussion about the collection of genomic data, she argued that it is important to capture both race and ancestry, because race data can provide information on the phenotypic risk of the experience of discrimination, while ancestry may provide information on biological risk.

Carlos noted that there are opportunities for building data capacity within all of these streams of work. In the case of cancer care delivery trials, it becomes important to understand both the clinic- and system-level characteristics and practices, and capture that information in a way that makes it possible to analyze patient outcomes within specific practice types. With patient-reported outcomes, the challenge is to develop ways to relay the information back to the clinician in a manner that ensures that it is received and is actionable. In the area of health equity, capacity could be enhanced by capturing evolving patient-specific insurance design features, capturing ZIP+4 as part of the address information and translating that into measures of structural inequity, and decreasing barriers to data extraction from electronic medical records to be able to obtain data such as allostatic load.

Carlos said that the complexity of the data types and location, as well as the need for equity, transparency, and regulatory compliance, underpinned by strong ethical principles in collection, access, and use, can rapidly seem daunting. This highlights the need to choose actionable potential targets for phased implementation that will ultimately expand data capacity for patient-centered outcomes research (PCOR).

The potential and the challenge of building data capacity for PCOR, according to Carlos, are highlighted by the "four Vs" of big data: *volume, variety, velocity,* and *veracity*. She argued that a fifth V worth adding is *value,* to characterize data in the context of priorities, such as that of providing actionable information.

Laura Esserman, University of California, San Francisco, said that electronic health records (EHRs) can play a role in accomplishing the goals laid out by previous speakers. EHRs help with organizing information in one place, bill for services, and keep orders and messages collated. Esserman said that learning health systems require another layer of functionality. She explained that EHRs, as they are usually designed and used, do not facilitate the reuse of data for multiple purposes in real time; rather, their unstructured nature makes it difficult to share data, tools, and processes across institutions. Additionally, she said the prevalence of unstructured data in EHRs makes it difficult to use those data for decision support and quality improvement in clinical settings. She noted that current versions of EHRs do not support registries or trials, although they could.

Esserman argued that to realize the vision of shared data, it is necessary to reimagine the process of generating clinical data. As an example, she discussed her work on the OneSource project in collaboration with the UCSF-Stanford Center of Excellence in Regulatory Science and Innovation.

Esserman noted that one challenge associated with how data are captured in EHRs is that the notes that are produced are unstructured and can be contradictory. However, it is possible to imagine a more integrated approach, she said, one where each clinician is responsible for capturing the pieces of data that were important to them in a structured format. Such an approach could contribute high-quality information to "a single source of truth" that could be consistently used for secondary purposes.

After examining source data from EHRs, Esserman and colleagues concluded that there is a disconnect between the data needed for clinical research and what clinicians record in their notes. She explained that EHR data could be more useful to health care providers, patients, and clinical investigators if a system was developed that focused on what data are already captured by clinicians, what is needed beyond that, and a way to integrate that into the clinical workflow. These considerations led to the idea of the OneSource checklist. Esserman noted that the goals of the checklist are to focus on data that are truly essential, determine when they need to be collected, and facilitate creation of a workflow that allows teams to work together to collect high-quality data. She said that the checklist could result in structured data that could be entered once over the course of care but used for multiple purposes.

As an example, Esserman discussed the I-SPY COVID-19 trial. For this study, Esserman and her colleagues began to think about workflow requirements and streamlining data capture before they opened the trial for enrollment. They developed a daily standardized checklist, which is integrated with the EHR, and includes items that clinicians wanted to capture routinely. The system automates the capture of demographics, medications, and laboratory results. It also supports decisions for both clinical care and research and sends daily checklist and trial reports back to the EHR system. Working groups, such as the safety working group, can easily access information on adverse events that have been reported. Researchers involved with the trial can track what is happening at every site, which makes it possible not only to troubleshoot but to keep the data clean as well. Esserman said the approach is generalizable across sites. It can be built once and then easily integrated into an existing system without an additional major investment.

Esserman noted that in the case of platform trials that can run several studies, centralized agreements can increase quality and efficiency, as well as facilitate collaboration around common approaches to data collection. A system such as OneSource can greatly simplify the workflow and processes and can generate data with the power to change practice. She argued that clinical research is just a special case of clinical care. In systems like OneSource, Esserman said, clinical care teams assemble essential data that support decisions, and by making the clinical trial summaries visible to clinicians, they make it possible to create more disciplined data collection in the clinic setting. That, in turn, improves the process for all patients.

Lesley Curtis, Duke University, began by describing two organizations that she has worked with, the National Institutes of Health (NIH) Healthcare Systems Collaboratory and the Patient-Centered Outcomes Research Institute's Patient-Centered Outcomes Research Network (PCORnet). The NIH Healthcare Systems Collaboratory's goal is to strengthen national capacity to implement large-scale cost-effective studies that engage health care delivery systems as research partners for clinical trials. Curtis noted that the coordinating center that she co-leads is involved with pragmatic trial demonstration projects designed to identify best practices and develop general knowledge and resources that are then made available to the research community. She said that the demonstration projects are required to make use of routinely collected EHR data. Curtis described PCORnet as a network of eight large clinical research networks that work together to answer clinical questions by using EHR data that are routinely refreshed, curated, and made accessible through a distributed research network.

Curtis next discussed some challenges and opportunities for improving the PCOR data ecosystem. She pointed out that complete outcomes data are essential for randomized trials. She also noted that the process of acquiring complete outcomes data requires negotiating several individual project-specific and site-specific data-sharing agreements and licenses. Obtaining complete data is often a cumbersome process, she said, because most potential research participants do not receive their care in a closed integrated delivery system.

Advances in privacy preserving record linkage (PPRL) solutions, Curtis said, have offered opportunities to access rich private data resources. However, in order to use those solutions researchers have to negotiate multiple network licenses, pay annual project fees, and access federal sources separately. Curtis also noted that those network license negotiations are time consuming, and she suggested that it would be beneficial to create a standard license for PPRL for federally funded projects to save time and money.

Echoing other speakers, Curtis said that Centers for Medicare & Medicaid Services (CMS) claims data are very useful for outcomes data and clinical trials. She noted that a significant challenge to using those data in clinical trials is that most clinical trials do not collect a Medicare beneficiary ID or social security number, which makes it difficult to link CMS claims data. She said that an additional challenge to using CMS claims data is that beneficiary IDs or social security numbers are usually stored in areas of EHRs that are separate from clinical data records and are difficult to access even with patient consent. She noted that a PPRL solution that could resolve these issues would be very helpful. Curtis also noted that Medicaid data are useful for PCOR and clinical trials but require researchers to negotiate with each individual state to access those data. She agreed with prior speakers that multistate coalitions of those states willing to share their Medicaid data for research would be beneficial to facilitate improved access.

Curtis argued that she would like to see an efficient and comprehensive PCOR data ecosystem that allowed participants to consent to their health data being used for research and allowed researchers to access all of those data without having to rely on the patient providing consent at multiple sites of care. She said that ideally this could be accomplished by the creation of a national identifier system. She noted that a barrier to such an idea is the current climate of misinformation and disinformation that has impacted patient trust in science and research. She underlined the need to develop strategies for disseminating information that emphasizes the value of research and science and combats misinformation.

Curtis concluded by highlighting the importance of standardized and structured data collection. She noted that increased access to raw U.S. Census data has the potential to be a source for social determinants of health (SDOH) data. However, she said use of those data for PCOR requires SDOH data expertise as well as specific skills for downloading and compiling raw Census data. She suggested that one solution could be to create a common set of important SDOH measures that are available as an extractable data package for researchers. She noted that currently researchers frequently must harmonize, clean, and integrate routinely collected data from multiple institutions to create high-quality research datasets. She emphasized that research and clinical care would benefit from structured and standardized data capture.

DISCUSSION

A key theme that emerged from the discussion also echoed the conversations from previous sessions about the disconnect between the data collected as part of clinical care and the data needed for research. The discussion surfaced concerns about the burden associated with capturing these data and the lack of incentives. Some of the presentations (discussed above) offered ideas for simplifying and streamlining the process of collecting clinical data, which could potentially make it easier to accommodate the need to collect additional data for research, if carefully designed to consider the implications for the resulting information.

Participants discussed ways of integrating data from sources other than medical records into clinical research studies. This could greatly expand research on SDOH, among other subjects. The need to establish data-use agreements was highlighted as a major challenge for sharing and linking data, especially in the case of collaborations that involve several institutions.

CONCLUSION

The session on clinical trial networks and collaborations illustrated the need for better integration between clinical care and research in ways that align differing interests and are mutually beneficial. Better integration can improve both the data available for patient care and the data needed for research.

CONCLUSION 4-1: Infrastructure investments could enhance the utility of data routinely generated in the course of care for clinical trials.

5

Public-Private Partnerships

Atul Butte, University of California, San Francisco (UCSF), discussed his experience within the University of California Health System (UC Health), a health enterprise that aims to become the single accountable care organization for the entire University of California system. UC Health combines 20 health professional schools, including six medical schools, 12 hospitals, and 1,000 care delivery sites.

UC Health has a centralized electronic health record (EHR) database that uses the Observational Medical Outcomes Partnership Common Data Model with data elements that are continuously being harmonized. The database includes EHRs from the six academic health centers: UCSF, UCLA, UC Irvine, UC Davis, UC San Diego, and UC Riverside. The database also includes additional information, such as California regulatory data, pathology and radiology text elements, and death index data.

Butte noted that initially the UC Health data are identifiable, and include geographic location, such as home address, as this information is needed for ensuring and improving the quality of medical care delivered. The address information can be linked to indices such as the Area Deprivation Index, Social Vulnerability Index, and the California Healthy Places Index, and contributes to an emerging understanding of social determinants of health. Butte also pointed out that all University of California academic medical centers make health data accessible to patients following federal standards such as Fast Healthcare Interoperability Resources.

Butte said that the database "pays for itself" because it benefits the health system's operations by improving the quality of care, decreasing specific unnecessary inpatient drug use, helping with managing costs in the self-funded health plans, and assisting with centralized population health management. The same database can also be used for research, once the data are de-identified. For example, UC Health recently conducted several COVID-19 related projects in collaboration with the Food and Drug Administration.[1]

The challenge highlighted by Butte to undertaking collaborations and data sharing is the competitive health care environment. While the benefits of data sharing are evident, health systems are cautious because the data can also potentially be used against them, leading to revenue loss. As an example, he mentioned Stanford University Medical Center health care workers' use of data on infection rates as a contract negotiation tactic. Butte argued that despite these concerns, leveraging scale for value (as in the case of UC Health) has clear advantages for health systems. Once a database is developed for operational purposes, the additional cost of making it available for research purposes can be relatively small.

Vincent Mor, Brown University, discussed his experiences with building a public-private data sharing cooperative focused on long-term care. The project was part of the National Institute on Aging (NIA) Imbedded Pragmatic Alzheimer's Disease and AD-Related Dementias Clinical Trials Collaboratory (IMPACT Collaboratory), which builds capacity to conduct pragmatic clinical trials of interventions embedded within health care systems for people living with dementia and their care partners.

Mor noted that COVID-19 has disproportionately affected long-term care residents, and the need for rich real-time data on nursing homes quickly became evident at the beginning of the pandemic. To respond to this need, Mor and his colleagues partnered with Genesis Health Care to obtain real-time data, and later expanded collaborations with the American Healthcare Association, Acumen LLC, and Exponent to build a data repository involving a broader range of nursing homes that have electronic medical records. Mor said that the database can become useful in monitoring future pandemics and policy changes. The database can also make it possible to selectively recruit facilities to participate in embedded randomized controlled trials of interventions.

Mor said that the initial Brown-Genesis COVID-19 partnership was possible because of prior collaborations that laid the foundation for this work. He echoed Butte's comments that trust between the partners is essential, particularly when there is a sharing of large volumes of real-time data. In the case of this project, there was also a need to access identifiable data

---

[1] R. Vashisht, A. Patel, B.O. Crews, O.B. Garner, L. Dahm, C. Wilson, and A.J. Butte. (2021). Age- and sex-associated variations in the sensitivity of serological tests among individuals infected with SARS-CoV-2, *JAMA Network Open* 4(2), e210337. doi:10.1001/jamanetworkopen.2021.0337.

to enable linkages to information that was not available from the electronic medical records. The researchers were sensitive to the risks for Genesis and have agreed to provide input focused on solving operational challenges as a priority over publications. However, the project also produced important research that contributed to knowledge on the COVID-19 outbreak.

Ultimately, the success of the initial collaboration led to the expansion of the project to include additional nursing home companies and partners. The resulting nursing home data-sharing collaborative now serves as the basis for several new studies, including randomized controlled trials, an analysis of vaccine effectiveness, and tracking breakthrough infections. Mor noted that the American Health Care Association, an industry association, played an important role in recruiting providers and negotiating agreements.

While researchers at Brown University and others who are part of the IMPACT Collaboratory will be the first users of the data, the data will later become available for other NIA investigators. The data from the electronic medical records can be particularly useful for recruiting facilities for trials and clinical research, while the electronic medical records data linked to claims data can further expand the possibilities to areas such as pharmaco-epidemiological research, public health surveillance research, and studies of the impact of treatments or policies.

Marc Overhage, Anthem, shared his perspectives on what makes public-private partnerships work based on his experience in a variety of settings, including academia, an academic medical center, an electronic medical records vendor, and currently a payer (Anthem). He emphasized that it is important to think of opportunities for collaboration as more than just data sharing, and consider the sharing of analytic techniques, computational resources, knowledge, and opportunities to commercialize and create value in other ways.

Overhage said that a typical public-private partnership might involve a collaboration between a government entity and a private organization, with the objective of building infrastructure or other services. The partners share the investment, the risks, and the rewards. He underscored the importance but also the challenge associated with establishing the mutual benefit in a partnership.

Overhage echoed previous comments about the particular concerns for private entities, including the potential disclosure of private, sensitive, or proprietary information; risks to brand reputation; and financial risks. He also highlighted the opportunity cost associated with the time invested in the collaboration. The fragmented nature of regulations, including state and local regulations that might apply to data sharing, also represents a risk. There are also security risks, both real and perceived.

Ethical risks were another area of concern Overhage discussed, specifically those associated with the loss of control over how the data might be used in the future. He said it is important to consider potential public perception, even if regulations permit data sharing. The public might have particular concerns about sharing data that involves both public and private entities, because their trust in the data being used appropriately has to extend beyond the original interaction. Overhage reiterated that the alignment of interests is especially important in these types of collaborations. He noted that while there is value in data, it is important to keep in mind the roles that domain knowledge, analytical expertise, and computational capabilities can play in partnerships.

The fact that data can be reused in ways that many other types of property cannot be raises additional ownership considerations, Overhage said. For example, analyzing the data in ways that someone else might not have analyzed them does not diminish the data's usefulness to someone else. This is important to consider, particularly for data that resulted from an effort that was publicly funded.

In summary, Overhage listed five key enablers that he believes can make public-private partnerships work:

- Achieving clear alignment of stakeholder interests at the outset of the partnership;
- Establishing responsible data governance;
- Putting processes in place to ensure that the insights that are created are accurate, unbiased, and, where appropriate, explainable;
- Providing decision makers with the tools, processes, and support to act on the insights resulting from the work; and
- Ensuring the long-term economic sustainability of the partnership.

DISCUSSION

A central theme of the discussions that followed the presentations was the risks associated with data sharing. Speakers noted that resistance to transparency is common among all types of entities. For example, despite recent regulations focused on price transparency, it is still not possible to compare costs across health care providers.

Participants also discussed ways of overcoming resistance to data sharing. A potentially compelling argument could be that there is a wealth of information in the various health datasets, and the organizations that own them do not have the capability to take full advantage of the data. Even in organizations with thousands of analysts, the demand for using the data to answer questions far exceeds the capacity to produce answers. Collaborations with academic groups, other commercial entities, government organizations, and others are necessary to take full advantage of the data, despite short-term risks, but the conversation further highlighted the important role trust plays in establishing collaborations that involve data sharing.

Finally, the challenges associated with navigating the process of establishing agreements were discussed, along with the challenges of coordinating with Institutional Review Boards across multiple institutions. At the same time, participants underscored how collaborations, once they are established, can lower data access barriers for early career researchers.

CONCLUSION

Discussions in this session echoed some of the themes that emerged in prior sessions, including barriers to accessing data. While the benefits of data sharing are clear, the workshop also highlighted some of the reasons behind reluctance to share and underscored the risks involved for the organizations providing the data. Successful data sharing agreements can be established when these factors are taken into consideration.

CONCLUSION 5-1: Successful partnerships across health care systems require participant trust, clear evidence of mutual benefit, and the ability to control risk.

6

Collaborations with Patient Groups

Pat Furlong of Parent Project Muscular Dystrophy (PPMD) highlighted the importance of data sharing and dataset linkage for rare disease research. She discussed PPMD's work to develop a clinical trial master protocol and network for research on Duchenne muscular dystrophy, a rare progressive neuromuscular disease. She noted that other rare diseases face similar challenges related to research, so PPMD's goal is to create a framework that could be replicated.

Furlong said that several organizations have conducted research studies and clinical trials to investigate treatments for Duchenne. She also noted that several past clinical trials for drugs to treat the disease have failed. Each of those clinical trials, she said, set up a significant data infrastructure, but when the trial failed, the infrastructure was dismantled, and frequently the data collected during the trial were lost. Furlong also noted that the data from failed clinical trials were not integrated into any other datasets. PPMD determined that this was a major barrier for progress and has been working on finding a mechanism to improve data sharing and linking for research.

Another challenge related to Duchenne research highlighted by Furlong was trial participation. Furlong noted that participation in a clinical trial requires time, money, and travel that are not always accessible to the patients and their families. She explained that any or all of those factors play a role in the decision to participate in such a trial. If a clinical trial master protocol were deployed at multiple sites, she suggested, this could increase the number of patients who could participate.

Furlong noted that PPMD's first action to improve data sharing for research was to work with the Critical Path Institute. In this work they developed a disease progression model for Duchenne muscular dystrophy, one that offers a central source for those data to be accessed by those involved in research. She explained that one of the data needs in research on this disease concerns its natural history and the effects of delayed treatment, data that could be culled from the placebo arms of clinical trials. PPMD is seeking to address this by creating a centralized database as part of its clinical trial master protocol. A key part of that infrastructure would be a mechanism for linking non-proprietary data from clinical trials that are using the master protocol. PPMD expects that this would result in larger datasets for analysis than are typically available for rare disease research. PPMD is also working on creating systems for standardizing data collection as part of its master protocol. Furlong concluded by emphasizing the importance of data sharing and improving stakeholder access to data for the benefit of patients.

James Lewis, University of Pennsylvania, spoke about his experiences with patient-centered outcomes research (PCOR) data in the context of his research on inflammatory bowel disease (IBD). He described several barriers related to the patient-centered component of PCOR, including the following:

- High expenses and time commitment needed,
- Low patient engagement,
- Reluctance among patients to be active research subjects, and
- Patient concerns about the safety of their data.

Lewis noted that in regard to the outcomes research component of PCOR, a barrier of note is that while outcomes research routinely measures processes or clinical outcomes, patients may have different priorities for information.

Lewis also discussed his experiences with the IBD Plexus program, which he described as a collection of ongoing and historical cohort studies from which they are working to build a centralized data warehouse. This data warehouse will be designed to link patients' electronic health records (EHR) data, biosample-derived data, and claims data to assist researchers in developing a full picture of the patient's experience with their disease. Lewis noted that an important component of this process was developing a SmartForm, one that could be integrated into Epic EHRs, to standardize how clinicians record patient data in the EHR. They have also engaged another tool in Epic EHRs that allows patients to report their symptom data for integration into the EHR in a standardized format. IBD Plexus is in the early stages of a study that involves a partnership with the Food and Drug Administration (FDA) to use the FDA MyStudies app to collect patient-reported data.

Lewis cited low data quality as one of the challenges with using data from EHRs and patient-reported data. He said these sources of data can be inaccurate or incomplete due to patients' misinterpreting or skipping questions or because of clinician time constraints. He noted that recently implemented Centers for Medicare & Medicaid Services rules around charting requirements may impact the amount of EHR data available for PCOR.

Lewis described possible solutions for filling data gaps. One of these solutions is to link EHR data, claims data, and patient-reported data, which allows researchers to develop a more holistic dataset for a patient, including information beyond what is captured by a single health care system. However, Lewis noted, concerns about confidentiality and data security among stakeholders—including patients, insurance companies, and researchers—are a challenge for data linkage. He also noted that some patients are concerned about whether their data are being used appropriately.

Finally, Lewis discussed natural language processing to convert free text that is entered in EHRs as another solution for filling in data gaps. However, he noted that given the large number of variables, that process often requires a significant time investment. Another potential solution he proposed was the creation of a neutral national organization to standardize, de-identify, and link data from major EHRs and major sources of claims data for use in research. Lewis concluded by highlighting the need to recognize the multidisciplinary nature of PCOR and the need for collaboration.

Marc Natter, Harvard University, said that early in his career he encountered difficulties finding longitudinal data for PCOR focused on childhood arthritis due to inadequate registries and data infrastructure. He noted that the Childhood Arthritis & Rheumatology Research Alliance (CARRA) and the CARRA Registry were developed to address this challenge. He explained that in the beginning, CARRA developed a registry that served as a federal data warehouse for data derived from studies of pediatric rheumatology diseases.

Natter said that over time the CARRA Registry evolved into a common data collection platform in addition to a research network. The platform includes a master data-use agreement and protocol that applies to all participating institutions, and to all identified and de-identified data, which flow bi-directionally between research sites, CARRA's Data Coordinating Center, and clinical centers. Natter explained that CARRA continues to build on its data infrastructure, which has facilitated a variety of pediatric rheumatology PCOR studies. He noted that he and his colleagues have also incorporated data infrastructure to facilitate collection of patient-reported outcome (PRO) data, including an application-based tool. He noted that they continue to research how best to collect and integrate PRO data.

Natter also highlighted some lessons that were learned as the CARRA registry and data platform have evolved. He noted that at some institutions they have faced challenges obtaining Institutional Review Board (IRB) approval for studies that include a patient-facing application platform. He suggested that the Department of Health and Human Services work to develop a set of universal guidelines for these patient-facing applications. He said that this would provide IRBs with clear standards to apply when evaluating proposals that include such applications. He also echoed points made by others about the need for researchers to communicate with patient and physician stakeholders to ascertain what information matters to them and to use that to guide how PCOR analytic results are presented.

Natter also noted that methods research needs more attention and the outcomes of that research should be incorporated into PCOR data standards. He said that validated disease metrics are needed to facilitate more effective use of advanced machine learning algorithms. He concluded by highlighting that as other speakers had noted, researchers need better access to large aggregated datasets that include claims data in order to conduct more robust PCOR data analysis.

DISCUSSION

The brief discussion after the presentations focused on the role patient organizations are best positioned to play in advancing PCOR. Participants highlighted patient organizations' ability to facilitate connections between researchers and people (patients and others) who are invested in the patient-centered aspect of PCOR. Participants also noted a potential role for patient organizations in facilitating patients' access to their own health data, including claims data. This would enable patients to contribute their information to research studies. Patient groups can also play an important role in providing input on outcome measures that matter most to people. Many of these ideas echoed the committee's conclusions from the first workshop.[1]

CONCLUSIONS

Collaborations with patient organizations can help in addressing patient concerns about participating in research studies and in building patient engagement, which are both important for achieving a patient-centered approach. Disease registries directed by patient groups can be a particularly useful additional source of data, providing information that would not be available to researchers otherwise.

---

[1] https://www.nap.edu/catalog/26297/building-data-capacity-for-patient-centered-outcomes-research-interim-report.

CONCLUSION 6-1: Patient groups can be helpful partners in all aspects of patient-centered outcomes research, including engaging patients in order to improve research participation and the impact of results.

CONCLUSION 6-2: Patient-directed disease registries can be a source of in-depth, longitudinal, prospective clinical and patient-reported data that are not available from other data sources.

Appendix A

Biographical Sketches of Committee Members

GEORGE ISHAM (NAM) (*Chair*) is a senior fellow at the HealthPartners Institute and a senior advisor for the Alliance of Community Health Plans. Previously, he served as a senior advisor to the board of directors and the senior management team of HealthPartners, and prior to that, he was HealthPartners' medical director and chief health officer, responsible for quality of care and health and health care improvement. He has been active in health policy, serving as a member of the Centers for Disease Control and Prevention's Task Force on Community Preventive Services, a member of the Agency for Healthcare Research and Quality's United States Preventive Services Task Force, a founding co-chair of the National Committee for Quality Assurance's committee on performance measurement, as well as founding co-chair of the National Quality Forum's Measurement Application Partnership. He has an M.D. from the University of Illinois at Chicago and an M.S. in preventive medicine and administrative medicine from the University of Wisconsin–Madison.

JOHN F.P. BRIDGES is professor and vice chair of academic affairs in the Department of Biomedical Informatics at The Ohio State University (OSU) College of Medicine. He is also a professor in the Department of Surgery and an adjunct professor in both the Division of Epidemiology at the OSU College of Public Health and Department of Health Behavior and Society at the Johns Hopkins Bloomberg School of Public Health. Prior to joining OSU he was on the faculty of the Johns Hopkins Bloomberg School of Public Health, the Department of Tropical Hygiene and Public Health within the University of Heidelberg School of Medicine, and the Department of

Epidemiology and Biostatistics within the Case Western Reserve University School of Medicine. He has previously held positions in the Department of Economics at the Weatherhead School of Management at Case Western Reserve University; the National Bureau of Economic Research; Center for Medicine in the Public Interest; and the Center for Health Economics, Research and Evaluation in Australia. He has a Ph.D. in economics from the City University of New York.

JULIE BYNUM is the Margaret Terpenning Professor of Medicine in the Division of Geriatric Medicine and vice chair for faculty affairs in the Department of Internal Medicine at the University of Michigan. She is also a research professor in the Institute of Gerontology, Geriatric Center Associate Director for Health Policy and Research, and a member of the Institute for Healthcare Policy and Innovation. She currently leads a portfolio of National Institutes of Health–funded research that examines the quality of care, diagnosis, and treatment of people with Alzheimer's disease and related dementia in the community, nursing homes, and assisted living and is the director of the Center to Accelerate Population Research in Alzhiemer's. She is currently a member of the National Academies of Sciences, Engineering, and Medicine's Forum on Aging, Disability, and Independence and was a member of a National Academies committee that authored *Vital Signs: Core Metrics for Health and Health Care Progress*. She has an M.P.H. from the Johns Hopkins University School of Hygiene & Public Health and an M.D. from the Johns Hopkins University School of Medicine.

ANGELA DOBES is vice president of the Crohn's & Colitis Foundation's IBD Plexus Program, a research-information exchange platform designed to centralize data and biosamples from diverse research initiatives to advance science, accelerate precision medicine, and transform the care of inflammatory bowel disease (IBD) patients. She has previously worked for clinical technology and pharmaceutical organizations, where she has led implementation of various technology solutions focused on business optimization and accelerating the delivery of new therapies to patients safely. She is currently serving as principal investigator on a study to enhance engagement, research participation, and collaboration through the IBD Partners Patient Powered Research Network. She has an M.A. in public health from the Icahn School of Medicine at Mount Sinai.

DEBORAH ESTRIN (NAE/NAM) is a professor of computer science at Cornell Tech where she holds the Robert V. Tishman founder's chair, serves as the associate dean for impact, and is an affiliate faculty at Weill Cornell Medicine. Her research activities include technologies for caregiving, immersive health, small data, participatory sensing, and public interest technology. Estrin was an Amazon Scholar, and before joining Cornell University she was founding director of the National Science Foundation's Center for Embedded Networked Sensing at the University of California, Los Angeles, pioneering the development of mobile and wireless systems to collect and analyze real-time data about the physical world. Estrin cofounded the nonprofit startup Open mHealth and has served on several scientific advisory boards for early-stage mobile health startups. She has a Ph.D. in electrical engineering and computer science from the Massachusetts Institute of Technology.

OLUWADAMILOLA FAYANJU is the Helen O. Dickens Presidential Associate Professor of Surgery at the Perelman School of Medicine at the University of Pennsylvania. She is also chief of breast surgery at Penn Medicine. Previously, she was associate professor of surgery and population health sciences in the Duke University School of Medicine and director of the Durham VA Breast Clinic. She was also associate director for Disparities & Value in Healthcare with Duke Forge, Duke University's center for actionable data science. In 2019, she was recognized by the National Academy of Medicine as an Emerging Leader in Health and Medicine Scholar. She received an M.A. in comparative literature from Harvard University and her M.D. and M.P.H.S. from the Washington University in St. Louis.

CONSTANTINE GATSONIS is the Henry Ledyard Goddard University Professor of Statistical Sciences, director of statistical sciences, and professor of biostatistics at Brown University. He was founding director of the Center for Statistical Sciences and founding chair of the Department of Biostatistics at Brown University. He is a leading authority on the evaluation of diagnostic and screening tests and has made major contributions to the development of methods for medical technology assessment and health services and outcomes research. He is a world leader in methods for applying and synthesizing evidence on diagnostic tests in medicine and is currently developing methods for comparative effectiveness research in diagnosis and prediction and radiomics. Since 2016 he has served as a statistical consultant for the *New England Journal of Medicine* and was the founding editor-in-chief of *Health Services and Outcomes Research Methods*. He has a Ph.D. in mathematical statistics from Cornell University.

ROBERT GOERGE is a senior research fellow at Chapin Hall at the University of Chicago. He is also a senior fellow and founder of the Master's Degree in Computational Analysis in Public Policy at the University of Chicago Harris School of Public Policy. His research is focused on improving the available data and information on children and families, particularly those who require specialized services related to maltreatment, disability,

poverty, or violence. At Chapin Hall, he is principal investigator for the Family Self-Sufficiency Data Center, the Linking Federal Data to Local Data project, and the National Survey for Early Care and Education. He currently serves on the National Academies of Sciences, Engineering, and Medicine's Committee on National Statistics. He has a Ph.D. in social policy from the University of Chicago.

GEORGE HRIPCSAK (NAM) is the Vivian Beaumont Allen Professor and chair of the Department of Biomedical Informatics at Columbia University. He is also the director of medical informatics services for New York Presbyterian Hospital. He is also a board-certified internist. He led the effort to create the Arden Syntax, a language for representing health knowledge that has become a national standard. As chair of the American Medical Informatics Association Standards Committee, he coordinated the medical informatics community response to the Department of Health and Human Services for the health informatics standards rules under the Health Insurance Portability and Accountability Act of 1996. His current research is on the clinical information stored in electronic health records. Using data mining techniques, he is developing the methods necessary to support clinical research and patient safety initiatives. He has an M.D. and an M.S. in biostatistics from Columbia University.

LISA IEZZONI (NAM) is professor of medicine at Harvard Medical School and the Health Policy Research Center at Massachusetts General Hospital, where she served as director in the past. She was previously co-director of research in the Division of General Medicine and Primary Care at Beth Israel Deaconess Medical Center in Boston. Her research focuses on risk adjustment methods for predicting cost and clinical outcomes of care, and on health care experiences and outcomes of persons with disabilities. She has served on the editorial boards of the *Annals of Internal Medicine*, the *Journal of General Internal Medicine*, *Health Affairs*, *Medical Care*, *Health Services Research*, and the *Disability and Health Journal*, among others. She has an M.D. from Harvard Medical School and an M.Sc. from the Harvard T.H. Chan School of Public Health.

S. CLAIBORNE JOHNSTON (NAM) is the inaugural dean of Dell Medical School, vice president for medical affairs, and the Frank and Charmaine Denius Distinguished Dean's Chair in medical leadership at The University of Texas at Austin. Previously, Johnston was associate vice chancellor for research at the University of California, San Francisco (UCSF). He also directed the Clinical and Translational Science Institute and founded the UCSF Center for Healthcare Value. His research is focused on clinical trials and health services research in stroke. He is also an expert in medical education, research administration, health care value, and population health. He has led several large-cohort studies of cerebrovascular disease and three international multicenter randomized trials. He has an M.D. from Harvard Medical School and a Ph.D. in epidemiology from the University of California, Berkeley.

MIGUEL MARINO is an associate professor with joint appointments in the School of Public Health Division of Biostatistics and the Department of Family Medicine at Oregon Health & Science University. His research focuses on the development and implementation of novel statistical methodology to address complexities associated with the use of electronic health records (EHRs) to study changes in policy; using EHRs to study health disparities; validation of EHRs as a reliable source for observational studies; pragmatic randomized trials; and preventive health maintenance. He was selected by the National Academy of Medicine as an Emerging Leader in Health and Medicine Scholar. He has a Ph.D. in biostatistics from Harvard University.

ELIZABETH McGLYNN (NAM) is vice president for Kaiser Permanente Research and executive director for the Center for Effectiveness & Safety Research at Kaiser Permanente. She is also interim senior associate dean for research and scholarships at the Kaiser Permanente Bernard J. Tyson School of Medicine. She is an internationally known expert on methods for evaluating the appropriateness and quality of health care delivery. She has led major initiatives to evaluate health reform options under consideration at the federal and state levels. She is the lead of Kaiser Permanente & Strategic Partners Patient Outcomes Research To Advance Learning (PORTAL) Network. She was a member of the Strategic Framework Board, which provided a blueprint for the National Quality Forum on the development of a national quality measurement and reporting system. She chaired the board of AcademyHealth, served on the board of the American Board of Internal Medicine Foundation, and served on the Board of Providence-Little Company of Mary Hospital Service Area in Southern California. She has a Ph.D. in public policy from RAND Graduate School.

DAVID MELTZER (NAM) is the Fanny L. Pritzker Professor in the Department of Medicine, chief of the section of Hospital Medicine and faculty in the Department of Economics and Harris School of Public Policy at the University of Chicago. He is also director of the Center for Health and the Social Sciences and of the Urban Health Lab at the University of Chicago. His research explores problems in health economics and public policy with a focus on the theoretical foundations of medical cost-effectiveness analysis and the cost and quality of hospital care. Since 1997, he has developed the inpatient general medicine services at the University of Chicago as a Learning Health Care System to produce knowledge on how to improve the care of hospitalized patients, mobilizing the clinical care process to generate and learn from diverse data from electronic health records, claims data, patient interviews, and bio-specimens on more than 100,000 patients. He is the lead of the University of Chicago network site as part of the Chicago Area Patient-Centered Outcomes Research Network. He has an M.D. and a Ph.D. in economics from the University of Chicago.

PAUL C. TANG (NAM) is an adjunct professor in the Clinical Excellence Research Center at Stanford University and an internist at the Palo Alto Medical Foundation. He was formerly chief innovation and technology officer at the Palo Alto Medical Foundation and vice president, chief health transformation officer at IBM Watson Health. He has more than 25 years of executive leadership experience in health information technology within medical groups, health systems, and corporate settings. He has directed innovation and technology teams in provider organizations, academic institutions, corporate research organizations, and product development organizations. Most recently, he led the creation, development, deployment, and evaluation of the application of artificial intelligence to physician point-of-care solutions integrated within an electronic health record system. He also led a corporate enterprise-wide design team. He has chaired numerous federal and private sector advisory and professional association groups related to health information technology and policy. He received an M.S. in electrical engineering from Stanford University and his M.D. from the University of California, San Francisco.

Appendix B

Workshop Agenda

Building Data Capacity for Patient-Centered Outcomes Research:
An Agenda for 2021 to 2030

Virtual Workshop 3: A Comprehensive Data Ecosystem for
Patient-Centered Outcomes Research

June 14, 2021, 11 am – 5 pm EDT

OBJECTIVES FOR THE WORKSHOP
- Discuss how research and data collaborations can evolve to meet PCOR and data capacity challenges, and how HHS can support effective research and data collaborations
- Identify barriers and potential solutions to the access and use of linked public data, and to the access and use of linked public and private/proprietary data
- Discuss the feasibility and utility of developing a phased-in approach to building the interoperable data capacity for patient-centered outcomes research with existing databases in HHS, other federal departments, and the private sector

11:00-11:05 am EDT	**Goals for the Workshop** GEORGE ISHAM (Committee Chair), HealthPartners Institute

11:05 am-12:50 pm EDT	**Federal Partners for PCOR** Moderators: JULIE BYNUM, University of Michigan, and GEORGE HRIPCSAK, Columbia University Speakers: MICKY TRIPATHI, Office of the National Coordinator for Health Information Technology ALLISON OELSCHLAEGER, Office of Enterprise Data & Analytics, Centers for Medicare & Medicaid Services MEAGAN KHAU, Office of Minority Health, Centers for Medicare & Medicaid Services MITRA ROCCA, Center for Drug Evaluation and Research, Food and Drug Administration ADI GUNDLAPALLI, Public Health Informatics Office, Centers for Disease Control and Prevention ALISON CERNICH, Eunice Kennedy Shriver National Institute of Child Health and Human Development JACOB KEAN, Salt Lake City VA Health Care System, Department of Veterans Affairs and University of Utah
12:50-1:00 pm EDT	Break
1:00-2:00 pm EDT	**State-Level Data and Data Collaborations** Moderators: ROBERT GOERGE, University of Chicago, and LISA IEZZONI, Massachusetts General Hospital Speakers: LYNN BLEWETT, State Health Access Data Assistance Center MARSHA LILLIE-BLANTON, George Washington University TODD GILMER, University of California, San Diego CLAUDIA STEINER, Kaiser Permanente Research

2:00-2:50 pm EDT	**Clinical Trial Networks and Collaborations** Moderators: DAVID MELTZER, University of Chicago, and CONSTANTINE GATSONIS, Brown University Speakers: RUTH CARLOS, University of Michigan LAURA ESSERMAN, University of California, San Francisco LESLEY CURTIS, Duke University
2:50-3:05 pm EDT	**Break**
3:05-4:00 pm EDT	**Public-Private Partnerships** Moderators: ELIZABETH MCGLYNN, Kaiser Permanente Research, and MIGUEL MARINO, Oregon Health & Science University Speakers: ATUL BUTTE, University of California, San Francisco VINCENT MOR, Brown University MARC OVERHAGE, Anthem
4:00-4:50 pm EDT	**Collaborations with Patient Groups** Moderators: JOHN F.P. BRIDGES, The Ohio State University, and ANGELA DOBES, Crohn's & Colitis Foundation Speakers: PAT FURLONG, Parent Project Muscular Dystrophy JAMES LEWIS, University of Pennsylvania MARC NATTER, Harvard University
4:50-5:00 pm EDT	**Wrap-up** GEORGE ISHAM (Committee Chair), HealthPartners Institute

Appendix C

Biographical Sketches of Workshop Speakers

LYNN BLEWETT is the director of the State Health Access Data Assistance Center (SHADAC), a research and policy center that supports state efforts to monitor and evaluate programs and reforms to increase access to needed health care. She is also a professor of health policy in the School of Public Health, University of Minnesota. Her research includes Medicaid payment reform, the evolving health care safety net, and measures to monitor population health outcomes. She brings expertise in state and federal health data resources, including federal surveys such as the Current Population Survey, the American Community Survey, the National Health Interview Survey (NHIS), and the Behavior Risk Factor Surveillance System, which are all accessible through SHADAC's interactive online Data Center. She also heads up a project funded by the Robert Wood Johnson Foundation to provide expertise in the use of data analytics to inform and monitor implementation of the Patient Protection and Affordable Care Act and was instrumental in establishing the University of Minnesota-based Census Research Data Center, which focuses on health services research and policy. She is also principal investigator of the Integrated Health Interview Series, a project funded by the Eunice Kennedy Shriver National Institute of Child Health and Human Development to harmonize and integrate more than 50 years of the NHIS and make it accessible through a web portal for academic and policy research. She earned an M.A. degree in public affairs and a doctorate degree in health services research from the University of Minnesota.

ATUL BUTTE (NAM), M.D., Ph.D., is the Priscilla Chan and Mark Zuckerberg Distinguished Professor and inaugural director of the Bakar

Computational Health Sciences Institute at the University of California, San Francisco. He is also the chief data scientist for the entire University of California Health System, the 10th largest health system by revenue in the United States, with 20 health professional schools, six medical schools, six academic health centers, 10 hospitals, and more than 1,000 care delivery sites. He has been continually funded by the National Institutes of Health for 20 years, is an inventor on 24 patents, and has authored more than 200 publications. His research has repeatedly been featured as well in the *New York Times*, *Wall Street Journal*, and *Wired Magazine*. He was elected into the National Academy of Medicine in 2015, and in 2013 he was recognized by the Obama Administration as a White House Champion of Change in Open Science for promoting science through publicly available data. Butte is also a founder of three investor-backed data-driven companies: Personalis (IPO, 2019), which provides medical genome sequencing services; Carmenta (acquired by Progenity in 2015), which discovered diagnostics for pregnancy complications; and NuMedii, which finds new uses for drugs through open molecular data. He trained in computer science at Brown University, worked as a software engineer at Apple and Microsoft, received his medical degree at Brown University, trained in pediatrics and pediatric endocrinology at Children's Hospital Boston, and then received his Ph.D. from Harvard Medical School and the Massachusetts Institute of Technology.

RUTH CARLOS is a professor of radiology and serves as the assistant chair for clinical research at the University of Michigan. Her work encompasses cost-effectiveness analysis, patient preference measurement, and meta-analysis and systematic reviews in diagnostic imaging. Her research also seeks to understand the effectiveness of maternally directed interventions to improve vaccine uptake in adolescent daughters. She brings her specific expertise in evaluating cultural barriers to adolescent HPV vaccination in African-American mothers and developing and pilot-testing tailored interventions directed at these cultural barriers. She also co-directs the Program on Women's Health Care Effectiveness Research in the Department of Obstetrics and Gynecology at the University of Michigan Medical School and currently chairs the GE Association of University Radiologists Research Radiology Academic Fellowship, a national program supporting early-stage investigators in health services research and care delivery. She received her medical degree from and completed her diagnostic radiology residency at the University of Chicago, and did a fellowship at the University of Michigan in Ann Arbor, joining the faculty at the University of Michigan in 1998. She also holds a master's degree from the School of Public Health at the University of Michigan.

ALISON CERNICH is the deputy director of the Eunice Kennedy Shriver National Institute of Child Health and Human Development (NICHD). In this role, she assists the NICHD director in overseeing the institute's programs supporting research on child development, developmental biology, nutrition, HIV/AIDS, intellectual and developmental disabilities, population dynamics, reproductive biology, contraception, pregnancy, and medical rehabilitation. Prior to this position, she was the director of NICHD's National Center for Medical Rehabilitation Research (NCMRR), where she managed a $72 million research portfolio aimed at improving the health and well-being of people with disabilities. As NCMRR director, she led the development and revision of the congressionally mandated National Institutes of Health Research Plan on Rehabilitation, an effort that included coordination with 17 institutes and centers and multiple external stakeholders. Before joining NICHD, she served as deputy director of the Defense Centers of Excellence for Psychological Health and Traumatic Brain Injury at the U.S. Department of Veterans Affairs (VA), where she coordinated prevention, education, research, and clinical care efforts for service members and veterans diagnosed with traumatic brain injury. Prior to her 10 years with the VA, she was the traumatic brain injury liaison to the Department of Defense, the chief of neuropsychology and director of the Polytrauma Support Clinic at the VA Maryland Health Care System, and a funded investigator through the VA Rehabilitation Research and Development Service. She received her doctoral degree in clinical psychology from Fairleigh Dickinson University and completed postdoctoral training in cognitive neuroscience at the National Rehabilitation Hospital in Washington, D.C.

LESLEY CURTIS is professor and chair of the Department of Population Health Sciences at the Duke University School of Medicine. A health services researcher by training, she is an expert in the use of Medicare claims data for health services and clinical outcomes research and a leader in national data quality efforts. She serves as co-principal investigator of the Food and Drug Administration's (FDA's) Sentinel Innovation Center, co-investigator of the Data Core for the FDA's Sentinel Initiative to monitor the safety of FDA-regulated medical products, and chair of the Data Quality Subcommittee for the National Evaluation System for health Technology Coordinating Center, which generates real-world evidence for health technology and medical devices. She also serves as co-investigator of the coordinating center for the Patient-Centered Outcomes Research Institute's National Clinical Research Network (PCORnet), working with health systems and patient networks to develop a harmonized network infrastructure that leverages health systems and electronic health records data for robust observational and interventional research. She received her Ph.D. from the University of Rochester.

LAURA ESSERMAN is a surgeon and breast cancer oncology specialist practicing at the University of California, San Francisco (UCSF) Breast Care

Center. She directs the UCSF Clinical Breast Cancer Program and co-leads the Breast Oncology Program. She is a professor of surgery and radiology at UCSF as well as a faculty member at the UCSF Helen Diller Family Comprehensive Cancer Center. Her research has focused on tailoring treatment to biology, which requires the integration of translational science, bioinformatics, medical and clinical informatics, systems integration, and clinical care delivery. She has led the I-SPY Trials, a collaboration among the National Cancer Institute, the Food and Drug Administration, more than 28 cancer research centers, major pharmaceutical and biotech companies, and the not-for-profit sponsor, Quantum Leap Healthcare Collaborative. Additionally, she led the creation of the University of California-wide Athena Breast Health Network, a learning system designed to integrate clinical care and research as it follows 150,000 women from screening through treatment and outcomes. As part of the network, she has spearheaded the development of the WISDOM study to learn how to improve breast cancer screening by examining the effectiveness of a personalized screening strategy informed by each woman's breast cancer risk and preferences, in comparison with the standard of annual screening. She recently collaborated with her pulmonary and critical care colleagues to launch the I-SPY COVID-19 Trial, to rapidly screen agents to improve outcomes for critically ill COVID-19 patients. She earned her undergraduate degree at Harvard University and completed her medical and surgical training at Stanford University. She completed a postdoctoral fellowship in breast oncology at Stanford and later earned an M.A. degree from the Stanford Graduate School of Business.

PAT FURLONG is the founding president and chief executive officer of Parent Project Muscular Dystrophy, the largest nonprofit organization in the United States solely focused on Duchenne muscular dystrophy (Duchenne). Its mission is to improve the treatment, quality of life, and long-term outlook for all individuals affected by Duchenne through research, advocacy, education, and compassion. She is the mother of two sons who lost their battle with Duchenne in their teenage years. She has served on the boards of the Genetic Alliance and the Muscular Dystrophy Coordinating Committee of the U.S. Department of Health and Human Services. She has also served on the data safety monitoring board for both the Rare Diseases Clinical Research Network and the Cooperative International Neuromuscular Research Group. She was a member of the Institute of Medicine's Committee on Accelerating Research and Development for Rare Diseases and Orphan Products. She graduated from Mt. St. Joseph College in Cincinnati, Ohio, with a B.S. in nursing, and attended graduate school at The Ohio State University.

TODD GILMER is professor and chief, Division of Health Policy, in the School of Public Health at the University of California, San Diego. His research has focused on four areas: health insurance, risk adjustment in Medicaid, cost-effectiveness of diabetes care, and mental health services. He specializes in research design and data analysis; the use of large datasets including those from Medicare, Medicaid, and commercial health plans, national surveys and census data; mixed methods that combine analysis of health insurance claims with qualitative interviews and focus groups; and the evaluation of community-based interventions to improve the health of vulnerable populations. His recent work has examined the comparative effectiveness of supporting housing programs for persons with serious mental illness who are homeless and the importance of the fidelity of these programs to the Housing First model of permanent supported housing; the effectiveness of behavioral health integration and complex care management in Medicaid managed care; the use of peer providers in mental health programs designed for transitional-age youth; and service use after first episode of psychosis. He leads teams of health services researchers to provide data analysis and performance monitoring for San Diego County Behavioral Health Services and in studying innovative service delivery models in San Diego and Los Angeles counties. He received his Ph.D. in economics from the University of Washington.

ADI GUNDLAPALLI is the chief public health informatics officer of the Center for Surveillance, Epidemiology, and Laboratory Services at the Centers for Disease Control and Prevention (CDC). In this role, he leads an interdisciplinary team to meet the evolving data and information needs of public health, thereby enhancing informatics capability. Prior to coming to the CDC, he was the chief health informatics officer for the Salt Lake City Veterans Affairs Health Care System and an infectious diseases staff physician in Utah. He was a tenured professor of internal medicine at the University of Utah School of Medicine and a physician at the University of Utah Hospitals and Clinics. He is board certified in internal medicine, infectious diseases, and clinical informatics. His clinical and research interests include infectious diseases, clinical immunology, bio-surveillance (and biodefense), preparedness for public health emergencies, infection prevention and hospital epidemiology, and health care for vulnerable populations. He received his medical degree from the Madras Medical College in Madras (now called Chennai), India. He received further training at the University of Connecticut Health Center, where he earned a Ph.D. in immunology and completed an internal medicine residency. In Utah he completed a 3-year clinical and research fellowship in infectious diseases at the University of Utah School of Medicine and an M.A. degree (with a thesis) in biomedical informatics.

JACOB KEAN is a research scientist with the Department of Veterans Affairs (VA) Informatics and Computing Infrastructure of the Salt Lake City

VA Health Care System and an associate professor in health system innovation and research in the Department of Population Health Sciences at the University of Utah. He was previously a research scientist at the Regenstrief Institute and on the faculty at Indiana University School of Medicine. Kean served as a visiting scientist at the Boston University Rehabilitation Outcomes Center, a visiting scholar at the Center for Rehabilitation Research Using Large Datasets at the University of Texas Medical Branch, and a VA Career Development Awardee. His expertise lies at the nexus of the creation and operation of research networks and the evaluation of network care practices using patient-centered outcomes. He is the director of the Population Health Science–U Health Learning Health System; principal investigator (PI) of the Cerebral Palsy Research Network Data Coordinating Center; PI of the Department of Defense-funded Optimizing Rehabilitation InterventiONs (ORION) for Cognition Following Complex Traumatic Brain Injury network; and co-PI of the VA-funded Brain Injury Data Sharing Project—all of which are electronic health records–based learning health systems focused primarily on the care of persons with acquired neurological disorders. He has a Ph.D. from Indiana University Bloomington in speech and hearing sciences. He also completed the National Institutes of Health Training Institute for Dissemination and Implementation Research in Health and a post-doctoral master's degree in measurement, evaluation, statistics, and assessment at the University of Illinois–Chicago.

MEAGAN KHAU is the director of the Data and Policy Analytics Group (DPAG) at the Centers for Medicare & Medicaid Services (CMS) Office of Minority Health (OMH). DPAG conducts research, data collection, and analyses to identify targets to reduce health disparities and improve quality of care, care transitions, access to care, and beneficiary satisfaction for vulnerable populations. DPAG is also involved in developing and implementing initiatives and data analyses to support cross-component/cross-agency collaborations to improve data collection, analysis, and reporting of race and ethnicity, primary language, disability, gender, and other characteristics associated with health disparities. Prior to joining CMS OMH, she was the deputy director of the Division of Pharmacy at the Center for Medicaid and Children's Health Insurance Program Services, managing the operations of the Medicaid Drug Rebate Program, supporting system developments, ensuring program compliance, and implementing new policies and regulations. She received her master's degree in health administration from the University of Southern California and her B.A. in sociology from the University of California, Irvine.

JAMES LEWIS is a professor of medicine and epidemiology, a senior scholar at the Center for Clinical Epidemiology and Biostatistics, and an associate director of the Inflammatory Bowel Disease (IBD) Program at the University of Pennsylvania's Perelman School of Medicine in Philadelphia, Pennsylvania. He has been actively involved in clinical research related to IBDs, medication safety, and optimizing medical therapies for more than 20 years. More recently, he has focused on the impact of diet on the gut microbiome and the course of IBD. His work has been funded by the National Institutes of Health, the Department of Health and Human Services Agency for Healthcare Research and Quality, the Patient-Centered Outcomes Research Institute, the Centers for Disease Control and Prevention, and numerous foundations and corporate sponsors. He previously served as the chair of the National Scientific Advisory Committee and as a member of the National Board of the Crohn's & Colitis Foundation. Lewis is currently the lead scientist for the Foundation's IBD Plexus Research Collaborative and co-principal investigator of SPARC-IBD, a multicenter prospective cohort study of patients with inflammatory bowel disease. He received his M.D. and his M.S. in clinical pharmacoepidemiology from the University of Pennsylvania School of Medicine.

MARSHA LILLIE-BLANTON is associate research professor in the Milken Institute School of Public Health at George Washington University. She is a public health professional with more than 30 years of experience working on health and health care access issues facing vulnerable populations. Her professional career has woven together opportunities to pursue scholarship and teaching in academia with efforts as a practitioner grounded in the realities that confront marginalized communities. She previously served as the chief quality officer and director of the Division of Quality and Health Outcomes at the Center for Medicaid and Children's Health Insurance Program (CHIP) Services at the Centers for Medicare & Medicaid Services (CMS). With a budget of $500 million over 6 years, she had responsibility for establishing a health care quality measurement and reporting program for Medicaid and CHIP, oversight of state contracts for annual external quality reviews of Medicaid managed care organizations, developing the state-federal partnership in quality improvement activities, and conducting the first-ever nationwide survey of Medicaid beneficiaries' experiences of care. Prior to her position with CMS, she held senior-level positions with the Henry J. Kaiser Family Foundation and the U.S. Government Accountability Office. She holds a bachelor's degree from Howard University and a master of health science and doctorate degrees from the Johns Hopkins University Bloomberg School of Public Health.

VINCENT MOR (NAM) is the Florence Price Grant professor of community health at the Brown University School of Public Health and a research health scientist at the Providence Veterans Administration Medical Center.

He has been principal investigator of more than 40 National Institutes of Health (NIH)-funded grants focusing on the use of health services by and outcomes for frail and chronically ill people. He has evaluated the impact of programs and policies including Medicare funding of hospice, changes in Medicare nursing home payment, and the introduction of nursing home quality measures. He coauthored the congressionally mandated Minimum Data Set (MDS) and was architect of an integrated Medicare claims and clinical assessment data structure used for policy analysis, pharmacoepidemiology, and population outcome measurement. He developed summary measures using MDS data to characterize residents' physical, cognitive, and psychosocial functioning. These data resources are the heart of Mor's National Institute on Aging (NIA)–funded program project grant, Changing Long-Term Care in America, which examines the impact of Medicaid and Medicare policies on long-term care. These data are also at the core of a series of large, pragmatic cluster randomized trials of novel nursing home-based interventions led by Mor. He received a MERIT award from NIA at NIH, a Robert Wood Johnson Health Policy Investigator award, and the Distinguished Investigator award from AcademyHealth. He received his Ph.D. at the Florence Heller School for Advanced Studies in social welfare, Brandies University.

MARC NATTER is a pediatric rheumatologist and researcher in bioinformatics at the Boston Children's Hospital Computational Health Informatics Program whose research is centered on the development and implementation of scalable software platforms that enable new ways of collecting and sharing data for research into chronic diseases. He is the chief informatics architect of the multi-site Childhood Arthritis & Rheumatology Research Alliance Registry for pediatric rheumatic diseases, leads the development of patient-facing technology for the Harvard Medical School-led Scalable Collaborative Infrastructure for Learning Healthcare System Clinical Data Research Network, and coordinates data integration and patient-facing technology for the PARTNERS Patient Powered Research Network and other projects. He received his M.D. from S.U.N.Y. at Stony Brook School of Medicine.

ALLISON OELSCHLAEGER is the chief data officer and director of the Office of Enterprise Data & Analytics at the Centers for Medicare & Medicaid Services (CMS). In this role, she focuses on maximizing the value and impact of CMS data for internal and external users. She oversees CMS's data and information product portfolio and directs efforts to make CMS datasets available to external organizations. She also manages the development of advanced analytics using CMS data that help inform policy decisions and evaluate programs. Before joining CMS, she worked at the Lewin

Group, where she specialized in program evaluation and data analysis. She is a graduate of Georgetown University.

MARC OVERHAGE (NAM) is the chief health information officer for Anthem, Inc., and previously served as the chief medical informatics officer for Cerner and Siemens Health Services. He is an internationally recognized expert in health information modeling, standards, and interoperability as well as clinical decision support, health services research, and implementation science. Previously, Overhage was the director of medical informatics and a research scientist at the Regenstrief Institute, Inc., and professor of medicine and Regenstrief professor of medical informatics at the Indiana University School of Medicine. He also is a member of the medical staff of the Wishard Memorial Hospital. His research has focused on the use of informational interventions to modify provider behavior, including computerized provider order entry, clinical decision support systems, and other forms of feedback. These systems require clinical data to drive them and have led him to begin developing approaches to health information exchange. To facilitate this work, he has engaged in developing clinical information standards, advising the federal government on policy-guiding health information technology, and developing sustainable models for providing health information services. He received his B.A. in physics from Wabash College and an M.D. in medicine and a Ph.D. in biophysics from the Indiana University School of Medicine.

MITRA ROCCA is associate director of medical informatics, Office of Translational Science, Center for Drug Evaluation and Research (CDER), at the Food and Drug Administration (FDA). She joined the FDA in 2009 as the senior medical informatician responsible for developing the health information architecture of the Sentinel System. Rocca serves as the lead for the FDA CDER Health Information Technology (IT) Board, focusing on the use of health IT to enhance regulatory decision making. She also serves as the FDA CDER lead to Health Level Seven (HL7), responsible for the review of HL7 draft standards. Prior to joining FDA, she served as the associate director of health care informatics at Novartis Pharmaceuticals Corporation, focusing on the reuse of electronic health records in clinical research. She served as the co-chair of the HL7 Clinical Interoperability Council from 2012 to 2018. She is a fellow of the American Medical Informatics Association and holds an advanced degree in medical informatics from the University of Heidelberg in Germany.

CLAUDIA STEINER is the executive director of the Institute for Health Research at Kaiser Permanente Colorado. She served as director for the Division of Healthcare Delivery Data, Measures and Research, in the

Center for Delivery, Organization, and Markets within the Agency for Healthcare Research and Quality (AHRQ) until February 2017. There she led the division's development and dissemination of data and software tools for use in research, policy analysis, quality improvement, and public reporting, with a particular focus on the Healthcare Cost and Utilization Project and the AHRQ Quality Indicators. She has conducted research on the influence of ambulatory surgery on standards of care, utilization, and clinical outcomes; the epidemiology of infectious diseases, including health care–associated infections; the prevalence and factors associated with readmissions to the acute care setting; and the use and impact of new medical technologies. She was a practicing internal medicine physician for 25 years with the Johns Hopkins Community Physicians and continues to serve as a practicing internist for adult patients with the Colorado Permanente Medical Group. She earned her medical degree and completed residency training in internal medicine at the University of Colorado Health Sciences Center. Subsequently, she obtained a master's of public health at the Johns Hopkins School of Hygiene and Public Health while completing a research fellowship through the Department of Medicine at Johns Hopkins University.

MICKY TRIPATHI is the national coordinator for health information technology at the U.S. Department of Health and Human Services, where he leads the formulation of the federal health information technology (IT) strategy and coordinates federal health IT policies, standards, programs, and investments. He has more than 20 years of experience across the health IT landscape. Tripathi most recently served as chief alliance officer for Arcadia, a health care data and software company focused on population health management and value-based care; as project manager of the Argonaut Project, an industry collaboration to accelerate the adoption of Fast Healthcare Interoperability Resources; and as a board member of HL7, the Sequoia Project, the CommonWell Health Alliance, and the CARIN Alliance. He served as the president and chief executive officer of the Massachusetts eHealth Collaborative, a nonprofit health IT advisory and clinical data analytics company. He was also the founding president and chief executive officer of the Indiana Health Information Exchange (HIE), a statewide HIE partnered with the Regenstrief Institute; an executive advisor to the investment firm LRVHealth; and a fellow at the Berkman-Klein Center for Internet and Society at Harvard University. Prior to receiving his Ph.D., he was a presidential management fellow and a senior operations research analyst in the Office of the Secretary of Defense in Washington, DC, for which he received the Secretary of Defense Meritorious Civilian Service Medal. He holds a Ph.D. in political science from the Massachusetts Institute of Technology, a master's degree in public policy from Harvard University, and an A.B. in political science from Vassar College.

Appendix E

Office of the Secretary
PCOR Trust Fund Project Portfolio

Project Title	Description	Implementing Agency	FY Funded	Status	Functionality Addressed*
Using Machine Learning Techniques to Enable Health Information Exchange to Support COVID-19-Focused Patient-Centered Outcomes Research (PCOR)	This project will implement data standardization, machine learning techniques for preserving data privacy, and application programming interfaces (API) to support the use of health data obtained from health information exchanges (HIEs) for research.	ONC	2021	Active	1, 4
Building Infrastructure and Evidence for COVID-19 Related Research, Using Integrated Data from National Center for Health Statistics (NCHS) Data Linkage Program	This project will reduce barriers to accessing linked datasets for PCOR by developing publicly available synthetic linked data products. These products will integrate data on social determinants of health (SDOH), health-related data, and administrative data while protecting participant privacy. Additionally, the product will allow for more timely access of COVID-19 pandemic data. The project will also develop a public-facing dashboard with information generated from the linked data.	NCHS-CDC	2021	Active (no start date noted)	3, 4
Multistate Emergency Medical Services (EMS) and Medicaid Dataset (MEMD): A Linked Dataset for Patient-Centered Outcomes Research	This project will develop the Multistate EMS and MEMD. This first-of-its-kind dataset will allow researchers to conduct PCOR related to Medicaid beneficiaries' health outcomes following their encounter with EMS.	ASPE-BHDAP, NHTSA EMS	2021	Active (no start date noted)	3, 4
Making Medicaid Data More Accessible Through Common Data Models and FHIR APIs	This project seeks to increase data capacity or infrastructure that will support research that will guide decisions about the efficacy of health interventions utilized in Medicaid and Children's Health Insurance Programs.	FDA, NIH/NLM	2021	Active	1, 2, 3

Project	Description	Funder	Year	Status	Notes
Understanding COVID-19 Trajectory and Outcomes in the Context of Multiple Chronic Conditions (MCC) through e-Care Plan Development	This project expands the previously funded project, the clinician and patient-facing electronic care (eCare) plan applications and Fast Healthcare Interoperability Resources (FHIR) implementation guide. It updates and exchanges health data for patients with multiple chronic conditions. This expansion will also add data elements for COVID-19 and post-acute sequelae of COVID-19 (PASC). The project will also develop a new unpaid-caregiver-facing application that includes COVID-19 and PASC data.	AHRQ, NIH/NIDDK	2021	Active	1, 2, 3
Dataset on Intellectual and Developmental Disabilities: Linking Data to Enhance Person-Centered Outcomes Research	This project will create a dataset by linking state-level data sources from four to six states. The state-level data will include the National Core Indicators In-Person Survey, Supports Intensity Scale, Medicaid claims, and other relevant state data sources. The resulting dataset will allow researchers to analyze relationships between several key variables and person-centered outcomes for individuals with intellectual disabilities or developmental disabilities before and during the COVID-19 pandemic.	ASPE-BHDAP	2021	Active (no start date noted)	3, 4
CURE ID: Aggregating and Analyzing COVID-19 Treatments from Electronic Health Records (EHRs) & Registries Globally	This project will update the CURE ID online platform and mobile application by adding the capacity to collect case reports for drug repurposing in the treatment of COVID-19. The update will also add automated extraction and manual data collection abilities to obtain data from EHRs and clinical disease registries.	FDA, NIH, Implemented through NCATS	2021	Active (no start date noted)	3, 4

Project Title	Description	Implementing Agency	FY Funded	Status	Functionality Addressed*
Severe Maternal Morbidity and Mortality EHR Data Infrastructure	This project will establish a primary infrastructure for EHRs that will enable PCOR on maternal morbidity and mortality. The anticipated final outcome will be a "Health Level Seven (HL7)® FHIR® Implementation Guidance encompassing pregnancy, pregnancy outcomes, and pregnancy-related conditions, co-morbidities, and procedures."	NIH, ONC, CDC	2021	Active	1, 3, 4
MAT-LINK2: Expansion of MATernaL and Infant NetworK to Understand Outcomes Associated with Treatment for Opioid Use Disorder during Pregnancy	This project will expand on MAT-LINK, a previously funded data platform, and associated standardized elements for collecting maternal and infant data for women treated for opioid use disorder (OUD) during pregnancy. The update will create a more robust and representative data repository by including data from additional clinical sites and collect data on infants through age 6 to allow for additional assessment of development impacts.	CDC	2021	Active	1, 3, 4
Enhancing Surveillance of Maternal Health Clinical Practices and Outcomes with Federally Qualified Health Centers' (FQHCs) Electronic Health Records Visit Data	This project will enhance and expand National Ambulatory Medical Care Survey data collection procedures from 2021 for maternal health visits to FQHCs to 2022 and increase the sample of FQHCs included. The project will also evaluate the feasibility of creating new data linkages to National Death Index (NDI) and U.S. Department of Housing and Urban Development (HUD) administrative data sources.	CDC	2021	Active	1, 3, 4

339

Project	Description	Agency	Year	Status	
Data Linkage: Evaluating Privacy Preserving Record Linkage Methodology and Augmenting the National Hospital Care Survey with Medicaid Administrative Records	This project will evaluate different methods for privacy preserving record linkage and expand on existing data resources to create new linked datasets for PCOR across the continuum of care.	CDC	2020	Active	3, 4, 5
Developing a Multi-State Network of Linked Pregnancy Risk Assessment Monitoring System (PRAMS) and Clinical Outcomes Data for Patient-Centered Outcomes Research	This project will build on the existing PRAMS infrastructure by linking survey data with additional data such as hospital discharge data and Medicaid claims.	CDC	2020	Active	3, 5
Data Capacity for Patient-Centered Outcomes Research through Creation of an Electronic Care Plan for People with Multiple Chronic Conditions 2.0: Development of the Patient-Facing Application	This project builds on the eCare plan 1.0 by creating additional patient-use resources and adding capabilities based on feedback from the pilot.	NIDDK, AHRQ	2020	Active	1, 2, 3, 4
Childhood Obesity Data Initiative (CODI): Integrated Data for Patient-Centered Outcomes Research Project 2.0	This project continues work done for the CODI 1.0 project. It will expand existing CODI infrastructure to accommodate linking individual pediatric data from diverse sources for PCOR. The resulting CODI 2.0 project is expected to improve the initiative's technical capabilities and sustainability.	CDC	2020	Active	1, 3, 4

Project Title	Description	Implementing Agency	FY Funded	Status	Functionality Addressed*
Training Data for Machine Learning to Enhance Patient-Centered Outcomes Research (PCOR) Data Infrastructure	This project will create high-quality training datasets for use in training algorithms for machine learning that will result in improving the ability of researchers to use artificial intelligence in PCOR. The project will also develop and disseminate machine learning algorithms and implementation guides for use in PCOR.	ONC, NIH/NLM	2019	Active	4
A Synthetic Health Data Generation Engine to Accelerate Patient-Centered Outcomes Research	This project will convene a technical expert panel to develop five to seven priority use cases for development of new synthetic data modules to enhance the synthetic data that Synthea can generate. Synthea is an open-access software program that generates large volumes of high-quality and realistic synthetic patient records for use in research, including PCOR.	ONC	2019	Active	5
Validating and Expanding Claims-Based Algorithms of Frailty and Functional Disability for Value-Based Care and Payment	This is a 4-year-long project that will increase data capacity for conducting PCOR with attention to patient functional risk and functional status data. The project is developing validated and refined algorithms that use Medicare and/or Medicaid claims data that identify patient functional risk. These algorithms will be publicly available through the Chronic Conditions Warehouse (CCW). The project will also draft EHR-modified algorithms and a guidance report about extracting patients' functional status data from the EHR.	ASPE, AHRQ, CDC, CMS	2019	Active	3, 4, 5

341

Bridging the PCOR Infrastructure and Technology Innovation through Coordinated Registry Networks (CRN) Community of Practice	This project will improve CRN's ability to capture standardized data and patient-generated data related to medical devices and link that data to other data sources.	FDA	2019	Active	2, 3
Surveillance Network: Maternal, Infant, and Child Health Outcomes Following Treatment of Opioid Use Disorder (OUD) During Pregnancy	This project will adapt and use the lessons learned from development of the Centers for Disease Control and Prevention (CDC) USZPIR (a surveillance system for monitoring pregnant women with a laboratory-confirmed Zika virus infection and their infants) for MAT-LINK. MAT-LINK will develop a surveillance network and data platform to collect linked data about maternal, infant, and child health following treatment for OUD during pregnancy.	CDC	2019	Active	1
Linking State Medicaid and Child Welfare Data for Outcomes Research on Treatment for Opioid Use Disorder and Other Behavioral Health Issues	This project seeks to link records from state level Medicaid and child welfare systems in a sample of states to create a dataset of patient-level data that includes Medicaid enrollment, diagnoses, services, claims, and child welfare outcomes. This project will result in improved data infrastructure and greater data availability for PCOR targeted at parents with children in the child welfare system with a focus on those needing treatment for OUD, other substance abuse disorders, or behavioral health diagnoses.	ASPE ACF/ OPRE	2019	Active	3, 4

Project Title	Description	Implementing Agency	FY Funded	Status	Functionality Addressed*
Augmenting the National Hospital Care Survey (NHCS) Data through Linkages with Administrative Records: A Project	This project links 2016 NHCS data with 2016 Centers for Medicare & Medicaid Services (CMS) Medicare Fee-for-Service claims data and HUD federal housing assistance program data. The new data linkage will improve data infrastructure to support PCOR that incorporates investigation of differences in intervention efficacy for previously unexamined subpopulations.	CDC	2019	Active	3
Identifying Co-Occurring Disorders among Opioid Users Using Linked Hospital Care and Mortality Data: Capstone to an Existing FY18 OS-PCORTF Project	This project will develop algorithms for use on the linked data from the FY18 project to identify hospital encounter records and death records of patients treated for an OUD that also have a diagnosis of another substance use or mental health disorder. The FY18 and FY19 projects will create linked files that allow researchers to examine data for patients for 1 year following their discharge from the hospital for an opioid-use-related event.	CDC	2019	Active	3, 4, 5
NIDA's AMNet: An Addiction Medicine Network to Address the United States Opioid Crisis	This project is using data from the American Psychiatric Association's (APA) clinical data registry (PsychPRO), APA members, and the American Society of Addiction Medicine to develop a new practice-based research network and electronic patient registry called the Addiction Medicine Network (AMNet).	NIH/NIDA	2019	Active	2, 3, 4

Data Capacity for Patient-Centered Outcomes Research through Creation of an Electronic Care Plan for People with Multiple Chronic Conditions	This project is developing an interoperable eCare plan by enabling aggregation of critical patient data from across the multiple settings where a patient with multiple chronic conditions receives care and sharing that data with all of the patient's health team members.	AHRQ, NIDDK	2019	Active	3, 4
Making Electronic Health Record (EHR) Data More Available for Research and Public Health	This project is developing an application that uses existing data and exchange standards to facilitate data exchange between differing EHRs, research, and public health record systems in real time.	CDC	2019	Active	1

Project Title	Description	Implementing Agency	FY Funded	Status	Functionality Addressed*
SHIELD - Standardization of Lab Data to Enhance Patient-Centered Outcomes Research and Value-Based Care	This project is building on the work of the Systemic Harmonization and Interoperability Enhancement for Laboratory Data (SHIELD) collaborative by creating and disseminating code-mapping manuals to ensure that the same LOINC (Logical Observation Identifiers Names and Codes) are used for the same in-vitro diagnostic device (IVD) in EHRs across different laboratories. This project seeks to improve semantic interoperability across systems. The SHIELD collaborative is a multi-agency/stakeholder network consisting of the Food and Drug Administration (FDA), CDC, National Institutes of Health (NIH), Office of the National Coordinator for Health Information Technology (ONC), CMS, U.S. Department of Veterans Affairs (VA), IVD manufacturers, EHR vendors, laboratories, College of American Pathologists, standards developers, Pew Charitable Trusts, National Evaluation System for Healthcare Technology, and academia.	FDA	2019	Active	3, 5

Enhancing Patient-Centered Outcomes Research (PCOR): Creating a National Small-Area Social Determinants of Health Data Platform	This project is developing a set of standardized and consolidated national databases focused on valid and reliable SDOH factors at the small-area and other geographic levels, using existing federal agency databases, including those from the Agency for Healthcare Research and Quality (AHRQ), Health Resources and Services Administration (HRSA), CDC, Assistant Secretary for Planning and Evaluation (ASPE), and NIH.	AHRQ	2019	Active	1, 3
Assessing and Predicting Medical Needs in a Disaster	This project is creating a data platform to facilitate the reporting and analysis of data related to medical encounters during a public health emergency or disaster. The platform will be able to collect and share medical encounter data during a disaster in real time. The platform will also facilitate disaster-response-and-recovery-specific PCOR.	AHRQ, ASPR	2018	Active	4
Capstone for the Outcomes Measures Harmonization Project	This project is creating a tool that links clinical data to two different patient registries and then facilitates the exchange of data between the patient registries and EHRs at the clinical sites. The resulting instructions and pieces of code are expected to assist researchers and registry developers to integrate clinical EHR systems and registries to facilitate PCOR.	AHRQ	2018	Active	3, 4

Project Title	Description	Implementing Agency	FY Funded	Status	Functionality Addressed*
Emergency Medicine Opioid Data Infrastructure - Key Venue to Address Opioid Morbidity and Mortality	This project created an OUD Data Dictionary to facilitate capture of relevant data from EHRs. It also created and conducted a pilot test of a mobile app for patients to use to complete post-discharge electronic surveys.	NIH/NIDA	2018	Completed	1, 2, 3
Childhood Obesity Data Initiative (CODI): Integrated Data for Patient-Centered Outcomes Research Project	This project is linking pediatric clinical EHR data, weight-management program intervention data, and census information to improve availability of that data for PCOR focused on childhood obesity.	CDC	2018	Active	1, 3, 4
Strengthening the Data Infrastructure for Outcomes Research on Mortality Associated with Opioid Poisonings	This project is redesigning the Medical Mortality Data System (MMDS) to capture and electronically code specific drug information found in the text fields of death certificate records. It is also developing and conducting a pilot test of an FHIR© API to facilitate data exchange between medical examiner and coroner case management systems and states' Electronic Death Registration System. This project is also establishing an NCHS Board of Scientific Advisors advisory committee to ensure that changes to the MMDS match the needs of end users.	CDC	2018	Active	3, 4

Project	Description	Agency	Year	Status	Ref
Enhancing Identification of Opioid-Involved Health Outcomes Using Linked Hospital Care and Mortality Data	This project is linking data from the NHCS, the NDI, and the National Vital Statistics System restricted use mortality files for drug overdose deaths to create a merged dataset for PCOR. This project includes an investment in infrastructure for improved hospital data collection and reporting and to disseminate information to promote use of the merged dataset.	CDC	2018	Active	1, 4
Technologies for Donating Medicare Beneficiary Claims Data to Research Studies	This project modified the CMS Blue Button platform to allow Medicare beneficiaries to allow access to their claims data for research purposes. Additionally, the project resulted in an application that allows researchers to view patient data from the CMS Blue Button platform and clinical data and an application that lets developers access CMS Blue Button data.	CMS, NIH	2017	Completed	3, 5
Developing a Strategically Coordinated Registry Network (CRN) for Women's Health Technology	This project created a CRN by linking existing and new women's health technology registries with established major data networks. The project created the necessary infrastructure for PCOR focused on evaluations of medical devices with clinical application unique to women.	FDA, NIH/NLM, ONC	2017	Completed	1
Harmonization of Various Common Data Models and Open Standards for Evidence Generation	The project developed a Common Data Model (CDM) to organize data from diverse clinical setting sources, including EHRs, insurance billing claims, and patient registries. The resulting CDM created an enhanced data infrastructure for PCOR.	FDA, NIH/NLM, NIH/NCI, NIH/NCATS, ONC	2017	Completed	1, 3, 4

Project Title	Description	Implementing Agency	FY Funded	Status	Functionality Addressed*
Enhancing Data Resources for Researching Patterns of Mortality in Patient-Centered Outcomes Research	This project is working to link the NDI data to NHCS inpatient and ED claims data, CMS Master Beneficiary Summary File (MBSF), and CMS CCW. The project also seeks to develop a long term strategy to support access of the NDI for PCOR.	CDC, FDA, CMS	2017	Active	3, 4, 5
Advancing the Collection and Use of Patient-Reported Outcomes (PROs) through Health Information Technology (IT)	This project created technical tools to standardize PRO data integration into EHRs and other health IT solutions to facilitate easier sharing of that information for PCOR.	AHRQ, ONC	2017	Completed	2, 4
PCOR: Privacy and Security Blueprint, Legal Analysis and Ethics Framework for Data Use, & Use of Technology for Privacy	This project created a legal and ethical framework for use of data and developed a best practices white paper for use of consent technology in research.	CDC, ONC	2015	Completed	1, 2, 3, 4
Use of the ADAPTABLE Trial to Strengthen Methods to Collect and Integrate Patient-reported Information with Other Data Sets and Assess Its Validity	This project built on lessons learned from Aspirin Dosing: A Patient-centric Trial Assessing Benefits and Long Term Effectiveness (ADAPTABLE) to develop a Patient-Reported Data Assessment tool that allowed researchers to compare patient-reported data with data from EHRs.	NIH	2016	Completed	1, 2, 3, 4

Project	Description	Agency	Year	Status	
Standardization and Querying of Data Quality Metrics and Characteristics for Electronic Health Data	This project created and implemented standards for metadata and a querying system to determine the quality, fitness for use, and completeness of electronic health data.	FDA	2016	Completed	4, 5
Utilizing Data from Various Data Partners in a Distributed Manner	This project developed a new open-source software application that allowed for researchers to perform distributed regression analyses of health data that were carried out at different institutions without also sharing associated potentially identifiable information across those different sites.	FDA	2015	Completed	4, 5
Improving the Mortality Data Infrastructure for Patient-Centered Outcomes (PCOR)	This project improved on existing infrastructure to facilitate more timely delivery of state death records to the NDI database and linked NDI data to hospital datasets collected at the national level. This created a more robust source for PCOR.	CDC	2015	Completed	1, 3
Development of a Natural Language Processing (NLP) Web Service for Public Health Use	This project created a publicly available NLP web service to assist researchers to convert unstructured clinical information to structured data with standardized coding.	CDC, FDA	2016	Completed	4, 5
Security and Privacy Standards for Patient Matching, Linking and Aggregation	This project developed the Patient Data Demographic Quality Framework to improve patient data standardization and matching across different organizations. It also developed a security tool that allows patients to control how their data is shared.	ONC	2015	Completed	3, 4

Project Title	Description	Implementing Agency	FY Funded	Status	Functionality Addressed*
Harmonization of Clinical Data Element Definitions for Outcome Measures in Registries	This project created an Outcomes Measures Framework to develop standardized outcome measures for clinical practice and PCOR. It also created a library of common data definitions for use in EHRs that will facilitate collection of standardized outcome data.	AHRQ	2016	Completed	1, 3
Source Data Capture from Electronic Health Records: Using Standardized Clinical Research Data	This project created a framework for development of systems used for electronic source data capture in regulated clinical investigations.	FDA	2016	Completed	1, 4
Creation of LOINC Equivalence Classes	This project used the LOINC coding system for laboratory tests and clinical observations to develop a mechanism to facilitate interoperable HIE between different health IT systems.	NIH	2016	Completed	1
Cross Network Directory Service	This project developed an open source interoperable service that facilitates data partner participation across multiple data research networks. The services allow researchers to search across multiple data networks, as well as share knowledge and analytic capabilities.	FDA	2015	Completed	5
Collection of Patient-Provided Information through a Mobile Device Application for Use in Comparative Effectiveness and Drug Safety Research	This project created the infrastructure for a mobile application to collect patient-generated health data (PGHD) and link that data to a data partner participating in the Sentinel distributed network.	FDA	2015	Completed	2, 3

Conceptualizing a Data Infrastructure for the Capture and Use of Patient-Generated Health Data	This project developed a policy framework for use of PGHD for research and delivery of care. It also conceptualized the development process for the data infrastructure required to facilitate patient sharing of data with health care providers, other caregivers, and researchers.	ONC	2015	Completed	1, 2
Improving Beneficiary Access to their Health Information through an Enhanced Blue Button Service	This project was a conceptual redesign of the CMS Blue Button platform to standardize data on the platform for acceptance by multiple applications and allow Medicare beneficiaries using the platform to make decisions on participation in research based on their preferences. It also made it easier for researchers to selectively pull Medicare claims data based on the needs of their study.	CMS	2016	Completed	5
Improving Beneficiary Access to Health Information: A Plan to Enhance "Blue Button"	This was an initiative to develop a plan to update the CMS Blue Button platform. The project defined functional requirements for improved functionality by engaging federal stakeholders, private sector developers, and third-party services. The project also developed campaign materials to raise consumer awareness about Blue Button.	CMS	2014	Completed	2, 4
Strengthening and Expanding the Community Health Applied Research Network (CHARN) Registry to Conduct Patient-Centered Outcomes Research (PCOR)	This project expanded and updated the CHARN data warehouse and improved the data infrastructure. It also created a data access plan to facilitate access to the CHARN data warehouse by researchers outside the network.	PCOR, HRSA	2014	Completed	1, 4

352

Project Title	Description	Implementing Agency	FY Funded	Status	Functionality Addressed*
Creating the Foundational Building Blocks for the Learning Health Care System: Data Access Standards for Electronic Health Records (EHRs)	This project created an API that facilitated standardized extraction of data from EHRs for PCOR.	ONC	2013	Completed	5
Creating the Foundational Blocks for the Learning Health Care System: Structured Data Capture (SDC)	This project developed technical and functional specifications needed to enable an EHR to retrieve and display standardized health data, enter that data in a structured form or template, then store and/or submit that to an outside data repository.	ONC	2013	Completed	1, 5
Expanding Data Collection for the National Program of Cancer Registries (NPCR) for Comparative Effectiveness Research (CER)	This project enhanced existing cancer registries by extending longitudinal data collection and creating tools that facilitated greater reporting of data from EHRs to central cancer registries for CER.	CDC	2013	Completed	1, 4
Comparative Effectiveness Research (CER) Inventory	This project was originally designed to develop a web-based tool to categorize and catalogue federal and non-federal CER activities. However, during the project, rapidly evolving technology allowed existing web-based search engines to surpass the CER tool under development and it was retired.	ASPE	2012	Completed	3, 5

Beta Testing the Multi-Payer Claims Database (MPCD)	This project was a beta test of the MPCD to determine whether it could be used as a data source for CER.	ASPE	2012	Completed	3, 5
Maintenance and Support of the Chronic Conditions Warehouse (CCW) for Comparative Effectiveness Research (CER)	This project maintained the CCW and increased opportunities for PCOR researchers to conduct projects through the CCW Virtual Research Data Center.	CMS	2012	Completed	3, 5
Development of Data Infrastructure for Use of Electronic Health Records (EHRs) in Comparative Effectiveness Research (CER)	This project created the Common Data Elements (CDE) Repository which was designed to allow access to the structured human- and machine-readable definitions of data elements that are required or recommended by NIH for use in research.	ONC, NLM	2012	Completed	1, 5

Functionalities:
1 - Standardized Collection of Standardized Clinical Data
2 - Collection of Participant Provided Information
3 - Linking of Clinical and Other Data for Research
4 - Use of Clinical Data for Research
5 - Use of Enhanced Publicly Funded Data Systems for Research

SOURCE: https://aspe.hhs.gov/collaborations-committees-advisory-groups/os-pcortf/explore-portfolio.